SCHOOL NUTRITION AND ACTIVITY

Impacts on Well-Being

SCHOOL NUTRITION AND ACTIVITY

Impacts on Well-Being

Edited by

Areej Hassan, MD

APPLE ACADEMIC PRESS

Apple Academic Press Inc.
3333 Mistwell Crescent
Oakville, ON L6L 0A2
Canada

Apple Academic Press Inc.
9 Spinnaker Way
Waretown, NJ 08758
USA

Printed in the United States of America on acid-free paper

International Standard Book Number-13: 978-1-77188-107-4 (Hardcover)

Library of Congress Control Number: 2014953390

Library and Archives Canada Cataloguing in Publication

School nutrition and activity : impacts on well-being / edited by Areej Hassan, MD.

Includes bibliographical references and index.
ISBN 978-1-77188-107-4 (bound)
1. School children--Nutrition. 2. School children--Health and hygiene. 3. Exercise for children--Health aspects. 4. Health promotion. 5. Obesity in children--Prevention. 6. Obesity in adolescence--Prevention. I. Hassan, Areej, editor

LB3475.S36 2015 371.7'16 C2014-906983-9

Apple Academic Press also publishes its books in a variety of electronic formats. Some content that appears in print may not be available in electronic format. For information about Apple Academic Press products, visit our website at **www.appleacademicpress.com** and the CRC Press website at **www.crcpress.com**

ABOUT THE EDITOR

AREEJ HASSAN, MD

Areej Hassan MD, MPH, is an instructor in pediatrics at Harvard Medical School as well as an attending physician at Boston Children's Hospital. She completed her pediatric residency at Hasbro Children's Hospital prior to training in adolescent medicine at Boston Children's. In addition to primary care, her clinical interests include reproductive endocrinology and international health. She also maintains an active role in medical education and has particular interest in building and developing innovative teaching tools through open educational resources. She currently teaches, consults, and is involved in pediatric and adolescent curricula development at multiple sites abroad in Central America and Southeast Asia.

CONTENTS

ACKNOWLEDGMENT AND HOW TO CITE

The editor and publisher thank each of the authors who contributed to this book. The chapters in this book were previously published in various places in various formats. To cite the work contained in this book and to view the individual permissions, please refer to the citation at the beginning of each chapter. Each chapter was read individually and carefully selected by the editor; the result is a book that provides a nuanced study of school nutrition. The chapters included examine the following topics:

- Chapter 1 provides a good overall review of the obesity epidemic. It gives a solid rationale for the research that follows in the rest of the book.
- Chapter 2 is an example of some extremely relevant research, and these two programs can have a huge impact on childhood obesity. Research like this should shape school and government policy to better address the powerful connections between school and the obesity epidemic.
- The interesting study in Chapter 3 succeeded in conducting a randomized controlled trial of intervention over a year's time. The results speak to how difficult it is to get kids to exercise; even with a well-developed intervention in place, there was still little change in physical activity levels, even though other positive impacts were seen.
- The research premise in Chapter 4 is a novel one. As an American clinician, I always encourage exercise, but outdoor-versus-indoor exercise is not one that I've previously considered. Since this is a British study, it perhaps reflects a cultural difference between the United States and the UK when it comes to awareness of the joys of outdoor exercise. Although urban children have less access to green spaces, most children seem to naturally love the outdoors, and this study indicates that this may be a successful way to motivate children to exercise.
- The extremely well-thought-out study in Chapter 5 is a randomized controlled trial with an impressive three-year follow-up. It offers a feasible intervention that can be replicated, with a wide range of outcome measures to assess all aspects of health. Disappointingly, the long-term effects (other than staying involved in aerobic fitness) were not sustainable. This speaks to the fact that school-based programs need to be funded so that students can take part during all of their years in school.

- Chapter 6 offers surprising but important negative findings, which underline the fact that obesity interventions have to involve more than only school programming. Schools play an important role, but family and community interventions are still necessary. One of the authors, Tracy Richmond, is at the forefront of research into the impact of school and neighborhoods on obesity.
- The small but feasible intervention in Chapter 7 makes use of built-in free time during the school day. Less-active children benefit from having staff working with them to increase physical activity.
- Although Chapter 8 includes an anti-smoking intervention as well, it offers excellent research that can be applied specifically to obesity interventions. Planet Health is one of the most effective school-based interventions, which offers clear direction to schools, policymakers, and researchers.
- Although Chapter 9 does not study a specifically school-based intervention, it does show the important role schools can play in helping to assess factors that contribute to obesity. Ninety-two British schools agreed to take part in the SPEEDY study (Sport, Physical activity and Eating behavior: Environmental Determinants in Young people), which allowed the investigators to collect important data relating to a range of obesity-related variables.
- Chapter 10 is a well-done review that offers specific recommendations. It puts together a wide range of obesity research, and then uses the results to develop three practical, take-home bullet-point messages.
- Again, as an American clinician, I feel it is good to look past US boundaries at ideas that may be unfamiliar and yet prove to be useful. The concept of "foodscapes" in Chapter 11 offers good talking points to get us thinking in new ways about the obesity epidemic. The recent updates to the original article make this research even more relevant and convincing.
- Often, interventions that have a positive effect in one setting are not always feasible to implement successfully in other settings. Chapter 12 looks at a small successful program that has been taken to the next level and rolled out in a larger way. The larger-scale program proved to not only be feasible but continued to show positive impact.
- Chapter 13 concludes this compendium with a comprehensive, excellent paper that provides a detailed overview, synthesis, and interpretation of existing literature. It then goes on to build concrete recommendations from this detailed foundation.

LIST OF CONTRIBUTORS

Stephen W. Banspach
Centers for Disease Control and Prevention, Atlanta, Georgia, United States of America

Jo Barton
School of Biological Sciences, University of Essex, Colchester, Essex, United Kingdom

Hans-Peter Brunner-La Rocca
Department of Cardiology, Maastricht University Medical Center, Maastricht, The Netherlands

Meghan M. Casey
School of Health Sciences, Federation University Australia, Ballarat, Australia

Aedín Cassidy
Department of Nutrition, Norwich Medical School, University of East Anglia, Norwich, UK

Margaret O. Caughy
University of Texas School of Public Health, Dallas, Texas, United States of America

Daniel Cohen
Instituto de Investigaciones, Escuela de Medicina, Universidad de Santander, Bucaramanga, Santander, Colombia

Geri A. Dino
Prevention Research Center, Robert C. Byrd Health Sciences Center, West Virginia University, Morgantown, WVa.

Rochelle M. Eime
School of Health Sciences, Federation University Australia, Ballarat, Australia and Institute of Sport, Exercise and Active Living (ISEAL), Victoria University, Melbourne, Australia

Marc N. Elliott
Statistics, RAND Corporation, Santa Monica, California, United States of America

Division of Adolescent and School Health
National Center for Chronic Disease Prevention and Health Promotion

Dominique Ernst
University of Basel, Basel, Switzerland

Frank A. Franklin
Department of Maternal and Child Health, School of Public Health, University of Alabama at Birmingham, Birmingham, Alabama, United States of America

Adele L. Franks
Prevention Research Centers Office. MS-K45 DACH/NCCDPHP/CDC, 3005 Buford Highway, Atlanta, GA 30341, Phone: 413-587-0025, Email: vog.cdc@sknarfa.

Luisa Franzini
Division of Management, Policy, and Community Health, The University of Texas School of Public Health/Blue Cross and Blue Shield of Texas Research Program in Payment Systems and Policies, Houston, Texas, United States of America

Christina Fung
School of Public Health, University of Alberta, 6-50 University Terrace, 8303 - 112 St, Edmonton, AB T6G 2 T4, Canada

M. Janice Gilliland
Birmingham, Alabama, United States of America

Steven L. Gortmaker
Prevention Research Center on Nutrition and Physical Activity, Harvard University, Cambridge, Mass.

Simon J. Griffin
Centre of Excellence in Diet and Activity Research, MRC Epidemiology Unit, Cambridge, UK

Jack T. Harvey
School of Health Sciences, Federation University Australia, Ballarat, Australia

Helge Hebestreit
University Children's Hospital Würzburg, Wuerzburg, Germany

Kimberly A. Horn
Prevention Research Center, Robert C. Byrd Health Sciences Center, West Virginia University, Morgantown, WVa.

Jennifer Huberty
School of Nutrition & Health Promotion, Arizona State University, Phoenix, AZ 85004-0698, USA

Ian Janssen
School of Kinesiology and Health Studies, Queen's University, Kingston, Ontario, Canada and Department of Community Health and Epidemiology, Queen's University, Kingston, Ontario, Canada

Amy Jennings
Department of Nutrition, Norwich Medical School, University of East Anglia, Norwich, UK

Amar Kanekar
Department of Health Studies, East Stroudsburg University of Pennsylvania, East Stroudsburg, PA, USA

Sameera Karnik
Masters of Public Health Program, American Public University, East Stroudsburg, PA, USA

Ichiro Kawachi
Department of Social and Behavioral Sciences, Harvard School of Public Health, Boston, Massachusetts, United States of America

Steven H. Kelder
Center for Health Promotion and Prevention Research, University of Texas Health Science Center at Houston, Houston, Tex.

Susi Kriemler
Service of Endocrinology, Diabetes and Metabolism, Centre Hospitalier Universitaire Vaudoise, University of Lausanne, Lausanne, Switzerland and University of Basel, Basel, Switzerland

Stefan Kuhle
School of Public Health, University of Alberta, 6-50 University Terrace, 8303 - 112 St, Edmonton, AB T6G 2 T4, Canada

Allana G. LeBlanc
School of Kinesiology and Health Studies, Queen's University, Kingston, Ontario, Canada

Richard Lowry
Centers for Disease Control and Prevention, Atlanta, Georgia, United States of America

Connie Lu
School of Public Health, University of Alberta, 6-50 University Terrace, 8303 - 112 St, Edmonton, AB T6G 2 T4, Canada

Mary Marian
University of Arizona, Tucson, Arizona, USA

Ursina Meyer
Department of Human Movement Science, Maastricht University, Maastricht, The Netherlands and University of Basel, Basel, Switzerland

Bent Egberg Mikkelsen
Aalborg University, Copenhagen, Denmark,

Amanda Mooney
School of Education, Faculty of Arts & Education, Deakin University, Melbourne, Australia

Warren R. Payne
Institute of Sport, Exercise and Active Living (ISEAL), Victoria University, Melbourne, Australia

Jules N. Pretty
School of Biological Sciences, University of Essex, Colchester, Essex, United Kingdom

Nicole Probst-Hensch
University of Basel, Basel, Switzerland

Megan Purcell
School of Public Health, University of Alberta, 6-50 University Terrace, 8303 - 112 St, Edmonton, AB T6G 2 T4, Canada

Marg Schwartz
School of Public Health, University of Alberta, 6-50 University Terrace, 8303 - 112 St, Edmonton, AB T6G 2 T4, Canada

Katharine Reed
School of Biological Sciences, University of Essex, Colchester, Essex, United Kingdom

Tracy K. Richmond
Division of Adolescent Medicine, Boston Children's Hospital, Boston, Massachusetts, United States of America

Daniel W. Russell
Iowa State University, Department of Human Development and Family Studies, Ames, IA 50011, USA

Pedro F. Saint-Maurice
Iowa State University, Department of Kinesiology, Ames, IA 50011, USA

Gavin R. H. Sandercock
School of Biological Sciences, University of Essex, Colchester, Essex, United Kingdom

Jason Schaub
University of Arizona, Tucson, Arizona, USA

Christian Schindler
University of Basel, Basel, Switzerland

Mark A. Schuster
Department of Medicine, Boston Children's Hospital, Boston, Massachusetts, United States of America

Eduardo J. Simoes
Prevention Research Centers Program, CDC, Atlanta, Ga.

Kate Storey
School of Public Health, University of Alberta, 6-50 University Terrace, 8303 - 112 St, Edmonton, AB T6G 2 T4, Canada

Amanda Telford
School of Medical Sciences, Discipline of Exercise Sciences, RMIT University, Melbourne, Australia

Willem van Mechelen
Department of Public and Occupational Health and EMGO+ Institute, VU University Medical Center Amsterdam, Amsterdam, The Netherlands

Esther M.F. van Sluijs
Centre of Excellence in Diet and Activity Research, MRC Epidemiology Unit, Cambridge, UK

Paul J. Veugelers
School of Public Health, University of Alberta, 6-50 University Terrace, 8303 - 112 St, Edmonton, AB T6G 2 T4, Canada

Courtney E. Walls
Epidemiology, Decision Resources, Burlington, Massachusetts, United States of America

Jean L. Wiecha
Prevention Research Center on Nutrition and Physical Activity, Harvard University, Cambridge, Mass.

Ailsa A. Welch
Department of Nutrition, Norwich Medical School, University of East Anglia, Norwich, UK

Gregory J. Welk
Iowa State University, Department of Kinesiology, Ames, IA 50011, USA

Carly Wood
School of Biological Sciences, University of Essex, Colchester, Essex, United Kingdom

Lukas Zahner
Institute of Exercise and Health Sciences, University of Basel, Basel, Switzerland

INTRODUCTION

Childhood and adolescent obesity has emerged as a critical public health problem over the last decade. Today, more than one-third of youth are considered overweight and obese, with both short- and long-term consequences to their health and well-being. While there are many factors that play a role in the striking increase in obesity rates, two of the cornerstones of prevention and treatment are access to good nutrition and increased physical activity.

A growing body of literature documents that school health programs can have positive effects on health-risk behaviors and health outcomes. Since about 95 percent of children and adolescents are currently enrolled in schools for a minimum of about six hours a day, schools have many opportunities to counsel youth. As a result, school interventions are a natural fit for anti-obesity programs that focus on healthy eating and physical activity. In recent years, there has been much media attention on school initiatives, from decreasing the availability of sugar-sweetened beverages in vending machines to implementing comprehensive physical education programs to developing health education modules aimed at students, with many more initiatives being developed and studied.

This compendium assesses the research foundations behind these initiatives. It looks at the issue from three levels: first, the effects of unhealthy eating and lack of exercise on a number of health outcomes in children and adolescents; second, successful small- and large-scale school-based interventions; and finally, synthesis of current literature and translation into specific guidelines and recommendations. This research provides schools with a strong foundation for implementing policies and practices that support healthy eating and regular physical activity. In the process, educators will be ensuring the best possible chance for increasing students' academic success, improving both physical and mental health, and decreasing the risk for myriad chronic diseases.

Areej Hassan, MD

Childhood obesity is a major public health crisis nationally and internationally. The prevalence of childhood obesity has increased over few years. It is caused by imbalance between calorie intake and calories utilized. One or more factors (genetic, behavioral, and environmental) cause obesity in children. Physical, psychological, and social health problems are caused due to childhood obesity. Hence, effective intervention strategies are being used to prevent and control obesity in children. The purpose of Chapter 1, by Karnik and Kanekar, is to address various factors influencing childhood obesity, a variety of interventions and governmental actions addressing obesity and the challenges ahead for managing this epidemic. In order to collect materials for this review a detailed search of CINAHL, MEDLINE, ERIC, Academic Search Premier databases was carried out for the time period 1999-2011. Some of the interventions used were family based, school based, community based, play based, and hospital based. The effective school-based interventions were seen targeting physical activity along with healthy diet education. The major challenges faced by these intervention programs are financial, along with stigmatization of obese children. Governments along with other health care organizations are taking effective actions like policy changing and environmentally safe interventions for children to improve physical activity. In conclusion, childhood obesity can be tackled at the population level by education, prevention and sustainable interventions related to healthy nutrition practices and physical activity promotion.

The childhood obesity epidemic has left healthcare professionals and laymen alike questioning the best strategy to improve children's health in the future. To effectively combat childhood obesity, we must have a thorough understanding of the establishment and development of programs currently responsible for pediatric health. Chapter 2, by Schaub and Marian, explores the history of two influential programs affecting children's diet and physical activity levels in schools: the National School Lunch Program and physical education classes. It is revealed that the National School Lunch Program contributes to the overall school nutrition environment, including the presence of fast food and vending machines on campuses. The history of physical education is traced back to ancient Greece, and it is shown that the familiar sports-based curriculum is an advent of the 19th century, with the roots of physical education originating from the founders of preventive medicine. Select childhood obesity and health intervention studies are reviewed with a focus on identifying notable features pertaining to the effectiveness of these programs. Future directions and recommendations, based on the history of these programs as well as evidence from current pediatric health studies, outlining the basis for a modernized health-based physical education curriculum designed to address today's public health concerns, are further discussed.

In Chapter 3, Casey and colleagues evaluated the effectiveness of a school-community program on Health-Related Quality of Life (HRQoL; the primary outcome), physical activity (PA), and potential mediators of PA among adolescent girls living in low-socioeconomic rural/regional settings. The study was a cluster-randomized controlled trial. Twelve communities with the requisite sports clubs and facilities were paired according to relevant criteria; one of each pair was randomly assigned to the intervention or control condition. Eight schools per condition were randomly selected from these communities and the intervention was conducted over one school year (2011). Female students in grades 7–9 in intervention schools participated in two 6-session PA units—a sport unit (football or tennis) and a recreational unit (leisure centre-based). These were incorporated into physical education (PE) curriculum and linked to PA opportunities for participation outside school. Students were surveyed at baseline and endpoint, self-reporting impact on primary and secondary outcome measures (HRQoL, PA) and PA mediators (e.g. self-efficacy). Linear mixed models for two-group (intervention, control) and three-group (completers, non-completers, control) analyses were conducted with baseline value, age and BMI as covariates, group as a fixed effect and school as random cluster effect. Participants completing baseline and endpoint measures included: 358 intervention (baseline response rate 33.7%, retention rate 61.3%) and 256 control (14.1% and 84.0%). Adjustment for age and BMI made no substantive difference to outcomes, and there were no cluster effects. For HRQoL, after adjustment for baseline scores, the intervention group showed significantly higher scores on all three PedsQL scores (physical functioning: $M \pm SE = 83.9 \pm 0.7$, $p = .005$; psychosocial: 79.9 ± 0.8, $p = .001$; total score: 81.3 ± 0.7, $p = .001$) than the control group (80.9 ± 0.8; 76.1 ± 0.9 and 77.8 ± 0.8). The three-group analysis found intervention non-completers had significantly higher PedsQL scores

(84.0±0.8, p=.021; 80.4±0.9, p=.003; 81.7±0.8, p=.002;) than controls (80.9±0.8, 76.1±0.9 and 77.8±0.8). There were no significant differences for any PA measure. Intervention completers had significantly higher scores than non-completers and controls for some mediator variables (e.g. self-efficacy, behavioural control). Positive outcomes were achieved from a modest school-community linked intervention. The school component contributed to maintaining HRQoL; students who completed the community component derived a range of intra-personal and inter-personal benefits.

Exercising in natural, green environments creates greater improvements in adult's self-esteem than exercise undertaken in urban or indoor settings. No comparable data are available for children. The aim of Reed and colleagues in Chapter 4 was to determine whether so called "green exercise" affected changes in self-esteem; enjoyment and perceived exertion in children differently to urban exercise. The authors assessed cardiorespiratory fitness (20 m shuttle-run) and self-reported physical activity (PAQ-A) in 11 and 12 year olds (n = 75). Each pupil completed two 1.5 mile timed runs, one in an urban and another in a rural environment. Trials were completed one week apart during scheduled physical education lessons allocated using a repeated measures design. Self-esteem was measured before and after each trial, ratings of perceived exertion (RPE) and enjoyment were assessed after completing each trial. They found a significant main effect ($F(1,74)$, = 12.2, $p<0.001$), for the increase in self-esteem following exercise but there was no condition by exercise interaction ($F(1,74)$, = 0.13, $p = 0.72$). There were no significant differences in perceived exertion or enjoyment between conditions. There was a negative correlation ($r = -0.26$, $p = 0.04$) between habitual physical activity and RPE during the control condition, which was not evident in the green exercise condition ($r = -0.07$, $p = 0.55$). Contrary to previous studies in adults, green exercise did not produce significantly greater increases in self-esteem than the urban exercise condition. Green exercise was enjoyed more equally by children with differing levels of habitual physical activity and has the potential to engage less active children in exercise.

School-based intervention studies promoting a healthy lifestyle have shown favorable immediate health effects. However, there is a striking paucity on long-term follow-ups. The aim of Chapter 5, by Meyer and colleagues, was therefore to assess the 3 yr-follow-up of a cluster-randomized controlled school-based physical activity program over nine month with beneficial immediate effects on body fat, aerobic fitness and physical activity. Initially, 28 classes from 15 elementary schools in Switzerland were grouped into an intervention (16 classes from 9 schools, n = 297 children) and a control arm (12 classes from 6 schools, n = 205 children) after stratification for grade (1st and 5th graders). Three years after the end of the multi-component physical activity program of nine months including daily physical education (i.e. two additional lessons per week on top of three regular lessons), short physical activity breaks during academic lessons, and daily physical activity homework, 289 (58%) participated in the follow-up. Primary outcome measures included body fat (sum of four skinfolds), aerobic fitness (shuttle run test), physical activity (accelerometry), and quality of life (questionnaires). After adjustment for grade, gender, baseline value and clustering within classes, children in the intervention arm compared with controls had a significantly higher average level of aerobic fitness at follow-up (0.373 z-score units [95%-CI: 0.157 to 0.59, p = 0.001] corresponding to a shift from the 50th to the 65th percentile between baseline and follow-up), while the immediate beneficial effects on the other primary outcomes were not sustained. Apart from aerobic fitness, beneficial effects seen after one year were not maintained when the intervention was stopped. A continuous intervention seems necessary to maintain overall beneficial health effects as reached at the end of the intervention.

Little is known about the contribution of school contextual factors to individual student body mass index (BMI). In Chapter 6, Richmond and colleagues set out to determine if school characteristics/resources: (1) are associated with student BMI; (2) explain racial/ethnic disparities in student BMI; and (3) explain school-level differences in student BMI. Using gender-stratified multi-level modeling strategies the authors examined the association of school characteristics/resources and individual BMI in 4,387 5th graders in the Healthy Passages Longitudinal Study of Adolescent Health. Additionally, they examined the association of race/ethnicity and individual BMI as well as the between-school variance in BMI before and after adding individual and school characteristics to test for attenuation. The school-level median household income, but not physical activity or nutrition resources, was inversely associated with female BMI (β = −0.12, CI: −0.21,−0.02). Neither school demographics nor physical activity/nutrition resources were predictive of individual BMI in males. In Black females, school characteristics attenuated the association of race/ethnicity and BMI. Individual student characteristics—not school characteristics/resources-reduced the between-school variation in BMI in males by nearly one-third and eliminated it in females. In this cohort of 5th graders, school SES was inversely associated with female BMI while school characteristics and resources largely explained Black/White disparities in female weight status. Between-school differences in average student weight status were largely explained by the composition of the student body not by school characteristics or programming.

A limitation of traditional outcome studies from behavioral interventions is the lack of attention given to evaluating the influence of moderating variables. Chapter 7, by Saint-Maurice and colleagues, examined possible moderation effect of baseline activity levels on physical activity change as a result of the Ready for Recess intervention. Ready for Recess (August 2009-September 2010) was a controlled trial with twelve schools randomly assigned to one of four conditions: control group, staff supervision, equipment availability, and the combination of staff supervision and equipment availability. A total of 393 children (181 boys and 212 girls) from grades 3 through 6 (8–11 years old) were asked to wear an Actigraph monitor during school time on 4–5 days of the week. Assessments were conducted at baseline (before intervention) and post intervention (after intervention). Initial MVPA moderated the effect of Staff supervision (β=−0.47%; $p<.05$), but not Equipment alone and Staff+Equipment ($p>.05$). Participants in the Staff condition that were 1 standard deviation (SD) below the mean for baseline MVPA (classified as "low active") had lower MVPA levels at post-intervention when compared with their low active peers in the control condition (Mean diff=−10.8±2.9%; $p=.005$). High active individuals (+1SD above the mean) in the Equipment treatment also had lower MVPA values at post-intervention when compared with their highly active peers in the control group (Mean diff=−9.5±2.9%; $p=.009$). These results indicate that changes in MVPA levels at post-intervention were reduced in highly active participants when recess staff supervision was provided. In this study, initial MVPA moderated the effect of Staff supervision on children's MVPA after 6 months of intervention.

Staff training should include how to work with inactive youth but also how to assure that active children remain active.

Establishing healthy habits in youth can help prevent many chronic health problems later in life that are attributable to unhealthy eating, sedentary lifestyle, and overweight. For this reason, many public health professionals are interested in working with school systems to reach children in school settings. However, a lack of familiarity with how schools operate can be a substantial impediment to developing effective partnerships with schools. In Chapter 8, Franks and colleagues describe lessons learned from three successful school health promotion programs that were developed and disseminated through collaborations between public health professionals, academic institutions, and school personnel. The programs include two focused on physical activity and good nutrition for elementary and middle school children—Coordinated Approach to Child Health (CATCH) and Planet Health—and one focused on smoking cessation among adolescents—Not-On-Tobacco (N-O-T). Important features of these school health programs include 1) identification of staff and resources required for program implementation and dissemination; 2) involvement of stakeholders (e.g., teachers, students, other school personnel, parents, nonprofit organizations, professional organizations) during all phases of program development and dissemination; 3) planning for dissemination of programs early in the development and testing process; and 4) rigorous evaluation of interventions to determine their effectiveness. The authors provide advice based on lessons learned from these programs to those who wish to work with young people in schools.

The rising prevalence of childhood obesity is a key public health issue worldwide. Increased eating frequency (EF) is one aspect of diet that has been beneficially associated with obesity, although the mechanisms are unclear. The aims of Jennings and colleagues in Chapter 9 were to determine whether increased EF was associated with improved adiposity in children, and if this was due to differences in dietary and activity behaviors. Cross-sectional data from 1,700 children aged 9–10 year were analyzed to examine the associations between EF, as estimated from diet diaries, measures of adiposity, and activity measured by accelerometer. Analyses were stratified by obesity status using waist-to-height ratio to define obesity as it has been shown to be a good predictor of adverse health outcomes. Mean EF was 4.3 occasions/day and after adjustment for underreporting, energy intake (EI), and activity significant relative mean differences of −2.4% for body weight ($P = 0.001$), −1.0% for BMI ($P = 0.020$), −33% for BMI z-score ($P = 0.014$), and −0.6% for waist circumference ($P = 0.031$) per increase in eating occasion were found in healthy-weight but not centrally obese children. Differences between the extreme quartiles of EF were observed for total fat intake at breakfast (−18%, $P < 0.001$), fruit and vegetables from snacks (201% healthy-weight and 209% centrally obese children, $P < 0.01$), and for healthy-weight children, vigorous activity (4%, $P = 0.003$). Increased EF was favorably associated with adiposity, diet quality, and activity behaviors in healthy-weight but not centrally obese children. Future obesity interventions should consider the mediating role of diet quality and activity in the relationship between EF and adiposity in children.

The purpose of Chapter 10, by Janssen and LeBlanc, was to: 1) perform a systematic review of studies examining the relation between physical activity, fitness, and health in school-aged children and youth, and 2) make recommendations based on the findings. The systematic review was limited to 7 health indicators: high blood cholesterol, high blood pressure, the metabolic syndrome, obesity, low bone density, depression, and injuries. Literature searches were conducted using predefined keywords in 6 key databases. A total of 11,088 potential papers were identified. The abstracts and full-text articles of potentially relevant papers were screened to determine eligibility. Data was abstracted for 113 outcomes from the 86 eligible papers. The evidence was graded for each health outcome using established criteria based on the quantity and quality of studies and strength of effect. The volume, intensity, and type of physical activity were considered. Physical activity was associated with numerous health benefits. The dose-response relations observed in observational studies indicate that the more physical activity, the greater the health benefit. Results from experimental studies indicate that even modest amounts of physical activity can have health benefits in high-risk youngsters (e.g., obese). To achieve substantive health benefits, the physical activity should be of at least a moderate intensity. Vigorous intensity activities may provide even greater benefit. Aerobic-based activities had the greatest health benefit, other than for bone health, in which case high-impact weight bearing activities were required. The following recommendations were made: 1) Children and youth 5-17 years of age should accumulate an average of at least 60 minutes per day and up to several hours of at least moderate intensity physical activity. Some of the health benefits can be achieved through an average of 30 minutes per day. [Level 2, Grade A]. 2) More vigorous intensity activities should be incorporated or added when possible, including activities that strengthen muscle and bone [Level 3, Grade B]. 3) Aerobic activities should make up the majority of the physical activity. Muscle and bone strengthening activities should be incorporated on at least 3 days of the week [Level 2, Grade A].

Chapter 11, by Mikkelsen, argues that the growth in obesity around the world necessitates finding new strategies that can counteract its development. The paper outlines some new ways of thinking about obesity and offering programs in schools.

In 2005, Fung and colleagues, the authors of Chapter 12, reported on the success of Comprehensive School Health (CSH) in improving diets, activity levels, and body weights. The successful program was recognized as a "best practice" and has inspired the development of the Alberta Project Promoting active Living and healthy Eating (APPLE) Schools. The project includes 10 schools, most of which are located in socioeconomically disadvantaged areas. The present study examines the effectiveness of a CSH program adopted from a "best practice" example in another setting by evaluating temporal changes in diets, activity levels and body weight. In 2008 and 2010, the authors surveyed grade 5 students from approximately 150 randomly selected schools from the Canadian province of Alberta and students from 10 APPLE Schools. Students completed the Harvard Youth/Adolescent Food Frequency Questionnaire, questions on physical activity, and had their height and weight measured. Multilevel regression methods were used to analyze changes in diets, activity levels, and body weight between 2008 and 2010. In 2010 relative to 2008, students attending APPLE Schools were eating more fruits and vegetables, consuming fewer calories, were more physically active and were less likely obese. These changes contrasted changes observed among students elsewhere in the province. These findings provide evidence on the effectiveness of CSH in improving health behaviors. They show that an example of "best practice" may lead to success in another setting. Herewith the study provides the evidence that investments for broader program implementation based on "best practice" are justified.

During the last 3 decades, the prevalence of obesity has tripled among persons aged 6--19 years. Multiple chronic disease risk factors, such as high blood pressure, high cholesterol levels, and high blood glucose levels are related to obesity. Schools have a responsibility to help prevent obesity and promote physical activity and healthy eating through policies, practices, and supportive environments. Chapter 13, a report put out by the U.S. Centers for Disease Control and Prevention, describes school health guidelines for promoting healthy eating and physical activity, including coordination of school policies and practices; supportive environments; school nutrition services; physical education and physical activity programs; health education; health, mental health, and social services; family and community involvement; school employee wellness; and professional development for school staff members. These guidelines, developed in collaboration with specialists from universities and from national, federal, state, local, and voluntary agencies and organizations, are based on an in-depth review of research, theory, and best practices in healthy eating and physical activity promotion in school health, public health, and education. Because every guideline might not be appropriate or feasible for every school to implement, individual schools should determine which guidelines have the highest priority based on the needs of the school and available resources.

PART I

OVERVIEW AND RATIONALE

CHAPTER 1

CHILDHOOD OBESITY: A GLOBAL PUBLIC HEALTH CRISIS

SAMEERA KARNIK AND AMAR KANEKAR

1.1 INTRODUCTION

Obesity is a major public health crisis among children and adults.[1,2] The range of weights for individuals if greater than the ideal weight, which is considered healthy for the particular height, is termed as either overweight or obese. Childhood-related obesity is an increasing concern with respect to the health and well-being of the child. Body mass index (BMI), a measure of weight with relation to height, is not only used as an outcome measure to determine obesity but also as a useful anthropometric index for cardiovascular risk.[3] For children between 2 and 19 years, BMI is plotted on the CDC growth chart to check for the corresponding age and sex related percentile. Childhood obesity is defined as a BMI at or above 95th percentile for children of same age and sex.[4] Classifications of obesity in children depend upon the body composition of the child, as it varies with respect to age and sex of the child.[4]

1.2 MAGNITUDE OF THE PROBLEM

The prevalence of childhood obesity is increasing in developed and underdeveloped countries.[5] The development in reducing the problem of obesity and overweight is monitored nationally by using data from National Health and Nutrition Examination Survey. The report presented by NHANES for the year 2007-2008 estimated that 16.9% of children and adolescent in the age group of 2-19 years were obese.[6] Childhood obesity prevalence among preschool children between age group of 2-5-year-old girls and boys has increased from 5.0 to 10% between 1976-1980 and 2007-2008 and it has increased from 6.5 to 19.6% among age group of 6-11 year olds.[6] The data collected for the same period shows that the adolescent (age group 12-19 years) obesity has increased from 5.0 to 18.1% [Figure 1, Table 1].[6]

TABLE 1: Prevalence of obesity among US children and adolescents aged 2-19, for selected years 1963-1965 through 2007-2008[6]

	Age (in years)			
	Total	2–5	6–11	12–19
NHANES 1963–1965 and 1966–1970	[3]	[3]	4.2	4.6
NHANES 1971–1974	5.0	5.0	4.0	6.1
NHANES 1976–1980	5.5	5.0	6.5	5.0
NHANES 1988–1994	10.0	7.2	11.3	10.5
NHANES 1999–2000	13.9	10.3	15.1	14.8
NHANES 2001–2002	15.4	10.6	16.3	16.7
NHANES 2003–2004	17.1	13.9	18.8	17.4
NHANES 2005–2006	15.5	11.0	15.1	17.8
NHANES 2007–2008	16.9	10.4	19.6	18.1

Note: Obesity defined as body mass index (BMI) greater than or equal to sex- and age-specific 95th percentile from the 2000 CDC Growth Charts

Healthy people 2010 have ranked obesity as number one health problem showing that prevalence of childhood obesity has increased over the years.[7] Increased prevalence of childhood obesity may have adverse morbidity and mortality implications in the adult life of the child.[8] Childhood obesity concern has increased worldwide. There has been increased prevalence of childhood obesity in England, especially among school children over last few decades.[9] Childhood obesity is common in United Kingdom and according to the health survey conducted in 2004, obesity among 2-10-year olds was 14% and among 11-15-year olds was 15%.[5]

1.3 METHODS

In order to collect materials for this review a detailed search of CINAHL, MEDLINE, ERIC, Academic Search Premier databases was carried out for the time period 1999-2011. A Boolean search strategy where the key words entered for search were "factors" and "childhood obesity" "interventions" and "governmental actions" and "economic problems" in differing orders were used to extract studies for this narrative review.

1.4 FACTORS INFLUENCING CHILDHOOD OBESITY

Childhood obesity is due to the imbalance between caloric intake of the child and the calories utilized (for growth, development, metabolism, and physical activities). Normally the amount of calories a child consumes through food or beverages, if not used for energy activities, leads to obesity.[10] Factors causing childhood obesity are genetic, behavioral, and environmental. Obesity can be multifactorial in children.

1.5 GENETIC FACTORS

There are certain genetic factors which may lead to obesity in children. These genetic factors increase the child's susceptibility for obesity.[10] Genetic factors may influence the metabolism, by changing the body fat content and energy intake and energy expenditure. Heritability of obesity from parents also influences obesity in children.[11]

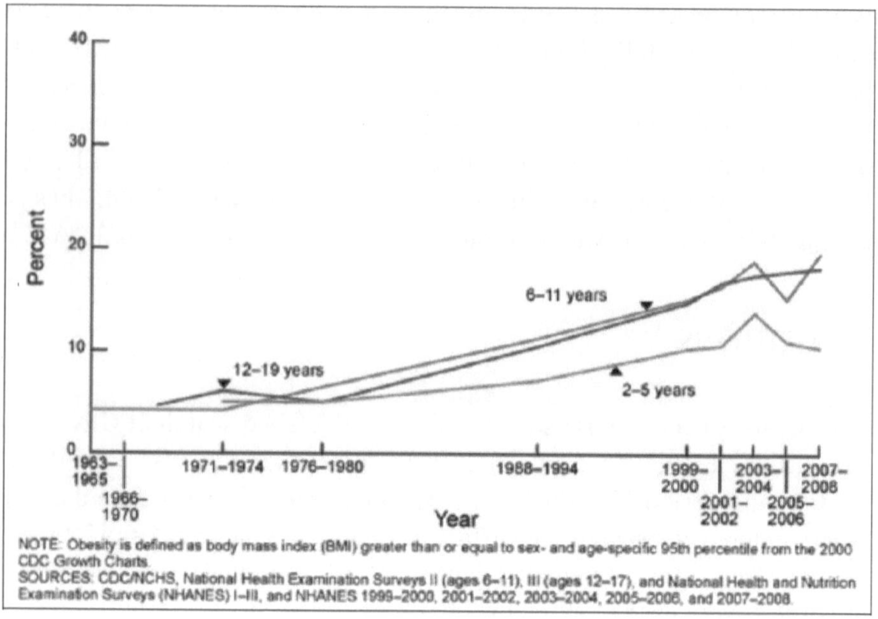

FIGURE 1: Graphically shows the increasing trend of obesity among children and adolescent population from 1963 to 2008. Source: CDC/NCHS, National Health Examination Surveys 11 (ages 6-11), 111 (ages 12-17), and National Health and Nutrition Examination Surveys (NHANES) 1-111 and NHANES 1999-2000, 2001-2002, 2003-2004, 2005-2006, and 2007-2008[6]

1.6 BEHAVIORAL FACTORS

There are some behavioral factors which can cause obesity. Sometimes children eat more or consume more energy via food and beverages which are not utilized appropriately.[10] Children may eat large portions of food, foods high in sugar, and energy-rich foods. Hence, energy intake is higher than energy expenditure. So this may lead to weight gain in children.[10]

Lack of physical activity also plays an important role in obesity. Energy gained should be properly balanced by energy expenditure. It is seen that children and teens nowadays lack the required amount of physical activity; hence the calories are not used properly and can lead to obesity.[10] In a recently conducted mixed-methods study conducted in Iran, lack of safe and easy-access place for physical activity and unsupportive family were the main barriers to physical activity among adolescents.[12]

It is seen that sedentary lifestyle is an important factor for obesity, as many children spend most of their time in front of television sets, play video games, and watch computers. Children snack more in front of television and spent most of their time sitting without any physical activity.[10] All these behavioral factors are in a vicious circle with one leading to another. Children are prone to sedentary lifestyle such as watching television, consuming more energy-dense foods or snacks with large portion sizes, and having reduced physical activity, giving rise to obesity. The television advertisements of energy-rich and sugar-rich foods influence children to make unhealthy choices. These unhealthy food choices may lead to weight gain and obesity.[10]

1.7 ENVIRONMENTAL FACTORS

Environmental factors are those that surround the children and influence their food intake and physical activity.[10] These factors are seen in various settings such as at home, in school, and in the community. At home, the parent-child interaction is very crucial as parents can influence children food choices and motivate them to have a healthy lifestyle. Children spend most of their time at school, so school can promote healthy food choices and physical activity among them.[10] Community's lack of accessibility and affordability of healthy food can affect the nutrition of these children. Their lack of physical activity may be because of lack of facilities like safe side walks, bike paths, and safe parks.[10]

1.8 CONSEQUENCES OF CHILDHOOD OBESITY

Much health-related problems are associated with obesity in children. Childhood obesity also leads to health risks in adulthood. Health problems related to obesity are not only physical but psychological and social as well.[13]

1.9 PSYCHOLOGICAL AND SOCIAL HEALTH ISSUES

Children who are obese have a negative body-image, which leads to lower self-esteem. Children feel depressed and are nervous about their obesity issue and this has a negative effect on their behavior. This may also reflect negatively on their academic and social progress. They feel socially discriminated and stigmatized by their peers and adults.[13,14]

1.10 OTHER HEALTH RISKS

Obese children have high risk of cardiovascular diseases, high blood pressure, and increased cholesterol levels.[13] Childhood obesity increases the risk of having insulin resistant type 2 diabetes.[14] Children may have high risk of having respiratory problems like asthma as well. Obesity causes shortness of breath and sleep apnea. The physical effects may also reflect on musculoskeletal system causing discomfort due to increased weight on joint, causing muscle and bone disorder.[14] Obesity may affect liver causing fatty degeneration of liver.[13]

1.11 BEHAVIORAL INTERVENTIONS

Childhood obesity is a major public health issue. The complications caused due to childhood obesity are severe and could continue to affect the health of a child even in adulthood.[13] Hence, there is need to address this problem at every possible step through effective interventions and motivation strategies.

1.12 FAMILY-BASED LIFESTYLE INTERVENTIONS

Family bonding is a strong structure in the behavioral molding of the child. Parents and siblings are the people around the child who can influence child behavior and lifestyle.[15] Hence, effective interventions in a family setting can be beneficial to change child's behavior of overeating and unhealthy choice of food. Physical activity can be improved by small strategies like parking cars away from stores so that kids can walk and to take stairs instead of elevators or escalators. It is essential that parents are aware of the potential risk the child is facing due to obesity and take actions to control the problem. Effective measures to prevent obesity in future can be promoted by these interventions.[14] These weight-control interventions can be achieved and sustained by providing good support and a variety of strategies to parents.[16]

1.13 SCHOOL-BASED INTERVENTIONS

Children spend most of their time in schools. Hence, school plays an important role in the life of the child. There are many school-based intervention strategies. Some interventions focus on nutrition-based or physical-based aspect of weight-control independently, while others jointly focus on both aspects of nutrition and physical activity to achieve the aim of weight control in children.[17] Children take at least one meal at school. Hence, schools can encourage kids to make a healthy food choice like reducing the intake of carbonated drinks or sugary foods, encourage kids to drink healthy fruit juices, water, vegetables, and fruits. Schools which provide meals can have healthy nutritious food items with emphasis on a balanced diet.[18] Schools can involve kids in physical activity by strategies like lengthening the time of physical activity; involving them in moderate to vigorous physical activity for short durations, encouraging them to walk or active commuting, and taking stairs instead of elevators. Kids should be encouraged to participate in various physical activities like games and dance groups with more emphasis on non-competitiveness. Some school-based programs along with the help of community members can help to promote physical education skills and healthy nutrition among children, with focus on implementing this education for maintaining long-term healthy behavior. Classroom-based health education can make older children and teens aware of eating nutritious diet and engaging in regular physical activity.[17]

1.14 COMMUNITY-BASED INTERVENTIONS

Community plays a crucial role in healthy lifestyle of children. The term "community" includes the environment around children along with other factors like geographic location, race, ethnicity, and socioeconomic status.[19] This resource can be effectively used to promote healthy nutrition and healthy behavior. Community support is invaluable in implementing interventions and organizing social events like healthy food festivals, harvest festivals, imparting healthy messages, and educating and encouraging people to adopt healthy lifestyle. Thus, community can help children to get affordable and accessible healthy food options and encourage healthy nutrition.[19] Community organizations along with parents can promote nutrition and physical activity-based programs for children, eg., walk to school. Community can make the neighborhood safe and accessible to children and motivate them to increase physical activity.[20] Other programs like providing play groups with safe play grounds and bike paths for kids to play outside will reduce their time spent in front of television sets. Community can provide children with easy accessible facilities like gymnasiums and supervised physical education with strategies such as music for physical activities. Community can influence media or local entertainment to promote healthy educational programs for parents and children. Hence, making them aware of healthy intervention programs via the community is important to reduce childhood obesity.[20]

1.15 PLAY-BASED INTERVENTIONS

Instead of just advising children what to eat they can appreciate nutrition-related education in a better way when it comes to them via fun activities like playing games. Some countries are using board games for children to make them understand about balanced diet and thus leading to knowledge gain.[17] Interactive multimedia can be used for interventions. Interactive multimedia like CD ROM can promote healthy nutrition in children with the help of virtual educational games. When these games are used in real-life situations children can make healthy food choices. They can promote decision making and self-esteem for healthy eating behavior. Thus, these programs can help and motivate children to make healthy food choices and also understand the benefits of making such choices.[17] These innovative interventions can encourage children to lead a healthy life.

1.16 CHILDHOOD-OBESITY PREVENTION INTERVENTIONS

Preventive programs are conducted to control obesity in children and to modify the social and behavioral aspect of developing obesity. Some of the preventive programs revolve around educating the general population about healthy nutrition and providing information about health problems caused due to childhood obesity.[15] Health care professionals can advise their patients, especially parents, about healthy child nutrition, tackling health problems due to childhood obesity, and benefits of breast feeding among newborn children to prevent weight gain.[21] Federal or state actions to deal with childhood obesity are directing all the food vendors to provide exact calorie readable labels on their products, mentioning calories upfront on menus, restricting advertisements of unhealthy foods, and promoting healthy food making among parents. Some of the other actions are to improve transportation facility for people and children, like providing bike paths, making sidewalks, and providing safe and clean surrounding for children to walk and play eg. no-car roads.[15]

1.17 HOSPITAL-BASED INTERVENTIONS

Laboratory investigations of children who are obese and at risk of complications are important. Children aged 7 years and younger with no secondary complications of obesity are advised weight management.[8] Weight-loss programs like dietary management (eating more of fiber-rich foods) and increasing physical activity are recommended for children above 7 years of age with risk of secondary complications. Pharmacological therapy for children with obesity above the age of 12 years can include drugs like orlistat (which blocks fat from the intestine thus giving negative energy balance).[8] Medical professionals are considering the benefits of bariatric surgery in extremely obese children to avoid complications of obesity in adulthood.[22]

1.18 POTENTIAL CHANGES

There may be some potential barriers to these interventions, which may make the task of promoting healthy behavior and improving physical activity in children challenging. Some of these challenges are:

1.19 FINANCIAL CHALLENGES

Financial investment in these interventions is very crucial. All the intervention-based programs need monitoring of progress and sustainability over many years, which may be costly. In today's world of economic problems funding for such programs is limited.[17] School-based intervention programs require much effort on budgeting and planning, as the cost of educating the teachers about the program, and providing facilities and infrastructure to conduct physical activities is enormous and prohibitive.[17] Communities also find it challenging to make the neighborhood safe for children to play, to organize events, and to provide adequate facilities.

1.20 STIGMATIZATION OF OBESE CHILDREN

Obese children are mostly discriminated due to their body image. This may lead to a potential challenge for these children to come forward and opt for healthy programs. Stigmatization of these children by their peers and by others acts as a mental barrier leading to negative body image and fear of food.[17]

1.21 LOGISTICAL ISSUES

Literature reviews of school-based interventions conducted in the past have shown mixed outcomes. According to a recent review about school-based interventions for obesity prevention, 17 out of 25 intervention studies were effective in reducing the body mass index.[23] Some interventions targeting physical activity through physical education along with nutritional education worked in reducing obesity. Interventions targeting physical activity education and television viewing were seen to be successful in this review study.[23] While another review addressed school-based interventions by conducting a meta-analysis, concluding that body mass index may not be a good outcome measure among school kids.[24]

1.22 US GOVERNMENTAL STRATEGIES TO REDUCE CHILDHOOD OBESITY

According to the Centers for Disease Control and Prevention, identifying effective intervention strategies that can target both improvements in physical activity and providing nutritious diet to reduce childhood obesity are important. These evidence-based programs can be effective in managing obesity in children.[21] Interventions encouraging mothers to breast-feed their babies can be effective in reducing the risk of obesity in children.[21] The United States government is changing the health policies involving transportation, land use, education, agriculture, and economics so that it can have an important impact on healthy environment and health of people in turn reducing obesity.[21] The United States government, along with other health organizations, is developing healthy environments like improving population access to healthy and fresh foods, building walk paths, bike paths, and playgrounds in underserved communities. State governments with the assistance of different health organizations are also getting involved in promoting healthy lifestyles for people. The First Lady has also initiated an obesity prevention and control program titled "Let's move." [21]

1.23 FUTURE IMPLICATIONS

Childhood obesity is a major public health problem. Hence, implementation of the available effective intervention programs is essential. Important data regarding evaluation of childhood obesity prevention schemes can be collected and can be used to make stronger and more effective strategies including policy building to reduce future childhood obesity rates.[25]

1.24 CONCLUSIONS

Childhood obesity has become a public health crisis, not just in the United States but all over the world. Childhood obesity problem can be reduced by educating children and parents about healthy nutrition and encouraging them to be physically active. There are effective interventions and government policies for prevention and control of childhood obesity. Sustainability of these interventions is a key factor, so that children can adopt these healthy behaviors as a lifelong practice and have a healthy life. This will lead to a nationwide healthy future for the kids.

REFERENCES

1. Centers for Disease Control and Prevention, Overweight and obesity; Defining overweight and obesity. [Last accessed on 2010]. Available from: http://www.cdc.gov/obesity/defining.html .
2. Theodore LA, Bray MA, Kehle TJ. Introduction to the special issue: Childhood obesity. Psychol Sch. 2009;46:693–4.
3. Ribiero RC, Coutinho M, Bramorski MA, Giuliano IC, Pavan J. Association of the waist-to-height ratio with cardiovascular risk factors in children and adolescents: The three cities heart study. Int J Prev Mednone. 2010;1:39–49.
4. Centers for Disease Control and Prevention, Overweight and obesity; Childhood overweight and obesity. [Last accessed on 2009]. Available from: http://www.cdc.gov/obesity/childhood/defining.html .
5. Reilly JJ. Childhood obesity: An overview. Child Soc. 2007;21:390–6.
6. Ogden C, Carroll M. Prevalence of obesity among children and adolescents: United States, trends 1963–1965 through 2007–2008. Retrieved from National center for health statistics, Center for Disease Control and Prevention. [Last accessed on 2010]. Available from: http://www.cdc.gov/nchs/data/hestat/obesity_child_07_08/obesity_child_07_08.pdf .
7. Tulchinsky TH, Varavikova EA. The new public health. 2nd ed. Burlington, MA: Elsevier academic press; 2009.
8. Singhal V, Schwenk WF, Kumar S. Evaluation and management of childhood and adolescent obesity. Mayo Clin Proc. 2007;82:1258–64.

9. Stamatakis E, Wardle J, Cole TJ. Childhood obesity and overweight prevalence trends in England: Evidence for growing socioeconomic disparities. Int J Obes (Lond) 2010;34:41–7.
10. Centers for Disease Control and Prevention, Overweight and obesity; childhood overweight and obesity, contributing factors. [Last accessed on 2009]. Available from: http://www.cdc.gov/obesity/childhood/causes.html .
11. Perusse L, Bouchard C. Role of genetic factors in childhood obesity and in susceptibility to dietary variations. [Last accessed on 2011 Sept 03];Ann Med. 1999 31:19–25. Available from: http://www.ncbi.nlm.nih.gov/pubmed/10342496 .
12. Kelishadi R, Ghatrehsamani S, Hosseini M, Mirmoghtadaee P, Mansouri S, Poursafa P. Barriers to physical activity in a population-based sample of children and adolescent in Isfahn, Iran. Int J Prev Med. 2009;1:131–7.
13. Centers for Disease Control and Prevention. Overweight and obesity; childhood overweight and obesity, consequences. [Last accessed on 2009]. Available from: http://www.cdc.gov/obesity/childhood/consequences.html .
14. Ben-Sefer E, Ben-Natan M, Ehrenfeld M. Childhood obesity: Current literature, policy and implications for practice. Int Nurs Rev. 2009;56:166–73.
15. Carraro R, García Cebrián M. Role of prevention in the contention of the obesity epidemic. Eur J Clin Nutr. 2003;57(Suppl 1):S94–6.
16. Pott W, Albayrak O, Hebebrand J, Pauli-Pott U. Treating childhood obesity: Family background variables and the child's success in a weight-control intervention. Int J Eat Disord. 2009;42:284–9.
17. Hutchinson G. Tackling obesity through school-based interventions. Br J Sch Nurs. 2010;5:335–7.
18. Rahman T, Cushing RA, Jackson RJ. Contributions of built environment to childhood obesity. Mt Sinai J Med. 2011;78:49–57.
19. Economos CD, Irish-Hauser S. Community interventions: A brief overview and their application to the obesity epidemic. J Law Med Ethics. 2007;35:131–7.
20. Tucker P, Irwin JD, Bouck LM, He M, Pollett G. Preventing paediatric obesity; recommendations from a community-based qualitative investigation. Obes Rev. 2006;7:251–60.
21. Centers for Disease Control and Prevention (2011) [Last retrieved on 2011 Feb 03];CDC grand rounds: Childhood obesity in the United States. Morbidity and Mortality Weekly Report. 60(02):42–46. Available from: http://www.cdc.gov/mmwr/preview/mmwrhtml/mm6002a2.htm?s_cid=mm6002a2_w .
22. Inge TH, Xanthakos SA, Zeller MH. Bariatric surgery for pediatric extreme obesity: Now or later? Int J Obes (Lond) 2007;31:1–14.
23. Doak CM, Visscher TLS, Renders CM, Seidell JC. The prevention of overweight and obesity in children and adolescents: A review of interventions and programmes. Obes Rev. 2006;7:111–36.
24. Kanekar A, Sharma M. Meta-analysis of school-based childhood obesity interventions in the U.K. and U.S. Int Q Community Health Educ. 2009;29:241–56.
25. Fussenegger D, Pietrobelli A, Widhalm K. Childhood obesity: Political developments in Europe and related perspectives for future action on prevention. Obes Rev. 2008;9:76–82.

CHAPTER 2

READING, WRITING, AND OBESITY: AMERICA'S FAILING GRADE IN SCHOOL NUTRITION AND PHYSICAL EDUCATION

JASON SCHAUB AND MARY MARIAN

> *Because of the increasing rates of obesity, unhealthy eating habits and physical inactivity, we may see the first generation that will be less healthy and have a shorter life expectancy than their parents.*
> —Former Surgeon General Richard Carmona, 2003 [1]

Childhood obesity in America has reached epidemic proportions. [2] According to the latest statistics from the Centers for Disease Control and Prevention (CDC), more than one-third of children in the United States aged 10–17 are overweight (18.2%) or obese (16.4%). [3] Recent findings conclude that compared with smoking, obesity is an equal or greater contributor of preventable death, indicating obesity has surpassed smoking as the leading cause of preventable death in America. [4]

Reprinted with permission from Sage Publications. Schaub J and Marian M. Reading, Writing, and Obesity: America's Failing Grade in School Nutrition and Physical Education. Nutrition in Clinical Practice, ***26****,5 (2011). doi: 10.1177/0884533611416820.*

The relationship between obesity and risk for chronic disease, such as cardiovascular disease (CVD), hypertension, and type 2 diabetes mellitus, has been established and is well documented. [5] Most chronic diseases develop over many years and, because 70%–80% of overweight and obese children will remain overweight their entire lives, [6] it is critical to understand why the childhood obesity rate is epidemic and develop effective strategies to reduce its incidence in the future. Over the past decade, numerous studies and programs have been developed to combat the growing obesity epidemic. Considering children spend the majority of their day in school, school-based programs have the potential to provide significant influence on a child's health.

The above quote, an excerpt from a statement by the former Surgeon General Richard Carmona titled *The Growing Epidemic of Childhood Obesity*, exemplifies how critical proper nutrition and physical activity are in maintaining health. This article provides an account of the historical and modern development of 2 programs responsible for nutrition and physical activity in American elementary, middle, and high schools: the National School Lunch Program (NSLP) and physical education (PE) classes. Because of the large amount of time children spend in school and on school campuses, a thorough understanding of these programs is essential when developing strategies to counter the childhood obesity epidemic.

2.1 SCHOOL NUTRITION PROGRAMS

The thought of school lunch likely conjures up many different memories of childhood. However, the foods offered today at elementary, middle, and high school campuses have changed considerably over the past 30 years. In the following section, a brief history of the NSLP and associated topics in school nutrition are presented.

2.1.1 SCHOOL NUTRITION PROGRAM HISTORY

The concept of a nationally funded school nutrition program was advocated through the 19th and 20th centuries by small-scale, independent welfare groups. The movement gained widespread consideration after World War I, when draft results identified a significant proportion of American men with malnutrition- and undernutrition-related conditions. [7] Rising rates of malnutrition during the Great Depression led to the first substantial assistance to school lunch programs from the federal government in 1932 under the umbrella of President Franklin D. Roosevelt's New Deal programs and the 1933 Agricultural Adjustment Act (AAA). The Reconstruction Finance Corporation and the Works Progress Administration also provided funds to schools to develop school meal programs, assist facility construction, and direct food service and preparation. [8] The New Deal programs stipulated that federal funds be spent on both food service as well as nutrition education in the classroom. [7]

In May 1941, at the request of President Roosevelt, a National Nutrition Conference for Defense was held to address the current status of nutrition in the United States. In a letter to the federal security administrator, Roosevelt stated, "Every survey of nutrition shows that here in the United States undernourishment is widespread and serious. . . . We do not lack, as we will not lack, the means of producing food in abundance and variety. Our task is to translate this abundance into reality for every American family." [9] Upon the closing of the conference, the first national Recommended Dietary Allowances (RDAs) for vitamins and minerals were constructed by a team from the U.S. Department of Agriculture (USDA) and the Food and Nutrition Board of the National Academy of Sciences. [7,10] Then, in 1943, the USDA published the National Wartime Nutrition Guide, which outlined the basic 7 food groups. This guide, revised in 1946 and renamed the National Food Guide, described a foundation diet that would provide the majority of the newly defined RDAs of vitamins and minerals to Americans.

On June 4, 1946, Congress passed the National School Lunch Program (NSLP) Act. Section 2 of the act states the purpose clearly: "It is hereby declared to be the policy of Congress, as a measure of national security, to safeguard the health and well-being of the Nation's children and to encourage the domestic consumption of nutritious agricultural commodities and other food, by assisting the States, through grants-in aid and other means, in providing an adequate supply of food and other facilities for the establishment, maintenance, operation and expansion of nonprofit school lunch programs." [11] The National School Lunch Program Act passed in

1946 was very similar to the New Deal programs it replaced with one important exception—the NSLP eliminated federal funds for nutrition education, designating nutrition education specifically as a state matter. [7,8]

The NSLP is administered through the Food and Nutrition Service (FNS) branch of the USDA and functions to provide meals containing one-third of the RDA of essential nutrients to students. In addition, schools must provide meals that conform to the joint Health and Human Services (HHS)–USDA Dietary Guidelines for Americans (DGA). Also, because one of the original intents of the act was to prevent nutrition deficits, participating schools must provide free or reduced-price meals to children who are unable to afford full-price meals. [12]

To cover operating costs, the act requires participating schools to match federal contributions to the program. Through the 1960s, most schools attempted to match federal contributions by balancing revenue from the sale of full-price meals with the cost of free or reduced-price meals. In turn, low-income school districts with relatively few students able to afford full-price meals could not match federal contributions and therefore could not participate in the NSLP. The inaccessibility of the program maintained malnutrition rates in low-income regions and eventually led to the rediscovery of hunger in America and President Lyndon B. Johnson's subsequent War on Poverty. [7]

Numerous congressional amendments have been made over the years to improve the accessibility of the program to those in need. The Child Nutrition Act of 1966 "extended, expanded and strengthened" the NSLP through grants-in-aid to states to "meet more effectively the nutritional needs of our children." [8] This included the integration of the Special Milk Program with the NSLP, and amendments made in 1968 expanded the NSLP to private, nonprofit, and service institutions.

Despite congressional efforts, budgeting issues remained, and in 1969, Secretary of Agriculture Orville Freeman deregulated the NSLP, allowing school districts to contract with private food service companies in an attempt to reduce costs. [7] A series of amendments followed, most notably those made in the 1970s allowing the sale of competitive foods, foods of minimal nutrition value (FMNV), and soft drinks and sports drinks in vending machines and snack carts. This resulted in a massive influx of new food offerings available to children. Student purchases of competitive foods increased, augmenting school revenue and reducing NSLP deficit, ultimately allowing for more free or reduced-price meals to be offered. [7] In fact, privatization of school meal service was so fiscally successful that, according to the CDC, in 2000, nearly 1 in 5 schools (20.2%) in America had brand-name fast-food services operating on campus. [12,14] Today the NSLP is operating in more than 101,000 public and nonprofit private schools—nearly 95% of schools in the United States. [12,15]

2.1.2 CURRENT NSLP MEAL COMPOSITION AND SCHOOL NUTRITION

The NSLP stipulates that meals must conform to the DGA, which includes standards for total fat (30%) and saturated fat (10%), as well as protein, vitamin A, vitamin C, iron, calcium, and calories. [12] However, recent evidence shows that on average, the current NSLP meal currently violates these limitations. Some recent findings include the following:

- Robinson-O'Brien et al [16] concluded that fruit and vegetable intake among NSLP participants in low-income regions is below recommended levels.
- Crepinsek et al [17] concluded from the third School Nutrition Dietary Assessment Study (SNDA III) that more than two-thirds of schools exceeded the recommended limit of saturated fat and total fat for NSLP lunches.
- Clark and Fox [18] also concluded from the SNDA III study, as well as from 24-hour diet recalls, that 80% of children had excessive saturated fat intake and 92% had excessive sodium intake.

In light of similar findings, the Institute of Medicine released a report in 2009 recommending the USDA modify menu standards for the NSLP to increase the amount and variety of fruits and vegetables, set minimum and maximum calorie levels, and reduce the levels of saturated fat and sodium. [19] Then, on February 9, 2010, President Barack H. Obama established the Task Force on Childhood Obesity, whose goal is to reverse the trend of childhood obesity within a generation through various interventions. [20] In response, the USDA has released a proposal to adopt these standards. [21]

In addition to the NSLP, the overall school nutrition environment also has been under review. In a report to Congress from the FNS in 2001, the USDA outlined the potential for competitive foods to affect "the viability" of the NSLP and pose diet-related health risks. [22] The School Health Policies and Programs Study (SHPPS) are national surveys performed periodically through the CDC on elementary, middle, and high school campuses. Results from the most recent SHPPS (2006) revealed that 32.7% of elementary schools, 71.3% of middle schools, and 89.4% of high schools had vending machines or snack bars where students could purchase a la carte foods or beverages. [23] Table 1 shows results from the 2006 SHPPS, listing the percentage of schools selling selected a la carte foods to students.

TABLE 1: Percentage of Schools Selling Select a la Carte Foods

Food Product	Elementary, %	Middle, %	High, %
1% or skim milk	4.2	12.9	20.2
100% fruit juice	16.8	41.1	64.7
Cookies, crackers, pastries not low in fat	12.0	27.6	58.3
Fruit or vegetables	4.2	8.7	17.9
Salty snacks, low fat	11.3	30.9	58.0
Salty snacks, not low in fat	11.6	30.4	61.4
Soda	16.4	45.0	76.8
Sports drinks	12.4	51.7	75.0

Data from the Centers for Disease Control and Prevention. [23]

Although the NSLP plays an integral role in student health, it is not independently responsible for student diet at school, primarily because not all students participate in the program. However, the NSLP indirectly affects nearly all students because a school's participation in the program can have considerable influence on the overall campus nutrition environment—chiefly through allowing commercial fast-food and soft-drink companies, vending machines, and foods of minimum nutrition value.

2.2 PHYSICAL EDUCATION (PE)

Likewise with school lunches, the thought of PE may also elicit early recounts of team sports and other competitive games, but unlike the NSLP, physical education has a long and extensive history dating back thousands of years. For much of that time, physical education was a natural pursuit of physicians, originating organically from their quest to achieve and maintain the health of their patients, a field known today as preventive medicine. As we will see, only recently has PE been so heavily focused on sports skills development.

2.2.1 HISTORY OF PHYSICAL EDUCATION

The modern physical education movement in America began during the turn of the 19th century, but the roots of PE can be traced back to the time of ancient Greece. Herodicus, a Greek physician who lived during the 5th century BC, has been attributed as one of the first to emphasize the relationship between physical activity and health. Herodicus practiced therapeutic gymnastics and believed exercise was "just as important to provide against disease in the healthy man as to cure him who was already attacked." [24] Historians believe that Herodicus's work on nutrition and exercise heavily influenced Hippocrates's theory on regimen in health, which outlines the importance both play in maintaining health and preventing disease. Hippocrates's work was further advanced in the 2nd century AD by Greek physician and philosopher Galen, whose theory on the relationship between the nonnaturals and health, later known as the Laws of Health, became the foundation of physical education for centuries to come. [24]

The Laws of Health are a set of variables Galen believed must be expressed in the proper balance to foster a harmonious environment for the body to exist free from disease. The variables—air, food and drink, motion and rest, sleep and wake, excretions and retentions, and passions of the mind—were called nonnatural because the expression of each is not controlled by nature but by the individual self. Galen collected his recommendations on exercise, nutrition, and the other disciplines in numerous works, most notably in his book titled *On Hygiene*. Written for the professional and layman alike, *On Hygiene* was one of the first books of preventive medicine to interest a diverse audience of readers. For centuries, living according to the Laws of Health was considered one of the most effective methods to prevent disease, and up until the mid-1800s, the term physical education was used to describe the teaching of these laws. [22,25]

2.2.2 PHYSICAL EDUCATION IN MODERN AMERICA

The first state legislation mandating that public schools provide regular instruction in physical education occurred in California in 1866. Supported by Superintendent of Public Instruction John Swett, the bill was passed to ensure attention was given to "such physical exercise for the pupils as may be conducive to health and vigor of the body, as well as the mind." [26(p362)] Understanding the importance of PE for students, in 1885, a group of likeminded medical doctors and physical educators founded the American Association for the Advancement of Physical Education (AAPE), whose objective was to achieve and maintain health through the teaching of the Laws of Health. [25] The name was changed to the American Physical Education Association in 1903 and later became the American Alliance for Health, Physical Education, Recreation and Dance (AAHPERD) after merging with the National Education Association in 1937. [27] Today the AAHPERD is one of the leading professional associations for physical educators.

In the early 1900s, a series of events dramatically changed the way physical education was taught and continues to influence many physical education curriculums today. One of the most influential of these events was the standardization of American medical education that took place in the first quarter of the 20th century. At the time, there was widespread discussion within the medical community on how to best adapt scientific advancements in theory and treatments to medical education. At the request of the Carnegie Foundation, Abraham Flexner undertook a project of immense proportion. Over a 2-year period, Flexner visited every medical school in the United States and Canada, uncovering widespread and considerable inconsistencies in all levels of operation among schools. His report, titled *Medical Education in the United States and Canada,* has been dubbed *The Flexner Report* because of the "epoch-making" status it gained when it galvanized the nation into medical education reform after its release in 1910. [25,26] In the report, Flexner outlined what would become the future of medical education in North America. [28]

Paramount to the report were findings related to the variance in admissions standards, testing, comprehension of basic tenets of the scientific method, and required clinical experience. Admission standards varied so greatly that Flexner was able to categorize schools into 3 groups: (1) schools that required 2 or more years of college coursework, (2) schools that required a high school degree, and (3) schools that "ask little or nothing more than the rudiments or the recollection of a common school education." [28] It was also discovered that the type of curriculum varied radically. For instance, some schools offered or required laboratory work, whereas others did not. In addition, some schools had no affiliation with a hospital, offering only didactic study. In light of these findings, a major conclusion of the report was that "a hospital under complete educational control is as necessary to a medical school as is a laboratory of chemistry or pathology." [28] As a result, not only was there a major overhaul of admissions criteria, curricula, training standards, and testing but also the closing altogether of some schools.

As Henry S. Pritchett, former president of the Carnegie Foundation, stated, "Progress for the future would seem to require a very much smaller number of medical schools, better equipped and better conducted than our schools now," and although fewer MDs would be produced, those that were would be "better educated and better trained." [28] The scientific foundation, as well as the integration of the now-standard clinical phase (residency) of modern MD programs, has been largely attributed to Flexner's efforts.

In addition to fewer new doctors being produced each year, another consequence of the *Flexner Report* was the heightening of the medical profession to a new level of elitism. More rigorous admissions and increased training came with a price, and many of the new generation of MDs chose to focus their work on researching and publishing advancements in modern medical science. Subsequently, the much-needed reform of American medical education resulted in the loss of physicians from the newly denigrated practice of traditional preventive medicine through physical education. [25,26,29]

Concurrent with the reformation of medical education in the early 20th century was the rise in popularity of competitive spectator sports, including football, baseball, and basketball. [25] The number of collegiate and youth sports teams also began to rise, and with the loss of physicians from the field, PE classes began to be taught primarily by school sports coaches. [26] The increasing prevalence of coaches teaching physical education, coupled with decreasing numbers of physicians involved in curriculum oversight, led to the shift of physical education curriculum from specifically health promotion to the more sports-skilled curriculum still prevalent today. [25]

The necessity for national youth physical fitness testing was realized in the early 1950s when reports published by Kraus and Hirschland revealed that European youth were more physically fit than American youth. [30] Subsequently, on July 16, 1956, president Dwight D. Eisenhower passed Executive Order 10673, establishing the President's Council on Youth Fitness. Then, together with the AAHPERD, the 1958 Youth Fitness Test was developed to quantify and track the physical fitness of young Americans. The testing battery consisted of general calisthenics and endurance trials, including sit-ups, pull-ups, distance runs, and aquatic tests. The battery has been modified over the years with relatively minor modifications. [30] In 1968, President Lyndon B. Johnson created the President's Physical Fitness Award and renamed the council the President's Council on Physical Fitness and Sports. The Youth Fitness Test was also renamed and became known as the President's Challenge. [31] The council was again renamed in 2010 by President Barack H. Obama to the President's Council on Fitness, Sports and Nutrition, emphasizing the importance of nutrition in fitness. [32]

2.2.3 CURRENT TRENDS IN PHYSICAL EDUCATION

Over the past 2 decades, there has been a significant decline in the number of students enrolled in PE classes. Data from the CDC's High School

Youth Risk Behavior Survey [33] showing the percentage of students who attended daily PE classes are presented in Figure 1. Over the 8-year time span from 1991 to 1999, the percentage of high school freshmen in daily PE classes dropped from 65.8% to 42.1%. During the same time period, sophomore PE enrollment dropped similarly, from 51.8% to 30.4%. There are numerous causes for the decline in PE class enrollment, many of which are beyond the scope of this article, but a major factor identified is reduced funding.

A recent statement by the National Association for Sport and Physical Education (NASPE) underscores this concern by outlining the case for PE to be recognized as an academic subject. The blueprint for the Elementary and Secondary Education Reauthorization Act released in 2010, commonly known as the No Child Left Behind Act, excludes PE from grants to core academic subjects, including English, science and technology, and math, as well as additional academic subjects, including art, foreign language, history and geography, economics, and other subjects. The NASPE believes that through the exclusion of physical education, the "Department of Education will once again send a strong message that PE is of marginal importance" and that "failure to include PE . . . will completely undermine the White House Task Force on Childhood Obesity's recommendation" to increase physical education for all students. [34]

2.3 CONCURRENT PEDIATRIC HEALTH ISSUES

With a historical perspective of physical education and school nutrition programs established, recent school-based obesity and health intervention studies will be reviewed. The studies have been selected for important differences in targets, methods, and applications, with the common goal of improving the health of children attending America's public schools. The different challenges each study addresses involving school-based health interventions will be discussed, with a focus on identifying the components essential to successful health promotion. Table 2 has been provided to serve as a quick reference guide for these studies.

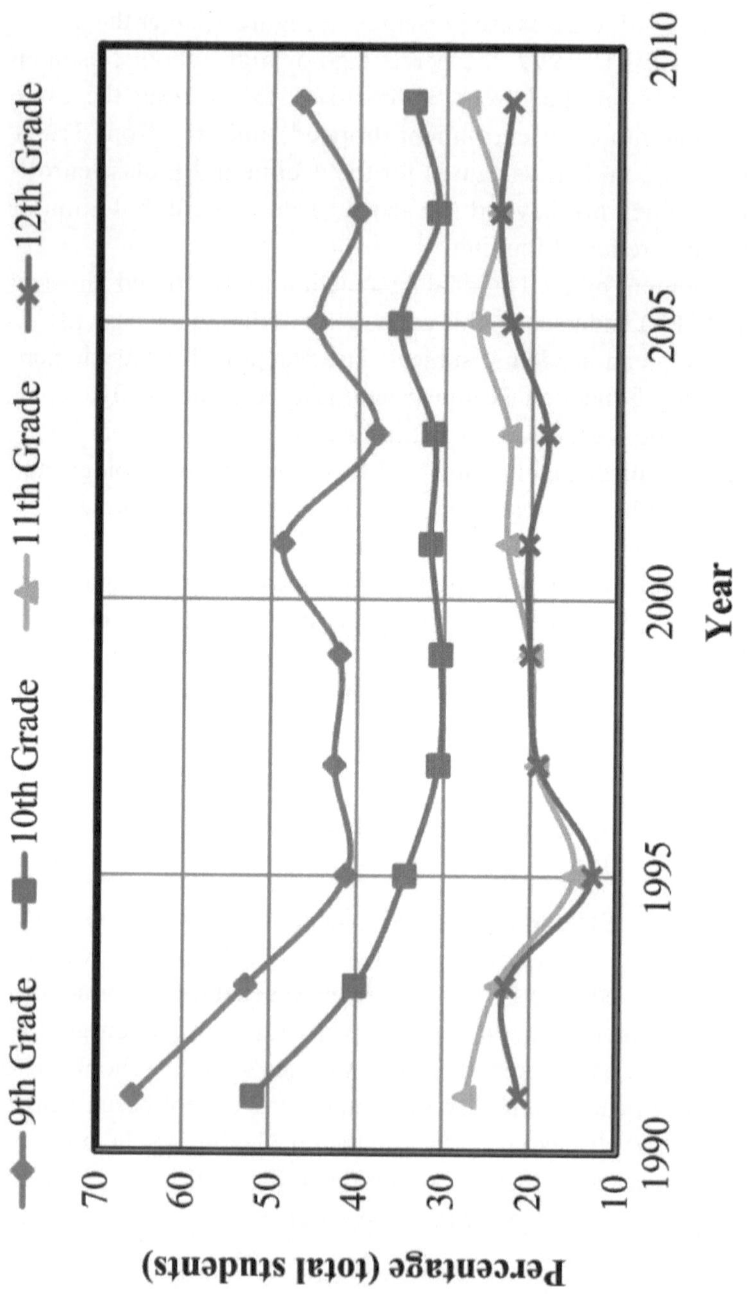

FIGURE 1: Percentage of students attending daily physical education (PE) classes, Centers for Disease Control and Prevention, Youth Risk Behavior Surveillance System.

TABLE 2: Select School-Based Pediatric Health Studies

Researchers	Publication	Intervention	Duration	Target	Methods	Results
Spiegel and Foulk [36]	*Obesity* 2006; 14(1)	Wellness, Academics and You, the WAY Program	1 year	BMI and academic performance	Classroom-based nutrition education, health education, physical activity, family outreach, behavior modification	2% reduction in BMI, incrased fruit and vegetable intake, increased physical activity
Harrell et al [38]	*J Pediatr* 1996; 128(6)	Cardiovascular Health in Children Study (CHIC)	8 weeks	Cardiovascular disease risk factor reduction	Classroom-based nutrition education, health education, smoking education, physical activity	Significantly greater health knowledge, significant increase in self-reported physical activity, reduction in serum total cholesterol level, reduction in body fat, increased aerobic power, smaller rise in diastolic blood pressure
McMurray et al [39]	*J Adolescent Health* 2002; 31(2)	Cardiovascular Health in Children and Youth Study II (CHIC II)	8 weeks	Cardiovascular risk factor reduction, focus on blood pressure and body fat reduction	Classroom-based nutrition education, health education, smoking education, PE curriculum modification	Intervention, particularly the combined treatment, resulted in less of an increase in skinfold measurements; intervention, particularly the exercise treatment, resulted in a decrease in blood pressure
Foster et al [41]	*Pediatric* 2008; 121(4)	School Nutrition Policy Initiative (SNPI)	2 years	Overweight and obesity	Classroom-based nutrition education, health education, nutrition environment modification, social marketing, family outreach	50% reduction in incidence of overweight; 35% reduction in prevalence of overweight; no change in incidence or prevalence of obesity
Cotts et al [42]	*Pediatr Cardiol* 2008; 29	Project Healthy Schools education program (PHS)	1 year	Cardiovascular risk factor reduction	Classroom-based nutrition education, health education, nutrition environment modification, family outreach	No significant change in BMI, systolic blood pressure, high-intensity exercise, or self-reported consumption of high-fat foods or sugary drinks; significant decrease in diastolic blood pressure, LDL cholesterol level, HDL cholesterol level, total cholesterol level and random blood glucose level; increased fruit and vegetable consumption

2.3.1 BEHAVIORAL AND MULTIDISCIPLINARY INTERVENTIONS: HEALTH EDUCATION CURRICULUM, PHYSICAL ACTIVITY, AND NUTRITION

Preventing the onset of overweight and obesity is a complex issue. Because of the highly diverse nature of the disease, the causes for weight gain can vary greatly from one individual to another. [35] Because obesity is most often caused by caloric imbalance due to excess energy intake coupled with insufficient energy expenditure, improving children's dietary and exercise routine remains the most logical preventive approach. However, the incidence of overweight and obesity in our society cannot effectively be reduced through constantly intervening in children's current daily routines with specialized nutrition and exercise training programs. Ultimately, the current routine must adapt to better meet the needs of the children.

Of critical importance to maintaining a healthy body weight is the development of healthy lifestyle behaviors that children can carry through life. A study by Spiegel and Foulk [36] used a program titled Wellness, Academics and You (WAY) that focused heavily on behavior modifications and lifestyle improvements to reduce body mass index (BMI) and increase academic performance. The title of the program is inspirational, evokes self-reflection, and invites the participants to consider the bigger picture rather than focusing only on weight loss or letter grades. Designed around the theory of reasoned action, the WAY program not only increased student knowledge but also developed positive attitudes and behaviors toward health, exercise, and nutrition through the use of specially designed activities. In addition to an engaging health education curriculum, the program also used a 10-minute aerobic exercise program during each session. The study resulted in a 2% decrease in BMI for the intervention group over the control group, which the authors attributed to changes in knowledge, attitudes, and behavioral intentions. Considering that no alterations to the school nutrition environment were made, this study suggests that well-designed health education, with an emphasis on attitudinal and behavioral intentions about food and exercise, can positively influence students' lifestyle. The development of positive attitudes and behaviors toward health may prove to be particularly important during times of increased stress attributed to the major life stage transitions from childhood through adolescence to young adulthood. [37]

In addition to BMI, other interventions have focused on reducing additional cardiovascular disease risk factors. The Cardiovascular Health in Children studies by Harrell et al [38] (CHIC-I) and McMurray et al [39] (CHIC-II) both used nutrition, health, and smoking education, as well as increased physical activity interventions to determine the effects on cardiovascular health. CHIC-I provided nutrition and health education to elementary school students twice a week for 8 weeks. In addition to any regularly scheduled PE classes, the intervention also provided 20 minutes of noncompetitive, lifestyle-type aerobic exercise activities per lesson. Children in the intervention had significantly lower total cholesterol, a minor but significant reduction in body fat, increased aerobic power, and increased health knowledge. The study design did not allow for lipoprotein subfractions to be measured. Knowledge was assessed using a modified Healthy Heart Knowledge test. The CHIC-II study was also 8 weeks, but the design stratified the experimental group into 3 subsets: exercise only, education only, and combined exercise and education. The exercise and nutrition components were similar to those implemented in the CHIC-I study. The results were also similar to those from CHIC-I, but more detailed information about the effectiveness of each mode of intervention was generated. The BMI of all groups increased, but the intervention groups resulted in less of an increase in skin folds. The combined exercise and education group appeared particularly protected from increases in skin fold, suggesting an increase in lean body mass.

The Cardiovascular Health in Children studies revealed 2 noteworthy features. First, they provide evidence that health-focused physical education programs can be successfully implemented in the school setting. Second, CHIC-II suggests that health education combined with physical activity provides the greatest resistance to increases in fat-tissue deposition. The increase in lean body mass is a significant feature of this study. The types of exercises used in this study are also important to note. The use of noncompetitive exercises with school-aged children was recently identified as an important factor in increasing child participation, citing that children's perceived confidence in their ability to perform the exercise can play a determining role in their participation. [37,40]

In addition to physical activity, the school nutrition environment is also likely a significant contributing factor to childhood obesity. As such, studies combining health education with a modified nutrition environment to investigate the effects on BMI have been performed. The School Nutrition Policy Initiative (SNPI) by Foster et al [41] was designed to counteract overweight and obesity through a comprehensive 6-component program. Participating schools modified their environments based on recommendations from the CDC School Health Index, using different strategies to improve the overall health environment such as limiting the use of food as a reward or punishment and advocating active recess. The program offered approximately 10 hours of staff training in nutrition and physical education. Student education was a primary focus, with 50 hours of interdisciplinary nutrition and health education revolving around personal behavior and health. Intervention school food options were adjusted in alignment with the DGA. Beverage options were limited to 100% fruit juice, low-fat milk, and water. Standards on snack foods were set, with limitations placed on saturated and total fat, sodium, and sugar, as seen in Table 3. In addition to health education and nutrition environment modifications, the SNPI also used social marketing and family outreach tools to reinforce the program's message. A cartoon character and a catchphrase slogan were developed, and nutrition educators held nutrition workshops and report card nights for parents.

TABLE 3: School Nutrition Policy Initiative Snack Food Standards [41]

Food Component	Limit Per Serving
Total fat, g	≤ 7
Saturated fat, g	2
Sodium, mg	360
Sugar, g	15

The results showed considerable effects on the incidence and prevalence of overweight. There was a substantial 50% decrease in the incidence of overweight, with 15% of children in control schools becoming overweight compared with 7.5% in the intervention schools. The prevalence of overweight decreased by 10.3% in intervention schools and increased 25.9% in control schools.

Interestingly, the SNPI produced no significant change in the incidence of obesity. This suggests that once children become obese, it is more difficult to lose weight than when children are at risk for overweight. This implies that obese children require more aggressive treatment to regain a healthy weight. Because the incidence and prevalence of overweight decreased in intervention schools, it is believed that the intervention protected students from becoming at risk for obesity.

The SNPI intervention successfully reduced the incidence and prevalence of overweight in elementary school-aged children. However, not all interventions using health education and nutrition environment modifications have been successful. A case in point is the 1-year Project Healthy Schools (PHS) program by Cotts et al. [42] The program was designed to reduce CVD risk factors among sixth-grade students and used health education modules focused on the following goals: increasing fruit and vegetable intake, decreasing intake of sugary beverages and fast food, increasing physical activity, and decreasing pursuits of sedentary behavior. The curriculum modules focused on teaching the importance of healthy lifestyle, including physical activity and nutrition. School food environment changes included the opening of a salad bar and healthy snack options. Noted food replacements were baked chips instead of fried chips and bottled water in place of soda.

In addition to a health questionnaire, anthropometrics, blood pressure, serum cholesterol, and random blood glucose were also recorded. Results indicated no statistically significant changes in BMI, reported intake of high-fat and fried-protein foods, reported intake of sugary beverages, reported frequency of high-intensity aerobic or strength-training activities, or systolic blood pressure. Students' total cholesterol levels decreased, but both low-density lipoprotein (LDL) and high-density lipoprotein (HDL) cholesterol decreased, with the reported drop in HDL being greater than LDL. There was a minor yet significant reduction in diastolic blood pressure and improvements in random blood glucose.

The SNPI and PHS interventions provide evidence-based information as to the types of strategies that are successful at improving the health of children in schools. Although it is acknowledged that improving health education and the nutrition environment of schools can have beneficial results, the methods and implementations used can have a significant impact on their effectiveness. These studies exhibit the important differences in implementation of multicomponent interventions that can have considerable influence on the overall success of the program.

One explanation for the variance between the SNPI and the PHS studies was the degree of nutrition environment modification. Schools participating in the SNPI modified all of their foods to meet the DGA standards with strict limitations on snack foods. Alternately, PHS did not undergo such expansive modifications, with no set limit on fat, saturated fat, or sodium in competitive foods. More important, although the PHS made healthier options available, the SNPI adjusted all NSLP meals in accordance to CDC recommendations, likely influencing a greater impact on children's overall diet. These results suggest that minor modifications—which appear to function to improve student health—can result in nonbeneficial outcomes, and more comprehensive nutrition modifications are necessary.

The extent of nutrition education also varied greatly between the SNPI and PHS programs. PHS provided nutrition education to students via 2 pathways: directly from PHS educators or from advisory teachers provided with a curriculum. Alternately, the SNPI provided education to children, teachers, and parents, which likely reinforced the program's initiative, leading to greater positive behavioral changes toward food and physical exercise. The use of social marketing and family outreach by the SNPI also likely contributed to the success of the program, particularly in today's world where children are commonly targeted as a customer base by food advertisers. In fact, in 2006, the Institutes of Medicine identified media advertisements promoting nutritionally poor foods to children as a significant contributor to the obesity epidemic. In response, there was an industry-wide agreement by food advertisers to set in place self-regulation policies to improve the nutrition quality of foods advertised to children, although evidence suggests that improvements have been negligible.43 The United Kingdom, also facing an obesity epidemic, has taken a more aggressive stance—banning advertisements of what they classify as obesogenic foods on television during children's programs. [44]

2.3.2 *SINGLE-MODE NUTRITION OBESITY INTERVENTIONS*

Single-mode interventions offer the benefit of being relatively low cost and simple to execute as compared to multidisciplinary interventions. In a study by Schwartz, [45] the effectiveness of a verbal prompt on fruit consumption was investigated in elementary school children participating in the NSLP. In the study, cafeteria food servers asked children, "Would you like fruit or juice?" with no further prompts. In the intervention group, 90% of children chose fruit, compared with 60% in the control group. In both groups, approximately 80% of children who chose fruit consumed the fruit. These results indicate that a simple verbal prompt can significantly increase fruit consumption among elementary school children. No long-term effectiveness was noted.

In a study by Hendy and colleagues, [46] the Kids Choice intervention program was investigated. The program used token reinforcement to persuade children to eat fruits and vegetables in exchange for prizes. It was concluded that the program effectively increased fruit and vegetable consumption, although a 7-month follow-up revealed that fruit and vegetable preferences had returned to preintervention levels.

Single-mode intervention studies, although likely not producing the same longer term behavioral changes as more comprehensive interventions have, are important in providing insight into the types of small changes that can be integrated relatively easily into normal school routines. The 2 studies presented here are provided simply to establish that relatively simple modifications can significantly affect students' fruit and vegetable consumption and that a comprehensive compilation and analysis of single-mode interventions is indicated.

2.4 SUMMARY

The NSLP was originally conceived for 2 purposes: the nutrition support of students for health, academic, and national security purposes and the financial support of the agriculture industry in response to hardships experienced by farmers during the Great Depression. Today, the NSLP acts primarily to support children's nutrition requirements while in school. Because the original structuring of the act made the program difficult or impossible for school districts in low-income areas to participate, a series of deregulations occurred in the late 1960s and 1970s to increase school revenue while allowing participation in the NSLP. These deregulations allowed for changes of considerable influence on the overall health and nutrition environment of schools. Prominent changes included allowing schools to contract with fast-food, soft drink, and vending machine companies, as well as the sale of competitive foods, including FMNV.

Historical evidence establishes that physicians have long acknowledged the importance of physical education programs. The concept and implementation of physical education to promote health, first recorded by Herodicus and later expanded by Hippocrates and Galen, eventually developed into the theory of preventive medicine as its basis. Continuing in this vein, physical education in modern America was established with the development of the AAPE by doctors and physical educators in 1885. However, the discipline was gravely affected by the eventual loss of medical doctors in the field, as a result of Abraham Flexner's 1910 report and the subsequent restructuring of American medical education. This, coupled with the rising popularity of organized competitive sports in the early 1900s, resulted in sports overtaking health as the dominant medium of physical education curriculums.

Today, America no longer faces an epidemic of undernutrition and widespread nutrient deficiency but rather an epidemic of obesity. [2,3,9] More than one-third of children are overweight or obese. [3] The danger obesity poses to health is significant. High blood cholesterol, high blood pressure, and glucose intolerance are all likely consequences of obesity and are primary risk factors for the development of atherosclerosis, liver disease, stroke, type 2 diabetes, and other chronic diseases. Fortunately, for the majority of the population, obesity is an entirely reversible and preventable disease.

Evidence suggests that properly designed health-based physical education is an effective mode of improving student health to combat excessive weight gain. As the interventions reviewed in this article indicate, these programs can be successfully implemented in the school setting. Combined with comprehensive school nutrition environment modifications, this model provides an avenue of great potential to implement the broad-scale, obesity-preventive techniques necessary to reduce the incidence of overweight and obesity in children across the country.

2.5 FUTURE DIRECTIONS

Schools are an ideal setting to teach children proper nutrition, exercise, and physical education practices they can carry through life. Programs including not just aerobic activity but also health and nutrition education, in combination with a school nutrition environment that promotes healthy eating habits, will likely be recognized as necessary steps to reduce the incidence of childhood overweight and obesity on a population-wide scale.

The current links between overweight, diet, and exercise are clear. Combined with knowledge built upon since Herodicus and Galen, physical education programs could be modernized to address the issues affecting children today. To be effective, such a curriculum should focus on several areas, including turning children on to lifelong healthy physical activities, integration of overall body health education, and the importance of nutrition and physical activity. Schools could support the new curriculum through improving the campus environment by adhering to stricter standards for foods sold on campus. Proposed recommendations for this modernized curriculum have been classified into the following 3 groups based on the core issues addressed.

2.5.1 DEVELOPMENT OF A HEALTH-BASED PHYSICAL EDUCATION CURRICULUM

Educating elementary-aged students on nutrition and exercise to improve health is complex, as interventions have resulted in mixed outcomes. As evident by the prevalence of childhood overweight and obesity, the current methods of physical education are ineffective at addressing the issues in pediatric health today. What is clear is that multidisciplinary curriculums, including health-based education designed to address underlying behavioral and attitudinal factors, can provide protection from weight gain. In addition, involving students, teachers, and parents likely provides reinforcement of core concepts. Nutrition education will be essential to the success of this new curriculum. The importance of this was recently signified when President Barack H. Obama renamed the council on physical fitness and sports the *President's Council on Fitness, Sports and Nutrition,* acknowledging the pivotal role of diet in health. Physical activity is also a key component, with evidence suggesting a benefit from focusing on noncompetitive, lifestyle-type exercises, particularly in combination with health-based physical education.

2.5.2 STRICT STANDARDS IMPOSED ON THE FOODS MADE AVAILABLE ON CAMPUSES

Health education programs coupled with nutrition environment modifications can provide a synergistic effect; however, changes to foods offered in schools should not be made haphazardly. Modifications using the latest evidence and made in accordance with the CDC's Guidelines to Promote Lifelong Healthy Eating and Physical Activity and the DGA, in addition to setting stricter nutrient limits on beverages and other a la carte snack foods, are proven methods at improving student diet. It is strongly recommended that the presence of commercial fast-food vendors on school campuses be reconsidered. Any efforts by parents, teachers, core curriculums, and intervention programs are undermined when schools provide highly processed, phytonutrient-poor foods as meals. In addition, the presence of commercial fast food, soda and sports drinks, and other nutritionally poor foods on campus may promote the consumption of these foods off campus.

2.5.3 ADEQUATE FUNDING TO ENSURE WIDESPREAD ADOPTION

As evident in Figure 1, there has been a significant decrease in the number of schools offering daily PE classes. Due primarily to reductions in funding, this issue is continuing today with most states redirecting resources toward what are considered core and additional academic subjects, as defined by the No Child Left Behind Act. To significantly affect the incidence of childhood overweight and obesity, a nationwide health-based physical education curriculum, as outlined above, coupled with school nutrition environment modifications, must be adequately funded to ensure widespread implementation.

2.6 CONCLUSION

The NSLP and physical education represent 2 components influencing pediatric health in America's public schools—nutrition and physical activity. The topics discussed in this article are designed to inform readers of the history and development of these 2 programs and explore their effect on student health today. The NSLP, originally designed to prevent malnutrition as undernutrition, now contributes to malnutrition as overnutrition by permitting a poor school nutrition environment. The focus of PE curriculums on sports rather than whole-body health is a relatively recent development, and as a model, it is clearly not meeting the needs of children today. The current school nutrition, health education, and physical activity environment is failing to meet the needs of children in the 21st century.

Facing an epidemic of obesity associated with a multitude of secondary complications, a logical approach for the future is the development of a revised health-based physical education curriculum. Rooted in the history of our science and developed using contributions from current evidenced-based research, a modernized physical education curriculum offers the potential to significantly improve the health of future generations. With this consensus, the next step is to determine how best to integrate the findings concluded from different interventions into a program that is financially feasible and applicable on a large scale.

The importance of health in life cannot be understated, particularly at times of increased stress often associated with transitional stages of maturation and education. As President Thomas Jefferson stated in 1790 in a letter to his cousin, John Garland Jefferson, discussing methods of studying law, reading should be done in the morning and evening, "leaving all the afternoon for exercise and recreation, which are as necessary as reading; I will rather say more necessary, because health is worth more than learning." [47]

REFERENCES

1. U.S. Department of Health & Human Services, Office of the Surgeon General. Speeches and presentations. http://www.surgeongeneral.gov/news/testimony/childobesity03022004.htm. January 8, 2007. Accessed February 16, 2011.
2. Centers for Disease Control and Prevention. CDC Grand Rounds: The Childhood Obesity Epidemic: Threats and Opportunities. http://www.cdc.gov/about/grand-rounds/archives/2010/06-June.htm. June 17, 2010. Accessed February 16, 2011.
3. Levi J, Vinter S, Laurent R, Segal L. F as in Fat 2010: How Obesity Threatens America's Future. Princeton, NJ: Robert Wood Johnson Foundation; 2010. http://healthyamericans.org/reports/obesity2010/Obesity2010Report.pdf. Accessed February 16, 2011.
4. Jia H, Lubetkin E. Trends in quality-adjusted life-years lost contributed by smoking and obesity. Am J Prev Med. 2010;38(2):138-144.
5. Centers for Disease Control and Prevention. Obesity and Overweight for Professionals: Health Consequences. http://www.cdc.gov/obesity/causes/health.html. August 19, 2009. Accessed February 16, 2011.
6. U.S. Department of Health & Human Services. The Surgeon General's Call to Action to Prevent and Decrease Overweight and Obesity: Overweight in Children and Adolescents. http://www.surgeongeneral.gov/topics/obesity/calltoaction/fact_adolescents.htm. January 11, 2007. Accessed February 16, 2011.
7. Levine S. School Lunch Politics: The Surprising History of America's Favorite Welfare Program. Princeton, NJ: Princeton University Press; 2008.
8. Gunderson G. The National School Lunch Program Background and Development. U.S. Department of Agriculture, Food and Nutrition Service. http://www.fns.usda.gov/cnd/lunch/AboutLunch/NSLP-Program%20History.pdf. May 27, 2009. Accessed February 16, 2011.
9. National Nutrition Conference for Defense. JAMA. 1941; 116(23):2598-2599.
10. Davis C, Saltos E. Dietary recommendations and how they have changed over time. In: America's Eating Habits: Changes and Consequences. Washington, DC: U.S. Department of Agriculture, Economic Research Service; 1999. http://www.ers.usda.gov/publications/aib750/aib750b.pdf. Accessed February 16, 2011.
11. PL 396, 79th Congress, June 4, 1946, 60 Stat. 231.
12. U.S. Department of Agriculture, Food and Nutrition Service. National School Lunch Program: fact sheet. http://www.fns.usda.gov/cnd/lunch/AboutLunch/NSLPFactSheet.pdf. January 28, 2011. Accessed February 16, 2011.
13. Electronic Code of Federal Regulations, Title 7, Part 210.11. GPO Access, U.S. Government Printing Office. http://ecfr.gpoaccess.gov/cgi/t/text/text-idx?c=ecfr&sid=02dde6ef8db07a90198929f18099722e&rgn=div5&view=text&node=7:4.1.1.1.1&idno=7#7:4.1.1.1.1.3.1.3. February 15, 2011. Accessed February 16, 2011.
14. Centers for Disease Control and Prevention. School Health Policies and Programs Studies 2000. Fact sheet, food service. http://www.cdc.gov/HealthyYouth/SHPPS/2000/factsheets/pdf/food_service.pdf. Accessed February 16, 2011.
15. Tray Talk, Communities for Healthy School Meals. Tray Talk, get the facts. http://www.traytalk.org/faqs/. 2011. Accessed February 16, 2011.

16. Robinson-O'Brien R, Burgess-Champoux T, Haines J, Hannan P, Sztainer D. Associations between school meals offered through the National School Lunch Program and the school breakfast program and fruit and vegetable intake among ethnically diverse, low-income children. J Sch Health. 2010;80(10):487-492.
17. Crepinsek M, Gordon A, McKinney P, Condon E, Wilson A. Meals offered and served in US public schools: do they meet nutrient standards? JADA. 2009;109(2)(suppl 1):s31-s43.
18. Clark M, Fox M. Nutritional quality of the diets of US public school children and the role of the school meal programs. JADA. 2009;109(2)(suppl 1):s44-s56.
19. Institute of Medicine of the National Academies. School Meals: Building Blocks for Healthy Children. http://www.iom.edu/Reports/2009/School-Meals-Building-Blocks-for-Healthy-Children.aspx. October 20, 2009. Accessed February 16, 2011.
20. The White House, Office of the Press Secretary. Presidential Memorandum—Establishing a Task Force on Childhood Obesity. http://www.whitehouse.gov/the-press-office/presidential-memorandum-establishing-a-task-force-childhood-obesity. Accessed March 1, 2011.
21. Barnes M. White House Task Force on Childhood Obesity: One Year Progress Report. Let's Move: America's Move to Raise a Healthier Generation. http://www.letsmove.gov/pdf/Obesity_update_report.pdf. February 2011. Accessed March 1, 2011.
22. Center for Science in the Public Interest. Foods Sold in Competition With USDA School Meal Programs: A Report to Congress. http://www.cspinet.org/nutritionpolicy/Foods_Sold_in_Competition_with_USDA_School_Meal_Programs.pdf. January 12, 2001. Accessed February 16, 2011.
23. Centers for Disease Control and Prevention. School Health Policies and Programs Studies 2006: Foods and Beverages Sold Outside of the School Meals Programs. http://www.cdc.gov/HealthyYouth/shpps/2006/factsheets/pdf/FS_FoodandBeverages_SHPPS2006.pdf. Accessed February 16, 2011.
24. Berryman J. The tradition of the "six things non-natural": exercise and medicine from Hippocrates through ante-bellum America. Exerc Sport Sci Rev. 1989;17(1):515-560.
25. Berryman J. Exercise is medicine: a historical perspective. Curr Sports Med Rep. 2010;9(4):195-201.
26. Hackensmith CW. History of Physical Education. New York: Harper & Row; 1966.
27. Alliance History. American Alliance for Health, Physical Education, Recreation and Dance. http://www.aahperd.org/about/upload/Alliance_History.pdf. 2011. Accessed February 19, 2011.
28. Flexner A. Medical Education in the United States and Canada. Second reproduction. Boston: Merrymount Press; 1972. http://www.carnegiefoundation.org/sites/default/files/elibrary/Carnegie_Flexner_Report.pdf. Accessed February 25, 2011.
29. Cox M, Irby D. American medical education 100 years after the Flexner Report. N Engl J Med. 2006;355:1339-1344.
30. Morrow J, Zhu W, Franks D, Meredith M, Spain C. 1958-2008: 50 years of youth fitness tests in the United States. Res Q Exerc Sport. 2009;80(1):1-11.
31. Department of Health and Human Services. The President's Council on Physical Fitness and Sports: About the Council. http://www.fitness.gov/about_history.htm. 2011. Accessed February 17, 2011.

32. President's Council on Fitness, Sports & Nutrition. Council History. http://www.fitness.gov/about-us/what-we-do/council-history/council-history.pdf. Accessed February 17, 2011.
33. Centers for Disease Control and Prevention. CDC-Youth Online-High School YRBS: home page. http://apps.nccd.cdc.gov/youthonline. Accessed January 18, 2011.
34. National Association for Sport and Physical Education. Physical Education Is an Academic Subject. http://www.aahperd.org/naspe/advocacy/governmentRelations/upload/PE-is-an-Academic-Subject-2010.pdf. 2010. Accessed February 17, 2011.
35. World Health Organization. Obesity: Preventing and Managing the Global Epidemic. WHO Technical Report Series 894. http://www.obesity.procon.org/sourcefiles/WHO_TRS_894.pdf. 1999. Accessed February 17, 2011.
36. Spiegel S, Foulk D. Reducing overweight through a multidisciplinary school-based intervention. Obesity. 2006;14(1):88-96.
37. Hills A, Okely A, Baur L. Addressing childhood obesity through increased physical activity. Nat Rev Endocrinol. 2010;6:543-549.
38. Harrell J, McMurray R, Bangdiwala S, Frauman A, Gansky S, Bradley C. Effects of a school-based intervention to reduce cardiovascular disease risk factors in elementary-school children: the Cardiovascular Health in Children (CHIC) study. J Pediatr. 1996;128(6):797-805.
39. McMurray R, Harrell J, Bangdiwala S, Bradley C, Deng S, Levine A. A school-based intervention can reduce body fat and blood pressure in young adolescents. J Adolesc Health. 2002;31(2):125-132.
40. Barnett L, Morgan P, Beurden E, Beard J. Perceived sports competence mediates the relationship between childhood motor skill proficiency and adolescent physical activity and fitness: a longitudinal assessment. Int J Behav Nutr Phys Activity. 2008;5:40.
41. Foster G, Sherman S, Borradaile K, et al. A policy-based school intervention to prevent overweight and obesity. Pediatrics. 2008; 121(4):e794-e802.
42. Cotts T, Goldberg C, Davis L, et al. A school-based health education program can improve cholesterol values for middle school students. Pediatr Cardiol. 2008;29:940-945.
43. Kunkel D, McKinley C, Wright P. The Impact of Industry Self-Regulation on the Nutritional Quality of Foods Advertised on Television to Children. Children Now. http://www.childrennow.org/uploads/documents/adstudy_2009.pdf. December 2009. Accessed February 17, 2011.
44. Kunkel D. Media research contributes to the battle against childhood obesity. Health Commun. 2010;25:595-596.
45. Schwartz M. The influence of a verbal prompt on school lunch fruit consumption: a pilot study. Int J Behav Nutr Phys Activity. 2007;4:6.
46. Hendy H, Williams K, Camise T. "Kids Choice" school lunch program increases children's fruit and vegetable acceptance. Appetite. 2005;45:250-263.
47. To John Garland Jefferson, June 11, 1790. In: Oberg BB, Looney JJ , eds. The Papers of Thomas Jefferson: Digital Edition. Charlottesville: University of Virginia Press, Rotunda; 2008.

PART II

EXAMPLES OF SCHOOL-BASED PROGRAMS AND THEIR EFFECTIVENESS

CHAPTER 3

EFFECTIVENESS OF A SCHOOL-COMMUNITY LINKED PROGRAM ON PHYSICAL ACTIVITY LEVELS AND HEALTH-RELATED QUALITY OF LIFE FOR ADOLESCENT GIRLS

MEGHAN M. CASEY, JACK T. HARVEY, AMANDA TELFORD, ROCHELLE M. EIME, AMANDA MOONEY, AND WARREN R. PAYNE

3.1 BACKGROUND

Participation in physical activity (PA) is important for physical and mental health [1]. Many adolescents, however, do not participate in sufficient levels of PA and fail to meet age-related PA recommendations to achieve health benefits [2,3]. PA levels generally decline markedly during adolescence, and gender, socioeconomic status (SES), and rurality are consistently associated with PA level. Specifically, girls are less active than boys [4,5], adolescents from socioeconomically disadvantaged communities have lower levels of PA [6], and regional living adolescents often have poorer access to services and facilities which negatively influences

PA behaviour [7]. The gender disparity in PA has highlighted the need to develop and evaluate interventions targeting at-risk youth to promote PA participation [8,9]. To date few PA interventions have specifically sought to target adolescents residing in low SES or rural communities [10].

The majority of PA promotion interventions for adolescent girls have been school-based without involvement of the family or community, implemented with a focus on increasing PA via physical education (PE) classes and/or health education strategies, and designed to facilitate participation in PA during school time and/or outside of school [9,11]. In recent years the number of school-based interventions focusing on PA for health has increased considerably, from 23 studies in the 1990s to '94 in the first decade of the 21st century [12]. These interventions have had some success, with short-term improvements in school-based PA, but limited evidence of positive effects on PA outside of school or during leisure time [11,13]. A multicomponent school-based study in Australian secondary schools reported no increase in PA, but reductions in self-reported screen time [14,15]. Consequently, multifaceted interventions that target multiple settings such as schools and communities are considered important for making positive changes to adolescent PA levels [13,16]. However, very few interventions to promote PA among adolescent girls have included a formal school-community link and more research is needed [8,17]. Two such studies which have resulted in positive PA outcomes for adolescent girls have included the Lifestyle Education for Activity Program (LEAP) and Trial of Activity for Adolescent Girls (TAAG) interventions. LEAP increased participation in vigorous-intensity PA; although it was unclear which components of the intervention (i.e. PE, health education, school environment, school health services, faculty/staff health promotion and family/community involvement) facilitated this change [17]. TAAG [8] was a 3-year intervention that linked schools and community agencies (e.g. local health clubs and community recreation centres) to develop and promote PA programs for girls. The TAAG intervention resulted in modest improvements in girls' PA, but only among girls who had been exposed to the intervention during their entire middle school years (6th to 8th grade) [8]. Both LEAP and TAAG were carried out in the United States and it has been suggested there is a "need for more interventions in different geographical and cultural contexts to have a wider evidence base" (p. 535) [16].

In contrast to the United States, where schools, colleges and universities play a dominant role in the provision of organised sport, in countries such as Australia, United Kingdom, Germany, France, and New Zealand community sporting clubs play a larger role in participation from the recreational to elite level. In Australia specifically, the school (PE, school sport) and the community (e.g. sports clubs, recreation centres) are the most common settings in which organised PA is delivered for adolescents. Further, many community sport and recreation organisations in Australia use the school setting to deliver and promote their sports programs, although few have formal, systematic or evidence-based strategies to link school-based sports programs with local community organisations to facilitate sustained participation opportunities [18]. In other contextual variations, demographic variables such as residential rurality and low SES have not been explored when researching the impact of school and community settings on PA behaviour [9].

This study sought to contribute to real-world evidence to better inform public policy and professional practice aimed at improving health and PA of adolescent girls living in low-SES rural and regional communities. The aim of the study was to evaluate the effectiveness of a school-community linked PA-promotion intervention program targeting adolescent girls living in low-SES Australian rural and regional communities on their Health-Related Quality of Life (HRQoL), levels of PA, and a range of potential mediators of PA (e.g. self-efficacy, perceived sport competence).

3.2 METHODS

3.2.1 INTERVENTION

The intervention involved a school-community linked program conducted over a 12-month period for adolescent girls in grade 7–9 living in low-SES Australian rural and regional communities. The intervention was designed in a collaborative manner by members of the research team who drew on the expertise and lived experiences of sports coaches from tennis and football, and community instructors from the YMCA. Ethics approval was obtained from the University of Ballarat Human Research Ethics

Committee, the Department of Education and Early Childhood Development (DEECD), and the Diocese of the Catholic Education Office. Details of the program design and implementation instructions have been previously published [19]. The program included a school PE component which incorporated student-centred teaching approaches and behavioural skill development. The PE component involved students participating in two 6-session units each designed as session per week during their 'normal' PE class time, which ranged from 57 to 100 minutes. The two units were a sport unit (tennis or football) and a recreational unit (YMCA). The PE classes were delivered in a collaborative manner by PE teachers with the relevant community fitness instructors, and tennis and football coaches, and were linked to a community component that was designed to address previously reported barriers to PA participation. Barriers such as skill level, competence, financial costs and teaching/coaching approaches were identified through ethnographic fieldwork and informed the design of the program [19-21]. The socio-ecological model [22] was the overarching theoretical framework that guided the development of the intervention. This was underpinned by: Social-Cognitive Theory (SCT), which involved incorporating self-management strategies to encourage adolescent girls to be independently active [23] and a capacity-building framework [24] to build the capacity of the teachers and coaches to deliver the program within the schools and community, respectively. Specific capacity building strategies included professional development to introduce the key principles of the planned curriculum and teaching approach. The curriculum and teaching approach drew on the principles of Game Sense [25], an Australian derivative of the Teaching Games for Understanding (TGfU) approach [26], and productive pedagogies [27] in curriculum development, which is further described in Casey et al. [19]. Game Sense was adopted as the pedagogical framework for each of the sports units (tennis and football) and saw the focus placed upon the tactical dimensions of the game, rather than skill performance [28]. Further this pedagogical approach was adopted in the school setting to align with recent developments in community sports club coaching contexts. Productive pedagogies include the dimensions of intellectual quality, connectedness, supportive classroom environment, and working with, and valuing, difference. Particular classroom practices that reflected the key tenets of the productive pedagogies framework were identified and signalled to teachers through the use of particular teaching and learning cues in the lesson plan resources [27].

3.2.2 SAMPLING DESIGN

Quantitatively, the study was a cluster-randomised trial with participants grouped by schools. There were two conditions (intervention and control) with data collected at baseline and endpoint (one year later). Including a control group was important, as whole-of-community approaches to improving physical activity have often not resulted in absolute improvements, but only in improvements relative to control groups [29].

Government and Catholic secondary schools in rural and regional communities in the Australian state of Victoria that met the following criteria were eligible for inclusion: 1) were below the Victorian median (i.e. 1009) for Socio-Economic Indexes for Areas Index of Relative Socio-economic Advantage and Disadvantage (SEIFA IRSAD) [30]; 2) classified by ARIA+ [31] as being inner or outer regional; and 3) had a local recreation facility, tennis club and football club. Following this, communities were matched on population size and Government and Catholic schools within these matched communities were eligible for inclusion. A total of twelve low-SES non-metropolitan communities had the requisite combination of sports clubs and leisure centres for delivery of the community component of the intervention. In one pair of communities, which consisted of the two largest regional cities in Victoria, three schools from each community were (subject to agreement by the schools) randomly chosen for inclusion in the study. For the other five pairs of communities, one school was randomly chosen (subject to agreement) from each community, with the exception that when in one control community no school agreed to participate, two schools were chosen from the closest matched control community. In summary, sixteen randomly chosen schools, eight located in six intervention communities and eight located in five control communities, were recruited into the study. The profiles of intervention and control communities ranged in size from 4,233 to 78,222 persons, were below the Victorian median for SEIFA IRSAD (range: 893 – 993), and were between 115 and 331 km from the state's capital city.

A cohort sampling design was used [17,32] with individuals' endpoint measures adjusted for their baseline values, potentially increasing the precision of the analysis [33]. The control condition involved schools going about their usual curricular and co-curricular programming and did not include any engagement strategy beyond those currently employed on a routine basis by the intervention program partners: Tennis Victoria, Football Federation Victoria and YMCA Victoria. Control schools received the intervention resources after end-point data collection.

Power analysis was based on the primary outcome HRQoL measures used in the study—PedsQL 4.0 [34]. For derived PedsQL scales, (explained later within measures) there is evidence that the differences between a healthy sample and a sample identified by parents as having a chronic health condition such as asthma, diabetes or attention deficit hyperactivity disorder or depression correspond to effect sizes in the range 0.52-0.81 [34]; that is medium (0.50) to large (0.80) effect sizes [35]. We conservatively specified a small effect size (0.20) for the difference between intervention and control groups. After adjusting for differences between the groups at the start of the study, assuming moderate correlation over time ($r=0.5$), $ICC=0.01$ and cluster size of 50 for school-level clustering effects, and an intervention:control allocation ratio of 2:1, with a significance level of 5% and 80% power, then based on an independent samples t test, the required sample size was $n=788$ (525 intervention and 263 control).

Based on recruitment and retention rates reported in similar international studies such as Pate et al. [17] and Simon et al. [32], tempered by the researchers' experience of low recruitment rates in the Australian context due to the ethics requirement to obtain explicit informed written consent from both participants and parents/carers, we assumed recruitment (take-up) rates of 40% (intervention) and 20% (control) and retention rates of 80% in both conditions. This led to a requirement for some 3280 girls (1640 in each condition) to be invited to participate in the study. An average of around 200 girls are enrolled in grade 7–9 in rural and regional secondary schools in Victoria; thus 16 secondary schools and their associated communities were recruited to participate in the research.

3.2.3 EVALUATION DESIGN

The RE-AIM framework [36] was used to examine the Reach, Effectiveness, Adoption, Implementation and Maintenance (RE-AIM) of the program. The extent to which the program reached the intended targets (Reach), the number of schools and students that adopted the program (Adoption), and the barriers and facilitators to the delivery of the intervention (Implementation) have been reported elsewhere [37]. This study addresses the effectiveness of the program.

Impact and outcome variables were measured at baseline and endpoint using available established reliable and valid self-report measures. The use of self-report to assess health behaviours such as physical activity is considered appropriate for the 12–15 year age group [38,39].

3.2.4 MEASURES

The self-report survey included several health and behavioural measures outlined below and was a paper-based survey administered by teachers during one school period (typically 45 mins). In most cases (unless stated), the measure used was the mean score on a set of related Likert scale items.

HRQoL was measured using the validated tool PedsQL 4.0 Generic Core Scales for Teens aged 13–18 [34,39]. Internal consistency reliability (Cronbach's α) for child self-report scores ranged from 0.80 to 0.88. HRQoL is related to an individual's health and includes the physical, mental and social health dimensions outlined by the World Health Organization [40]. The 23-item PedsQL includes questions on physical functioning (8 items, e.g. "It is hard for me to walk more than a block"), emotional functioning (5 items, e.g. "I feel sad or blue"), social functioning (5 items, e.g. "Other kids tease me") and school functioning (5 items, e.g. "It is hard to pay attention in class") which are used to derive summated scores for physical health, psychosocial health (emotional, social and school functioning) and a total score [41]. The summated scores were transformed to a 0–100 scale, with high scores indicating better HRQoL.

The concept of "level of PA" is multi-facetted [2]. We assessed the level of PA in three ways. First, self-reported general PA level was measured using a single 5-point Likert scale item: 'In general, how physically active would you say you are?'—'not at all', 'a bit', 'moderately', 'very', 'extremely' [42]. Single-item questions have been shown to be acceptable measures of PA when compared to accelerometry measures [43] and to multiple-item questions or diaries [44]. Second, respondents were also asked to report on how many out of the past seven days they had engaged in moderate (e.g. brisk walking, bike riding, dancing) to vigorous (e.g. activities that make you 'huff and puff' like netball, soccer, running, swimming) sport or recreational PA for a total of 60 minutes or more, in accordance with Australian Government's Physical Activity recommendations for 12–18 year olds [45]. We refer to these activities as leisure-time moderate to vigorous physical activity (LTMVPA). Finally, PA was measured using a 24-hr Previous Day Physical Activity Recall (PDPAR-24) questionnaire, which has been validated against 24-h step counts in a sample of Australian adolescents with validity coefficients (correlations) ranging from 0.29 to 0.34, $p<.05$ [46]. Self-report for PA provides low to moderate validity [47] and is considered appropriate to capture a large participant base at low costs [38]. The PDPAR-24 was modified slightly to reflect the Australian female context (e.g. inclusion of netball). Estimates of the rate of energy expenditure in metabolic equivalents (METs) were derived from the PDPAR data using the Compendium of Physical Activities [48]. MVPA was defined as any activity with a $\text{MET} \geq 3.0$. The number of 30-minute blocks of LTMVPA and hence the total LTMVPA (min) and total MET-weighted LTMVPA (MET-min) were derived from the responses for leisure-time activities in the PDPAR diary [48].

Perceived sports competence was measured using the items of Harter's Self-Perception of Athletic Competence scale [49], although the scale was modified to suit the format of the overall survey in this study. Our 5-point scale was similar to the 4-point scale of Wichstrøm [50] which had better reliability, convergent validity and factorial validity than the original scale. Participants were provided with five statements ('I do very well at all kinds of sports', 'I think I could do well at just about any new PA', 'I feel that I am better than others my age at sports', 'I don't do well at new sports', 'I do not feel that I am very athletic') with responses: 'Disagree a lot', 'Disagree', 'Neither', 'Agree' and 'Agree a lot'.

Self-management strategies (SMS) [51], perceived behavioural control (PBC) [52], outcome expectation and outcome expectancy-value [52] and self-efficacy were measured with items previously developed and used with adolescent girls, and which were based on contemporary PA behaviour change theories such as theory of planned behaviour and self-efficacy theory [53]. SMS were measured to determine the extent of behavioural and cognitive strategies adopted by respondents to participate in PA, as behaviour self-management underpinned the program design [19]. The scale included four items relating to cognitive strategies and four items relating to behavioural strategies [51]. A fifth item for behavioural strategies was developed by the research team to examine social support behavioural strategies ('I have a friend or family member who encourages me to do PA'). Participants responded on a 5-point scale ranging from 'Never' (1) to 'Very often' (5). PBC was measured using a question from Motl et al. [52]. Participants were asked to respond to one item ('For me to be physically active during my free time on most days would be…") on a 5-point scale ranging from 'Very hard' (1) to 'Very easy' (5); responses to the other three items (e.g. 'I have all the things I need to be physically active during my free time on most days') were on a 5-point scale ranging from 'Disagree a lot' (1) to 'Agree a lot' (5). Outcome expectation and outcome expectancy-value were assessed with questions consisting of: belief statements (e.g. If I were to be physically active during my free time on most days it would help me spend more time with friends) on 5-point scales ranging from 'Disagree a lot' (1) to 'Agree a lot' (5); and corresponding value statements (e.g. spending time with my friends is…), on 5-point scales ranging from 'Very unimportant' (1) to 'Very important' (5) [54]. The outcome-expectancy value items were formed as a product of the belief and corresponding value item scores [55].

Self-efficacy was measured using a question developed by Nigg [56] which includes 10 items with responses on a 5-point scale from 'Not at all confident' (1) to 'Extremely confident' (5) to measure confidence in the ability to persist with PA whenever conditions are not ideal. This measure includes five items specific to adolescents (e.g. 'How confident are you about participating in sport or PA in the next month when you have homework to do?') and five more generally applicable items (e.g. 'When you are tired').

Enjoyment of a range of activities at school and outside of school was also assessed. Participants were asked to indicate how much they liked participating in competitive sport or PA (e.g. basketball, netball), organised but non-competitive sport or PA (e.g. aerobics, 'Zumba', social tennis), and non-organised PA (e.g. walking, jogging, camping) both at school and outside of school. Enjoyment of a range of sedentary activities outside of school was also assessed including: talking on the phone, chatting, texting, watching TV or DVDs, playing computer games, listening to radio, CD, iPod, surfing the internet, and social networking. Responses to the 12 items were on a 5-point scale from 'Hate it' (1) to 'Love it' (5). A 'Don't know, never tried' (0) category was also provided. Two scores were derived, for PA enjoyment (six items) and sedentary enjoyment (six items).

Barriers to participation in sport and PA included nine items regarding personal barriers (e.g. 'I don't like being physically active because of my body shape') and seven items relating to organisational/environmental barriers (e.g. 'Cost of participation'). The list of items were derived from PA studies [57]. Participants were asked how often these barriers kept them from participating in sport and physical activity, and the items were scored on a 5-point scale from 'Never' (1) to 'Very often' (5).

The influence of family and friends on PA and sport participation was measured using a modified version of questions on family and peer influences which has demonstrated good reliability [57]. In terms of family influence, participants were asked to complete several items assessing social support (e.g. encouragement, role modelling, supervision) by indicating in the past month whether a member of their household had: 'Encouraged you to do physical activities or play sport'; 'Done a PA or played sport with you'; 'Watched you participate in physical activities or sport'; 'Told you that you are doing well in physical activities or sport'; or 'Been willing to assist you with travel to physical activities or sports after school or on weekends'. In terms of peer influence, participants were asked with respect to the past month 'Did you encourage your friends to do physical activities or play sports?', 'Did your friends encourage you to do physical activities or play sport?', 'Did your friends do physical activities or play sport with you?', 'Did your friends tell you that you are doing well in physical activities or sports?'. The family and peer influence items were scored on a 5-point scale from 'Never' (1) to 'Very often' (5).

Baseline body mass index (BMI) was calculated by dividing participant's self-reported weight (in kilograms) by the square of their self-reported height [kg/m^2]. Finally, baseline age was calculated as the duration from reported birthdate to reported date of completion of the baseline survey, expressed as decimal years.

3.2.5 ANALYSIS

'Intention-to-treat' principles were adopted in part. The usual intention-to-treat approach to loss to follow up is to make the "worst case" assumption that due to non-compliance the intervention treatment has not been experienced, and to carry forward the baseline value, thereby assuming no change in these cases. However, in the present study the first school-based stage of the intervention was mandatory, and the loss to follow up was due only to failure to comply with reporting requirements. Consequently, the carry-forward approach was considered inappropriate in this study, and so only complete cases were analysed. However, respondents who completed both baseline and follow-up surveys but who reported that they did not complete the second community-based stage of the intervention, were included in the analysis, which is in accordance with intention-to-treat principles.

Quantitative outcome measures and summated scales based on multiple Likert items, together with potential mediators, were initially analysed using linear mixed models (LMM), with the baseline value of the measure as a covariate, group as a fixed effect and school as a random effect in order to allow for the investigation of school-level cluster effects. Models were fitted with and without adjustment for age and BMI. Two sets of analyses were conducted. In the first set of analyses, the group factor was the condition of the study (intervention v control). In the second set of analyses, the intervention group was split into self-reported 'completers' (those who had participated in the both the in-school component and out-of-school community component) and 'non-completers' (those who had participated in the in-school component only) and a 3-group analysis was undertaken. This analysis was aimed at differentiating between the effects of the two components of the intervention (in-school v out-of-school community components). Paired t-tests were used to further examine the patterns of change from baseline to follow-up within each group. A similar suite of analyses were conducted on two dichotomous outcome measures using logistic regression models fitted by the method of generalised estimating equations, incorporating an examination of school-level cluster effects. No cluster effects were observed therefore results of ordinary logistic regression analyses are reported. McNemar chi-square tests were used to further examine the patterns of change from baseline to follow-up within each group. Analyses were conducted using SPSS version 18.0.

3.3 RESULTS

3.3.1 RESPONSE RATE

Eight schools (n=1755 Year 7–9 female student enrolment) accepted the invitation to participate as an intervention school; however one school withdrew part way through the intervention due to unsatisfactory experiences with a community sport and recreation provider and data from this school were excluded from analyses (n=264 students). A further eight schools accepted the invitation to participate as a control school (n=2208 enrolment).

Participants who completed both baseline and follow-up surveys included 362 intervention students (recruitment rate at baseline 33.7% of student enrolment, retention rate 61.3% of those recruited) and 259 control students (recruitment rate 14.1%, retention rate 83.4%). For analyses incorporating adjustment for age and BMI, participants who did not provide birthdate or estimates of height and weight were excluded. In accordance with the practice of excluding cases for which data are potentially statistically influential but probably spurious [58,59], those whose estimated BMI lay outside the extreme values for 13 year-old females recorded in accumulated data from direct measurements in 21 studies during the period from 1985–2008, incorporating 70,758 Australian children (Professor

Tim Olds, personal communication, 9 July 2009) were also excluded. This resulted in data from 263 intervention and 199 control participants being available for analysis of age and BMI.

For analysis associated with the PDPAR-24, participants whose diaries were incomplete were excluded. Cases with estimated MVPA of more than 256 mins/day (i.e. those who reported more than eight 30-minute blocks), which corresponds to the 99th percentile of responses in the 2007 Australian National Children's Nutrition and Physical Activity Survey (Prof Tim Olds, personal communication, 14 December 2011), were also excluded. This resulted in data from 136 intervention and 107 control participants being available for analysis of MET-mins and time spent in MVPA, of whom 106 intervention and 80 control participants also provided valid age and BMI data. To control for the possibility of systematic differences in PA levels on different days of the week, the PDPAR-24 measures were also adjusted for day of week, by multiplying each observation by the reciprocal of the ratio of the mean value for the particular day of the week to the grand mean value (the unweighted mean of the means).

3.3.1 PARTICIPANT PROFILE

Table 1 presents a summary of participant characteristics at baseline—including demographic data, health measures, PA measures, and indicators and potential mediators of PA—of respondents in intervention (completers and non-completers) and control groups. There was a consistent pattern of somewhat higher levels of all health and PA measures and indicators among completers compared to non-completers and controls. However, only three PA measures showed statistically significant differences. The proportion who reported meeting PA guidelines in the past seven days was higher among the intervention group than the control group ($p=.021$); and both the PDPAR measures (Mins of LTMVPA and MET-mins of LTMVPA) were significantly higher among program completers than controls ($p=.016$ and $p=.002$ respectively), and higher among controls than non-completers ($p=.028$ and $p=.010$ respectively). There were also significant differences between groups for three of the potential mediators: enjoyment of sedentary activities, which was significantly higher in the control group than the intervention group (p=.027); and perceived sport competence and outcome expectation, which were significantly higher among program completers than non-completers and controls (p=.001 and p=.039 respectively).

TABLE 1: Participant baseline characteristics

	Intervention: all n=362		Intervention: completers n=91		Intervention:non-completers n=271		Control n=259	
Characteristic	n	Mean ± SD or percent	n	Mean ± SD or percent	n	Mean ± SD or percent	n	Mean ± SD or percent
Demographics								
Age (yr)	350	13.4 ± 0.9	88	13.2 ± 0.9	262	13.4 ± 0.9	238	13.4 ± 0.9
BMI	263	19.9 ± 3.9	66	19.8 ± 4.1	197	20.0 ± 3.8	199	19.6 ± 3.5
Live in two parent households	362	78.7	91	74.7	271	80.1	259	74.5
Health								
General health – excellent or good	333	71.2	85	80.0	248	68.1	233	73.0
PedsQL physical functioning score	358	83.9 ± 13.0	90	85.7 ± 12.0	268	83.3 ± 13.2	248	84.5 ± 13.2
PedsQL psychosocial functioning score	357	80.6 ± 14.3	90	82.0 ± 12.9	267	80.1 ± 14.7	247	81.5 ± 13.6
PedsQL total score	357	81.8 ± 13.0	90	83.3 ± 11.7	267	81.2 ± 13.4	248	79.8 ± 15.4
Physical activity:								
MET-mins of LTMVPA (24-hr)	136	546.4 ± 489.1	27	955.2 ± 590.2	113	454.4 ± 413.6	107	624.5 ± 515.8
Mins of LTMVPA (24-hr)	136	79.2 ± 66.3	27	123.6 ± 77.6	113	69.2 ± 59.4	107	88.6 ± 67.1
Number of days in past seven with at least 60 min of LTMVPA	358	5.0 ± 1.8	90	5.3 ± 1.7	268	4.9 ± 1.8	259	4.8 ± 1.6
Met PA guidelines in past seven days1	358	11.2	90	12.2	268	10.8	259	5.8
Sport club/leisure centre member	358	55.0	90	61.1	268	53.0	256	59.4

TABLE 1: *Cont.*

Characteristic	Intervention: all n=362		Intervention: completers n=91		Intervention:non-completers n=271		Control n=259	
	n	Mean ± SD or percent	n	Mean ± SD or percent	n	Mean ± SD or percent	n	Mean ± SD or percent
Potential mediators:								
Perceived sports competence	349	3.37 ± 0.74	87	3.62 ± 0.62	262	3.29 ± 0.75	258	3.37 ± 0.74
Self-management strategies	347	3.42 ± 0.75	86	3.55 ± 0.7	261	3.38 ± 0.76	251	3.48 ± 0.77
Perceived behavioral control	358	3.92 ± 0.66	88	3.94 ± 0.64	270	3.91 ± 0.67	255	3.96 ± 0.59
Outcome expectation	351	36.54 ± 5.53	85	37.84 ± 5.02	266	36.12 ± 5.63	253	36.37 ± 5.37
Outcome expectancy-value	346	152.87 ± 48.21	84	161.73 ± 46.14	262	150.03 ± 48.6	246	152.63 ± 46.73
Self-efficacy	339	2.83 ± 0.72	82	2.87 ± 0.68	257	2.81 ± 0.73	244	2.79 ± 0.69
PA enjoyment	352	23.81 ± 5.65	89	24.88 ± 4.93	263	23.44 ± 5.84	250	24.04 ± 4.72
Sedentary enjoyment	351	4.64 ± 0.77	89	4.59 ± 0.74	262	4.66 ± 0.78	245	4.78 ± 0.70
Personal barriers	343	2.31 ± 0.77	90	2.18 ± 0.68	253	2.36 ± 0.8	246	2.39 ± 0.77
Organisation barriers	348	2.01 ± 0.73	88	2.01 ± 0.67	260	2.01 ± 0.75	243	2.02 ± 0.73
Family support	353	3.82 ± 1.00	89	3.91 ± 0.98	264	3.79 ± 1.01	251	3.82 ± 0.91
Friends support	357	3.43 ± 0.98	90	3.58 ± 0.91	267	3.38 ± 1	249	3.53 ± 0.91

[1]*PA guidelines: At least 60 min of LTMVPA each day (i.e. all of the past seven days).*

3.3.2 INTERVENTION EFFECTS

Table 2 presents the findings from analyses of 17 quantitative outcome measures: three HRQoL measures, two PA measures, and 12 potential mediators. The table includes results of 2-group analyses (condition: intervention vs control) and 3-group analyses (intervention completers i.e. school+community components, intervention non-completers i.e. school component only, control) on the differences between groups at follow-up with regard to each quantitative measure, with adjustment for corresponding baseline scores. For variables where significant differences were present, the direction and magnitude of significant pairwise group differences are also shown. In every case, when the analysis was repeated for the subsample who had provided weight and height data, with and without adjustment for age and BMI (results not tabulated), the adjustment made no substantive difference to the results. For most measures, there was no evidence of clustering of responses by school. However, personal and organisational/environmental barriers did provide significant clustering effects which were accounted for in the LMM.

3.3.3 HRQOL

The 2-group analysis (intervention vs control) showed that, after adjustment for baseline levels of PedsQL, the intervention group had significantly higher scores on all three PedsQL scores—physical functioning (adjusted M ± SE=83.9 ± 0.7, $p=.005$), psychosocial (79.9 ± 0.8, $p=.001$) and total score (81.3 ± 0.7, $p=.001$)—than the control group (80.9 ± 0.8; 76.1 ± 0.9 and 77.8 ± 0.8 respectively), suggesting that the program positively influenced quality of life. Differences in PedsQL were also present in the 3-group analysis (intervention completers, intervention non-completers and control), whereby the intervention non-completers had significantly higher scores (84.0 ± 0.8, $p=.021$; 80.4 ± 0.9, $p=.003$; and 81.7 ± 0.8, $p=.002$ respectively) than the control group (80.9 ± 0.8, 76.1 ± 0.9 and 77.8 ± 0.8 respectively). The lack of a significant difference between intervention completers and the control group may be attributed to a combination of two factors: the fact that the intervention completers group had higher PedsQL scores at baseline than the other groups (possible ceiling effect) and the smaller sample size of the intervention completers group. Paired t-tests of changes over time within each group revealed a further aspect of the differences between intervention and control groups. All PedsQL scores decreased significantly in the control group (physical functioning: $M=-3.3$, $p=.001$; psychosocial functioning: $M=-3.8$, $p<.001$; total score: $M=-3.6$, $p=.001$), while there were no significant changes over time in the intervention group (physical functioning: $M=-0.0$, $p=.992$; psychosocial functioning: $M=-0.3$, $p=.726$; total score: $M=-0.2$, $p=.791$).

3.3.4 PHYSICAL ACTIVITY

There was no statistically significant difference in either the 2-group or 3-group analysis for mins of LTMVPA, MET-mins of LTMVPA, or in the proportion meeting physical activity guidelines.

3.3.5 POTENTIAL MEDIATOR VARIABLES

There were no statistically significant differences between intervention and control groups among the potential mediator variables. However, the 3-group analyses showed that there were significant differences between groups on several potential mediator variables after adjustment for the corresponding measure at baseline. Specifically, intervention completers had significantly higher scores than both intervention non-completers and controls for perceived behavioural control (adjusted M ± SE: completers 4.05 ± 0.07; non-completers 3.84 ± 0.04; controls 3.87 ± 0.04, $p=.034$), outcome expectancy-value (completers 157.5 ± 5.3; non-completers 140.1 ± 3.0; controls 139.1 ± 3.4, $p=.008$), self-efficacy (completers 3.03 ± 0.08; non-completers 2.75 ± 0.05; controls 2.78 ± 0.05, $p=.006$) and family support (completers 3.90 ± 0.08; non-completers 3.67 ± 0.05; controls 3.63 ± 0.05, $p=.017$), and significantly higher scores than intervention non-completers, but not controls, for self-management strategies (completers 3.63 ± 0.07; non-completers 3.38 ± 0.04; controls 3.47 ± 0.04, $p=.10$), personal barriers (completers 2.57 ± 0.07; non-completers 2.38 ± 0.04; controls 2.56 ± 0.04, $p=.004$) and support of friends (completers 3.46 ± 0.08; non-completers 3.23 ± 0.05; controls 3.36 ± 0.05, $p=.048$). There were no significant differences with regard to enjoyment of PA or sedentary pursuits, perceived sports competence, or organisational/environmental barriers.

Table 3 presents the findings from logistic regression analyses of three dichotomous indicators: perceived level of PA (moderate or high v low), having met PA guidelines (at least 60 mins of MVPA per day) on each of the past seven days (yes v no) and sport club membership (member v non-member). The table includes results of 2-group analyses (condition: intervention vs control) and 3-group analyses (intervention completers i.e. school+community components, intervention non-completers i.e. school component only, control) on the differences between groups at follow-up, with adjustment for baseline values. For each indicator, when the analysis was repeated for the subsample who had provided weight and height data, with and without adjustment for age and BMI (results not tabulated), the adjustment made no substantive difference to the estimated group differences.

With regard to self-reported PA level and meeting PA guidelines, there were no statistically significant differences between intervention and control groups, nor between completers, non-completers and controls. With regard to sports club/leisure centre membership, after adjustment for baseline levels of sports club membership, the difference between intervention and control groups in the odds of belonging to a sports club/leisure centre were not quite statistically significant ($p=.056$), but there were significant differences between non-completers and controls ($OR=1.66$; $p=.021$), with the intervention non-completers group more likely to be members of sports clubs/leisure centres. Again, the lack of a significant difference between intervention completers and the control group can be attributed to a combination of two factors: the fact that the intervention completers group had higher percentage of sports club membership at baseline than the other groups (likely ceiling effect) and the smaller sample size of the intervention completers group. McNemar tests of changes over time within each group revealed that the percentage of sports club members decreased, though not significantly, in both the intervention completer group (baseline 60.2%; follow-up 56.8%; $p=.648$) and the control group (baseline 59.6%; follow-up 55.7%; $p=.220$), and increased significantly in the intervention non-completer group (baseline 53.2%; follow-up 60.3%; $p=.016$).

TABLE 3: Analysis of dichotomous variables for groups at follow-up, with adjustment for baseline category

Variable	Group	n	p-value	Odds ratio#	Group^	n	p-value	Odds ratio#
Self-reported PA level (moderate/high v low)	1. Intervention	358	0.977		1. Completers	90	0.578	
	2. Control (reference)	258			2. Non-completers	268	0.838	
	3. Control (reference)	258						
Met PA guidelines in past seven days	1. Intervention	351	0.772		1. Completers	89	0.466	
	2. Control (reference)	255			2. Non-completers	262	0.455	
	3. Control (reference)	255						
Sport club/leisure centre (member v non-member)	1. Intervention	355	0.057		1. Completers	88	0.878	
	2. Control (reference)	255			2. Non-completers	267	0.021*	1.66
	3. Control (reference)	255						

*#Significant odds ratios *p < 0.05.*
^Completers = school component + community component; Non-completers = school component only.

3.4 DISCUSSION

This study evaluated the effectiveness of a school-community linked PA-promotion intervention program on increasing HRQoL, PA, and a range of potential mediators of PA among adolescent girls living in low-SES regional and rural communities. Studies such as this which are realistic in their scope are important as they provide the real-world implementation evidence to inform public policy and professional practice. However, they are very challenging to implement as they require the engagement of multiple stakeholders with varying objectives and capacities over a considerable time period [60].

The program design was informed by learnings from similar randomised controlled trials [8,9]. The program included: formative research to inform the program design; the socioecological model as the overarching theoretical framework—underpinned by social cognitive theory, capacity building strategies and educational theory; and attempted to create direct links between school and community PA opportunities to sustain PA participation [19]. We know that studies consisting of both physical and cognitive components are more likely to have significant positive intervention results [12]. This study incorporated both of these elements and there were a number of significant positive results.

In terms of HRQoL, previous research has shown that HRQoL decreases during adolescence, especially among girls [61]. In this study, such a decrease was observed in the control group, while the intervention group maintained its baseline levels of HRQoL. The intervention may have had a protective effect on the intervention group's HRQoL, which is a positive outcome of the study. Specifically, the group difference between intervention and control for the three PedsQL scores ranged from +3.0 to +3.8, which is approaching minimal clinically important differences in PedsQL scores for youth without and with type 2 diabetes (+5.41 for total score) [62].

There were no significant changes in (self-reported) PA levels. Other multi-component interventions with school- and community strategies have resulted in only modest improvements in girls' PA and have suggested that the length of time girls are exposed to the intervention may affect PA [8]. A recent systematic review of PA interventions in the school setting [12] reported that medium-term studies (i.e. four to 12 months) reported significant differences in PA levels in favour of the intervention group more frequently (68.6%) than short-term (i.e. less than three months, 47.4%) or long-term studies (i.e. 13 or more months, 45.0%). However, long-term school-based interventions have also reported negative effects on student attitude towards PA [12]. In addition, interventions were likely to achieve positive PA outcomes if the intervention was delivered four or more times per week [12] and whole of school approaches have also been shown to be effective [9].

The length of the intervention in this study may have been insufficient to achieve changes in PA. The intervention in this study was modest and realistic in scope, and specifically focused on developing formal and evidence-based strategies to link schools and community organisations for sustained participation. The school component was implemented as two 6-session units delivered during the scheduled PE class time, generally one session per week for six weeks for each unit. Given this focus on the PE setting, the intervention was subject to timetable and curriculum constraints. Others have reported institutional barriers to the provision of PE in Australian schools including restricted timetabling of PE and lack of access to facilities, equipment and suitable teaching spaces [63]. In addition, PE is often organised with a predisposition towards team games and development of sport skills [64], and therefore, a limited range of physical activities, which are not necessarily lifelong activities [65,66]. The intervention in this study included a traditional team sport (football), a lifestyle sport (tennis) and a range of lifestyle physical activities (leisure centre activities) that were linked to local facilities and programs to add value to the existing school PE program, which has been recommended by others [67]. Further, at the conclusion of the intervention, only a quarter of students in the intervention group reported attending one of the community-based sports programs outside of school. Developing meaningful and sustained linkages between schools and community settings for PA across a range of PE curriculum and activity areas may result in the achievement of better outcomes.

In terms of becoming a sports club or leisure centre member, after adjustment for sports club/leisure centre membership at baseline, non-completers were more likely to belong to a sports club at follow-up, not only compared to controls, but also compared to completers. The latter counter-intuitive result may be attributable to a number of factors. There was a higher proportion of sports club/leisure centre membership at baseline among those who went on to complete the program than among non-completers. It may also be that the intervention raised awareness among the non-completer group about joining a sports club/leisure centre that was not linked to the intervention per se. The intervention was limited to two sports and one recreational organisation and as a consequence factors such as personal preference, access and peer influence may have affected this outcome. Again, the notion of developing a range of linkages between schools and community settings for PA in various PE curriculum and activity areas may result in the provision of student choice and potentially better outcomes.

The intervention also appeared to have positive effects on a range of intra-personal capacities (i.e. self-efficacy, self-management, perceived behavioural control, outcome expectancy-value) and inter-personal factors (i.e. support from family and friends), as improvements favoured intervention completers over non-completers, and to a lesser degree over controls. Few PA interventions have assessed mediators of PA behaviour among youth [68] and studies that examine the mediators of behaviour change in interventions are required [69]. Several studies have reported that mediators of PA, such as self-efficacy, partially mediate the effects of an intervention on PA [68,69]. In our study, while PA did not change, there were positive differences between intervention and control groups with regard to both HRQoL and previously identified PA mediators. These anomalous results may in part be attributable to lower power from the smaller sample sizes for the PDPAR variables, but may also reflect the existence of pathways to HRQoL in this intervention other than via the quantity of PA alone.

There were no significant changes with regard to enjoyment of PA or non-PA pursuits, perceived sport competence or perceived organisational/environmental factors. In terms of perceived sports competence, the sports of tennis and football adopted 'Game Sense' as the pedagogical approach to the intervention curriculum. Specifically, the intervention drew on Game Sense pedagogies to avoid traditional 'command-orientated' and 'teacher/coach-directed' pedagogies that tend to be more characteristic of masculine approaches to teaching [70] and were identified as a barrier in the ethnographic fieldwork [19]. Further, the ethnographic fieldwork highlighted that girls tended to have strongly entrenched ideas about their own physical ability, which shaped their attitudes towards, and participation in, PE and out-of-school sport [20]. Game Sense places participation in games as the foundation from which teaching and skill refinement proceeds [71] and has been shown to strongly impact on students' learning, especially among girls and low skill-level students [72]. Process evaluation of the implementation of the program revealed that the understanding of, and commitment to, the intention of a Game Sense approach varied among both teachers and coaches [37,73]. In particular, there was a widely held perception that fundamental motor skills were a prerequisite to game play, which indicates that in many cases the intervention may not have been implemented as intended. Whilst strategies such as professional development workshop and cooperative delivery model were employed to empower teachers and coaches further work is required in the provision of sport and physical activities for adolescent girls [73]. The research team acknowledge critiques of a multi-activity sports approach to physical education [74,75] and particularly for the decontextualized approach to skill learning, implementation of the intervention program relied on the cooperation of teachers and coaches. It was decided that a 'repackaging' of a unit of work in PE might help to identify the merits of such an approach that could potentially inform teaching and learning practices in the physical education program more broadly.

The lack of significant differences in PedsQL scores between completers and the control group may be a consequence of the fact that completers had higher PedsQL scores at baseline than non-completers and control groups, which may mean significant changes were harder to achieve. Specifically, the health and PA profiles of completers at baseline were comparable to population norms for PedsQL scores [76] and proportion of students meeting PA guidelines of MVPA for 60 minutes or more in the past 7 days [77]. In comparison, the control groups had lower scores compared to a healthy sample of children aged 5–18 years for all three PedsQL measures reported by Varni and colleagues (total score: 83.00 $\pm$ 14.79; Physical functioning 84.41 $\pm$ 17.26; and psychosocial functioning: 82.38 $\pm$ 15.51), whilst non-completers had lower PedsQL scores than the healthy sample for psychosocial functioning and total score, but not physical functioning [76].

Similarly, in terms of the proportion of students meeting PA guidelines at baseline, the intervention group (11.2%) were comparable to an Australian sample of students from 2005, in which 12.7% of students aged 12–13 and 12.1% of students aged aged 14–15 were engaged in at least

60 minutes of MVPA each day in the previous week [77]. In comparison, the control group had a very low proportion (5.8%) of students meeting PA guidelines [77].

The socio-ecological model was the overarching theoretical framework—underpinned by individual through to organisational strategies designed to develop linkages between school and community PA opportunities in order to improve PA participation [19]. Some aspects of the program were not fully implemented as intended, such as the student-centred pedagogical approach (Game Sense) and self-management strategies, which is likely to have had a negative impact on the intended dose of the intervention [37]. Program implementation barriers within the school setting were related to a perception that fundamental motor skills were a prerequisite to game play, a lack of experience among program deliverers with the teaching approach, and complex organisational barriers like school timetabling, and are discussed in detail elsewhere [37,73].

3.4.1 STRENGTHS AND LIMITATIONS

The strengths of this study include the prospective and controlled study design, which allowed the effects of the intervention to be assessed comparatively and longitudinally over time. With regard to limitations, studies of this population cohort are very hard to conduct, particularly in light of the ethics requirement of Australian education authorities to obtain specific 'opt-in' parental consent, which is exacerbated by the necessity to communicate with parents only indirectly in writing via the school and the students themselves. The research team were dependent on the efforts of teachers with many competing priorities to facilitate and promote recruitment and retention, amid the complexities of school operations and scheduling. Consequently, limitations to this study include moderate consent/recruitment and retention rates in the intervention group, and low consent/recruitment, albeit offset by a higher retention rate, in the control group. A potential consequence of the low to moderate recruitment rate is self-selection bias; if more physically active girls were more motivated to participate in the study, the study sample would not be representative of the whole population of adolescent girls. A potential effect on longitudinal analyses of moderate retention rates is the possibility of further bias due to less physically active participants being more likely to drop out of the study. A further consequence is reduced statistical power, due to failure to achieve the design target sample sizes. Despite (and perhaps because of) these unavoidable limitations, there have been few interventions and little evaluative research in this domain, particularly longitudinal research, and so our findings, interpreted with appropriate caution, are important.

Objective measures of PA would have strengthened the assessment of potential outcomes, as self-report measures provide low to moderate validity and participants may have difficulties recalling information [47]. The self-report approach was used because diaries are considered appropriate to capture a large participant base at low cost [38] and are relatively unobtrusive and quick to administer compared to objective measures. In addition, it was over-ambitious to attempt to fit the lengthy survey form, especially the PDPAR-24 component, into school timetable slots, which resulted in many incomplete diaries and hence loss of statistical power with regard to the measurement of LTMVPA and MET-weighted LTMVPA.

3.5 CONCLUSION

In conclusion, the school community-linked intervention resulted in a number of positive outcomes. These positive outcomes arose from what was effectively a modest intervention that was focused on formal strategies to link schools with community organisations for sustained participation. The school component of the program appeared to contribute to maintaining HRQoL; whilst those students who completed the community component developed a range of intra-personal capacities such as self-efficacy and inter-personal factors including support from family, which support participation in PA. It also appeared that the intervention increased awareness of sports clubs/leisure centres in the community, as the rate of membership of these community organisations significantly increased among non-completers. Developing meaningful and sustained linkages between schools and community settings for PA across a range of PE curriculum and activity areas may result in the achievement of better outcomes.

In summary, we observed a protective effect on HRQoL as a result of participation in this modest intervention program, which was independent of any change in PA. This was unexpected and may be attributed to an enhanced sense of control and self-efficacy developed in response to the intervention program that was designed to meet the needs of the participants.

REFERENCES

1. Janssen I, LeBlanc AG: Systematic review of the health benefits of physical activity and fitness in school-aged children and youth. Int J Behav Nutr Phy Act 2010, 7:1-16.
2. Eime R, Harvey J, Sawyer N, Craike M, Symons C, Polman R, Payne W: Understanding the contexts of adolescent female participation in sport and physical activity. Res Q Exerc Sport 2013, 84:157-166.
3. Dumith SC, Gigante DP, Domingues MR, Kohl HW: Physical activity change during adolescence: a systematic review and a pooled analysis. Int J Epidemiol 2011, 40:685-698.
4. Barnett TA, O'Loughlin J, Paradis G: One- and two-year predictors of decline in physical activity among inner-city schoolchildren. Am J Prev Med 2002, 23:121-128.
5. Olds T, Wake M, Patton G, Ridley K, Waters E, Williams J, Hesketh K: How do school-day activity patterns differ with age and gender across adolescence? J Adolesc Health 2009, 44:64-72.
6. Stalsberg R, Pedersen A: Effects of socioeconomic status on the physical activity in adolescents: a systematic review of the evidence. Scand J Med Sci Sports 2010, 20:368-383.
7. Gordon-Larsen P, Nelson M, Page P, Popkin B: Inequality in the built environment underlies key health disparities in physical activity and obesity. Pediatr 2006, 117:417-424.
8. Webber LS, Catellier DJ, Lytle LA, Murray DM, Pratt CA, Young DR, Elder JP, Lohman TG, Stevens J, Jobe JB, Pate RR: Promoting physical activity in middle school girls: trial of activity for adolescent girls. Am J Prev Med 2008, 34:173-184.
9. Camacho-Miñano MJ, LaVoi NM, Barr-Anderson DJ: Interventions to promote physical activity among young and adolescent girls: a systematic review. Health Educ Res 2011, 26:1025-1049.
10. Dudley DA, Okely AD, Pearson P, Peat J: Engaging adolescent girls from linguistically diverse and low income backgrounds in school sport: a pilot randomised controlled trial. J Sci Med Sport 2010, 13:217-224.
11. De Meester F, Van Lenthe F, Spittaels H, Lien N, De Bourdeaudhuij I: Interventions for promoting physical activity among European teenagers: a systematic review. Int J Behav Nutr Phys Act 2009, 6:1-11.

12. Demetriou Y, Höner O: Physical activity interventions in the school setting: a systematic review. Psych Sport Exerc 2012, 13:186-196.
13. van Sluijs EMF, McMinn AM, Griffin SJ: Effectiveness of interventions to promote physical activity in children and adolescents: systematic review of controlled trials. Brit Med J 2007, 335:703.
14. Lubans DR, Morgan PJ, Okely AD, Dewar D, Collins C, Batterham M, Callister R, Plotnikoff R: Preventing obesity among adolescent girls: one-year outcomes of the nutrition and enjoyable activity for teen girls (neat girls) cluster randomized controlled trial. Arch Pediatr Adolesc Med 2012, 166:821-827.
15. Dewar D, Morgan P, Plotnikoff R, Okely A, Collins C, Batterham M, Callister R, Lubans D: The nutrition and enjoyable activity for teen girls study: a cluster randomised controlled trial. Am J Prev Med 2013, 45:313-317.
16. Murillo Pardo B, García Bengoechea E, Generelo Lanaspa E, Bush PL, Zaragoza Casterad J, Julián Clemente JA, García González L: Promising school-based strategies and intervention guidelines to increase physical activity of adolescents. Health Educ Res 2013, 28:523-538.
17. Pate R, Ward D, Saunders R, Felton G, Dishman R, Dowda M: Promotion of physical activity among high-school girls: a randomized controlled trial. Am J Public Health 2005, 95:1582-1587.
18. Eime R, Payne W: Linking participants in school-based sport programs to community clubs. J Sci Med Sport 2009, 12:293-299.
19. Casey M, Mooney A, Eime R, Harvey J, Smyth J, Telford A, Payne W: Linking physical education with community sport and recreation: a program for adolescent girls. Health Promot Prac 2013, 14:721-731.
20. Mooney A, Casey M, Smyth J: "You're no-one if you're not a netball girl": rural and regional living adolescent girls' negotiation of physically active identities. Annals of Leis Res 2012, 15:19-37.
21. Smyth J, Mooney A, Casey M: Where has class gone to? The pervasiveness of class in girls' physical activity in a rural town. Sport Educ Soc 2014, 19:1-18.
22. McLeroy K, Bibeau D, Steckler A, Glanz K: An ecological perspective on health promotion programs. Health Educ Quart 1988, 15:351-377.
23. Corbin CB, Lindsey R: Fitness for Life. 4th edition. Scott Foreman: Glenview, IL; 1997.
24. Health NSW: A Framework for Building Capacity to Improve Health. Australia, NSW Health Department: Sydney; 2001.
25. den Duyn N, Australian Sports Commission: Game Sense: Developing thinking players. Belconnen, ACT: Australian Sports Commission; 1997.
26. Bunker D, Thorpe R: A model for the teaching of games in secondary schools. Bulletin of Phys Educ 1983, 18:5-8.
27. Hayes D, Mills M, Christie P, Lingard B: Teachers and Schooling Making a Difference: Productive Pedagogies, Assessment and Performance. Allen and Unwin: Crows Nest, NSW, Australia; 2006.
28. Light R, Fawns R: Knowing the game: Integrating speech and action in games teaching through TGfU. Quest 2003, 55:161-176.

29. Brown W, Mummery K, Eakin E, Schofield G: 10,000 steps Rockhampton: evaluation of a whole community approach to improving population levels of physical activity. J Phy Act Health 2006, 1:1-14.
30. Australian Burearu of Statistics (ABS): Socio-Economic Indexes for Areas (SEIFA) technical paper 2033.0.55.001. 2014. Retrieved June 4th 2014 from [http://www.ausstats.abs.gov.au/ausstats/subscriber.nsf/0/22CEDA8038AF7A0DCA257B3B00116E34/$File/2033.0.55.001%20seifa%202011%20technical%20paper.pdf]
31. Department of Health and Aged Care: Measuring remoteness: Accessibility/Remoteness Index of Australia (ARIA).. Adelaide: DHAC; 2001.
32. Simon C, Wagner A, Platat C, Arveiler D, Schweitzer B, Schlienger J, Triby E: ICAPS: a multilevel program to improve physical activity in adolescents. Diabetes Metab 2006, 32:41-49.
33. Stevens J, Murray D, Catellier D, Hannan P, Lytle L, Elder J, Young D, Simons-Morton D, Webber L: Design of the Trial of Activity in Adolescent Girls (TAAG). Contemp Clinical Trials 2005, 26:223-233.
34. Varni J, Burwinkle T, Seid M, Skarr D: The PedsQL 4.0 as a pediatric population health measure: feasibility, reliability, and validity. Ambul Pediatr 2003, 3:329-341.
35. Cohen J: A power primer. Psychol Bull 1992, 112:155-159.
36. Glasgow RE, Vogt TM, Boles SM: Evaluating the public health impact of health promotion interventions: the RE-AIM framework. Am J Public Health 1999, 89:1322-1327.
37. Telford A, Casey M, Smyth J, Harvey J, Eime R, Mooney A, Payne W: An evaluation of a school community-linked sport and recreation program for adolescent girls. J Sci Med Sport 2014, 16:e35.
38. Dollman J, Okely AD, Hardy L, Timperio A, Salmon J, Hills AP: A hitchhiker's guide to assessing young people's physical activity: deciding what method to use. J Sci Med Sport 2009, 12:518-525.
39. Varni J, Limbers C, Burwinkle T: How young can children reliably and validly self-report their health-related quality of life? An analysis of 8,591 children across age subgroups with the PedsQL™ 4.0 Generic Core Scales. Health Qual Life Outcomes 2007, 5:1-13.
40. World Health Organization: World definition of Health. Preamble to the Constitution of the World Health Organization as adopted by the International Health Conference, New York, 19–22 June, 1946; signed on 22 July 1946 by the representatives of 61 States Official Records of the World Health Organization, no. 2, p. 100) and entered into force on 7 April 1948. 1948. Retrieved from http://www.who.int/about/definition/en/print.html 1948
41. Varni J: Pediatric Quality of Life Inventory™ PedsQL™. Lyon, France: Mapi Research Trust; 2010.
42. Payne W, Harvey J, Eime R, Craike M, Symons C: Relationships between different self-report measures of physical activity. J Sci Med Sport 2010, 13:e96.
43. Milton K, Clemes S, Bull F: Can a single question provide an accurate measure of physical activity? Brit J Sport Med 2013, 47:44-48.
44. Weiss T, Slater C, Green L, Kennedy V, Albright D, Wun C: The validity of single-item, self-assessment questions as measures of adult physical activity. J Clin Epidemiol 1990, 43:1123-1129.

45. Department of Health: Australia's physical activity and sedentry behaviour guidelines, 2014. Retrieved 14 February 2014 from [http://www.health.gov.au/internet/main/publishing.nsf/content/health-pubhlth-strateg-phys-act-guidelines]
46. Trost SG, Marshall AL, Miller R, Hurley JT, Hunt JA: Validation of a 24-h physical activity recall in indigenous and non-indigenous Australian adolescents. J Sci Med Sport 2007, 10:428-435.
47. Kohl H, Fulton J, Caspersen C: Assessment of physical activity among children and adolescents: a review and synthesis. Prev Med 2000, 31:S54-S76.
48. Ainsworth BE, Haskell W, Herrmann S, Meckes N, Bassett JRD, Tudor-Locke C, Greer J, Vezina J, White-Glover M, Leon A: Compendium of physical activities: a second update of codes and MET values. Med Sci Sports Exerc 2011, 2011(43):1575-1581.
49. Harter S: The perceived competence scale for children. Child Dev 1982, 53:87-97.
50. Wichstrøm L: Harter's self-perception profile for adolescents: reliability, validity, and evaluation of the question format. J Pers Assess 1995, 65:100.
51. Dishman RK, Motl RW, Sallis JF, Dunn AL, Birnbaum AS, Welk GJ, Bedimo-Rung AL, Voorhees CC, Jobe JB: Self-management strategies mediate self-efficacy and physical activity. Am J Prev Med 2005, 29:10-18.
52. Motl RW, Dishman RK, Trost SG, Saunders RP, Dowda M, Felton G, Ward DS, Pate RR: Factorial validity and invariance of questionnaires measuring social-cognitive determinants of physical activity among adolescent girls. Prev Med 2000, 31:584-594.
53. Glanz K, Rimer BK, Viswanath K: Health Behavior and Health Education. San Francisco, CA: Jossey-Bass; 2008.
54. Lytle L, Murray D, Evenson K, Moody J, Pratt C, Metcalfe L, Parra-Medina D: Mediators affecting girls' levels of physical activity outside of school: findings from the trial of activity in adolescent girls. Ann Behav Med 2009, 38:124-136.
55. Ajzen I: The theory of planned behavior. Organ Behav Hum Dec 1991, 50:179-211.
56. Nigg C: Explaining adolescent exercise behavior change: a longitudinal application of the transtheoretical model. Ann Behav Med 2001, 23:11-20.
57. Sallis JF, Taylor WC, Dowda M, Freedson PS, Pate RR: Correlates of vigorous physical activity for children in grades 1 through 12: comparing parent-reported and objectively measured physical activity. Pediatr Exerc Sci 2002, 14:30-44.
58. Harvey J, Eime R, Payne W: Effectiveness of the 2006 Commonwealth Games 10,000 steps walking challenge. 2009, 41:1673-1680.
59. Tudor-Locke C, Bassett DJ: How many steps/day are enough? Preliminary pedometer indices for public health. Sports Med 2004, 34:1-8.
60. Proctor E, Silmere H, Raghavan R, Hovmand P, Aarons G, Bunger A, Griffey R, Hensley M: Outcomes for implementation research: conceptual distinctions, measurment challenges, and research agenda. Adm Policy Ment Health 2011, 38:65-79.
61. Williams JW, Canterford L, Hesketh KD, Hardy P, Waters EB, Patton GC, Wake M: Changes in body mass index and health related quality of life from childhood to adolescence. Int J Pediatr Obes 2011, 6:e442-e448.
62. Hilliard M, Lawrence J, Modi A, Anderson A, Crume T, Dolan L, Merchant A, Yi-Frazier J, Hood K: Identification of minimal clinically important difference scores

of the PedsQL in children, adolescents, and young adults with type 1 and type 2 diabetes. Diabetes Care 2013, 36:1891-1897.
63. Jenkinson KA, Benson AC: Barriers to providing physical education and physical activity in Victorian state secondary schools. Aust J Teacher Educ 2010, 35:1-17.
64. Marshall J, Hardman K: The state and status of physical education in schools in international context. Eur Phys Educ Rev 2000, 6:203-229.
65. Fairclough S, Stratton G, Baldwin G: The contribution of secondary school physical education to lifetime physical activity. Eur Phys Educ Rev 2002, 8:69-84.
66. Trost S: Public Health and Physical Education. In Handbook of Physical Education. Edited by Kirk D, O'Sullivan M, MacDonald D. London: Sage; 2006:163.
67. Faber L, Hodges Kulinna P, Darst P: Strategies for physical activity promotion beyond the physical education classroom. J Phys Educ Rec Dance 2007, 78:27-31.
68. Lubans DR, Foster C, Biddle SJH: A review of mediators of behavior in interventions to promote physical activity among children and adolescents. Prev Med 2008, 47:463-470.
69. Plotnikoff RC, Costigan SA, Karunamuni N, Lubans DR: Social cognitive theories used to explain physical activity behavior in adolescents: a systematic review and meta-analysis. Prev Med 2013, 56:245-253.
70. Light R, Kentel J, Kehler M, Atkinson M: Soft Pedagogy for a Hard Sport: Disrupting Hegemonic Masculinity in High School Rugby Through Feminist-Informed Pedagogy. In Boys' Bodies: Speaking the Unspoken. Edited by Kehler M, Atkinson M. New York: Peter lang Publishing Inc; 2010:133-154.
71. Metzler M: Instructional Models for Physical Education. 2nd edition. Scottsdale, Arizona: Holcomb Hathaway Publishers, Inc; 2005.
72. Mesquita I, Farias C, Hastie P: The impact of a hybrid sport education–invasion games competence model soccer unit on students' decision making, skill execution and overall game performance. Eur Phys Educ Rev 2012, 18:205-219.
73. Mooney A, Casey M: "Girls get going': Using Games Sense to Promote Physical Activity Amongst Adolescent Girls in Rural and Regional Contexts in Australia'. In Contemporary Developments in Games Teaching. Edited by Light R, Harvey S, Quay J, Mooney A. Milton Park, Abingdon: Routledge; 2014.
74. Ennis C: Creating a culturally relevant curriculum for disengaged girls. Sport Educ Soc 1999, 4:31-50.
75. Kirk D: Physical Education Futures. Milton Park, Abingdon: Routledge; 2010.
76. Varni J, Seid M, Kurtin P: PedsQL (TM) 4.0: reliability and validity of the pediatric of life inventory (TM) version 4.0 generic core scales in healthy and patient populations. Med Care 2001, 39:800-812.
77. Scully M, Dixon H, White V, Beckmann K: Dietary, physical activity and sedentary behaviour among Australian secondary students in 2005. Health Promot Int 2007, 22:236-245.

Table 2 is not available in this version of the article. To view this additional information, please use the citation on the first page of this chapter.

CHAPTER 4

A REPEATED MEASURES EXPERIMENT OF GREEN EXERCISE TO IMPROVE SELF-ESTEEM IN UK SCHOOL CHILDREN

KATHARINE REED, CARLY WOOD, JO BARTON,
JULES N. PRETTY, DANIEL COHEN, AND GAVIN R. H. SANDERCOCK

4.1 INTRODUCTION

The prevalence of mental ill health in UK children is rising; approximately 1 in 10 young people suffer from a diagnosable mental health disorder each year [1]. Self-esteem is one indicator of mental health and is defined as: "a person's positive or negative attitude towards the self in totality" [2]. Low self-esteem is a common occurrence in many forms of mental illness [3]; thus methods of improving self-esteem in children are important for mental health.

The positive relationship between exercise and mental health is widely evidenced [4], [5], with a moderate effect size (d = 0.51) for changes in children's self-esteem due to exercise [6]. However, approximately 23–

34% of males and 35–53% of females aged 11–15 years are failing to meet the daily recommendation of sixty minutes of moderate to vigorous physical activity [7]. Evidence also shows that exposure to nature can improve mental well-being in children; improving cognitive functioning and concentration and reducing psychological distress [8]–[9]. In adults, "Green Exercise" research suggests a synergistic health benefit for self-esteem of engaging in "physical activities in the presence of nature" [10]–[12]. Thus, "Green Exercise" might also be effective at improving self-esteem in children.

A multi-study analysis of green exercise in adults (ten studies, n = 1252) demonstrated significant improvements in self-esteem across many social groups, types of activity and green space [10]. The review also showed a u-shaped "dose-response curve" indicating that even short engagements with nature can have a positive impact. Activities of light intensity (walking, fishing etc) had a greater effect on self-esteem than vigorous activities (mountain biking, conservation activities etc.), although all intensities had positive effects. This suggests that green exercise can complement other approaches in making significant improvements to mental health [10]. While the findings are encouraging, showing a moderate combined effect size (d = 0.6), what cannot be determined from these data is if the changes in self-esteem following "green exercise" are greater than those one would expect to observe following another type of exercise intervention.

The benefits of Green Exercise for self-esteem may occur due to enhanced enjoyability of exercise in a natural environment. Green spaces may also encourage greater distractibility from daily stresses, helping people to feel better about themselves [13]. Instead of relying on music or television to provide distraction, findings from green exercise research imply that nature is inherently fascinating and may provide a driver for changes in self-esteem [11]. Outdoor natural environments may also provide a distraction from feelings of fatigue experienced during exercise; thus helping exercise to feel easier [14]. However, all of the above findings are from studies of adults and there are few data regarding the potential additive benefit that nature may have for children when exercise is performed in a green environment [12]. Young people are an important population to study as physical activity habits formed in youth may track into adulthood where adequate levels of activity are protective against many chronic diseases [12].

Much of young peoples' experience of physical activity comes from the physical education (PE) they receive at school [15] and enjoyment of PE is well correlated with children's overall levels of physical activity [16], [17]. Positive experiences gained during PE at school may also promote participation in physical activity during adulthood [18]. One of the aims of PE should be to offer enjoyable experiences that encourage extracurricular activities and promote a lifelong habit of healthy physical activity and experiences likely to create lifelong exercise adherence. Exercising in green environments is associated with reductions in perceptions of exertion [14] and greater enjoyment, satisfaction and positive engagement compared to indoor exercise [19]. Participants' intentions to repeatedly engage in exercise were also greater in the outdoor conditions, implying a better longer-term adherence rate. Therefore, green exercise activities during PE may enhance the self-esteem of children and offer attractive alternatives for children who are typically disengaged with sports and other competitive activities.

The primary aim of this experiment was to determine the effects of green exercise on self-esteem when compared with a control (outdoor, non-green urban area) exercise condition using a counterbalanced, randomised cross-over design. Secondary aims were to determine if there were differences in enjoyment and perceived exertion between exercise environments and how these might be affected by children's levels of fitness and physical activity.

We hypothesised that green exercise would increase self-esteem significantly more than the control condition. Our secondary hypothesis was that children would find green exercise more enjoyable and perception of effort would be lower in comparison to the control condition.

4.2 METHODS

4.2.1 ETHICS STATEMENT

The University of Essex faculty ethical review committee approved the study. Permission was granted by the school's head teacher and written parental consent and individual assent was gained for all children who volunteered to participate. Pupils from four year-7 classes took part in the runs, as they were performed as part of a compulsory PE class. However, only children who volunteered and provided consent for participation in the study completed the questionnaires and fitness test. Overall, n = 86 children (11–12 year old) from a local secondary school participated in the study. However due to drop-outs and absences the total number of children completing the study was n = 75.

4.2.2 MATERIALS

Each child completed the physical activity questionnaire for adolescents to provide an estimate of their habitual physical activity levels [20]. Each participant then completed a version of the 20 m shuttle-run; the FITNESSGRAM PACER test [21] which is a valid method by which to assess aerobic fitness (herein referred to as fitness) in this age group [22].

Immediately before and after each exercise condition, pupils completed the Rosenberg Self Esteem Scale (RSE) [23], reproduced on a single sheet of paper in a large, easy to read font. The RSE is widely used in green exercise research analysing the effects of acute exposure [10]. The instrument provides a self-reported one-dimensional measure of global self-esteem. It consists of 10 statements, each of which are scored on a four point likert scale from strongly agree (1) to strongly disagree (4). An overall self-esteem score is calculated ranging from 10 to 40, with a low self-esteem score representing fewer negative perceptions and thus a higher self-esteem.

Following exercise in both conditions, pupils provided retrospective ratings of perceived exertion using the Ratings of Perceived Exertion (RPE) scale [24]. This scale asks participants to rate how hard they perceive to be working on a scale from 6 (no effort) to 20 (extremely hard) and is designed for use during exercise. RPE was collected immediately at the end of each exercise bout, in order to ensure consistent timing of the scale between the two exercise bouts and so that an overall assessment of each run could be obtained. We also assessed their overall enjoyment of the exercise session using a visual-analogue scale. The scale comprised a line on which participants were asked: "Tell us how much you enjoyed the exercise you just did." The line was demarcated at either end with emoticons (sad face and happy face) and the line between emoticons was exactly 12 cm (120 mm). A score between zero and 120 was determined by measuring the exact distance of the mark from zero (sad face) in mm.

4.2.3 PROCEDURE

We visited the school on three separate occasions. On the initial visit, all pupils were weighed and their stature was assessed. Weight and stature were measured in order to obtain descriptive information about the participants. On the initial visit the study was also explained in full to the pupils. Whilst the study had been explained in detail in the consent form, the initial visit to the school was used to reiterate the key points. Participants were informed about the timings of questionnaires and the importance of completing the questionnaires individually and honestly. Participants were also told that the questionnaires were not being used to evaluate them as individuals and that all data would be anonymised. Furthermore, all pupils were invited to ask for assistance in completing questionnaires if there was anything they did not understand.

Each child was then asked to undertake two bouts of exercise (running) over a standard distance (1.5 miles). We chose this distance so that the exercise would take between 10 and 20 minutes. This exercise duration is effective in promoting positive changes in adult's mental state [25]. The experiment took place in the second week of the new school year (early September) and it was the first PE class of this type undertaken by all pupils. Conditions were randomised and counterbalanced by PE group. Two groups ($n = 42$) completed the control condition first and two groups ($n = 44$) completed the green condition first. A total of $n = 81$ participants completed the green condition and $n = 85$ completed the control condition; however only 75 participants completed all questionnaires. The runs were conducted at the same time of day, exactly one week apart.

The control condition was a 1.5 mile run of a one lap course around the school campus, on a relatively flat terrain (±2 m). The school is located within a moderate density housing estate on the outskirts of town. The local area has low-to-moderate levels of deprivation; situated at the 59th percentile of area-level deprivation [26] and predominant local land use is classified as urban according to DEFRA (Department for Rural Affairs) standard land-use classification [27].

The school itself is bounded on three sides by housing developments, office buildings and another school. One side of the school grounds is dominated by hard surface playing areas and a multi-use games area or "Astroturf" court. The route ran through the school campus and around the perimeters of the hard surface areas with some time spent on the school playing field, the field itself is, however bounded by housing.

The green condition was also a 1.5 mile run of a single lap course through the local country park. This area was located close to the school and pupils were escorted across the main roads to access the park. The park comprises woodland and dirt paths and the route also ran along the course of a stream. The course had an overall climb (and subsequent descent) of 46m and required participants to get wet feet and jump puddles. At no points in the route could participants see buildings, pylons or other manmade objects except one wooden footbridge used to cross the stream. The park is maintained to a high standard by the local council and volunteers and is largely litter free. In previous work this has been classed as a "rural pleasant green environment" [11].

In each condition, six researchers acted as stewards for both runs, guiding pupils' running direction with hand signals and verbal directions, but they were instructed not to encourage pupils or to provide information on performance or distance. PE staff were present during both conditions and acted as "sweepers" by running behind the last placed pupil to ensure all pupils returned to the start point. Pupils completed the self-esteem scale before each bout of exercise and during the immediate post-exercise period when pupils had returned to the PE department. Following both exercise conditions, we assessed pupils' RPE and enjoyment ratings.

4.2.4 STATISTICAL ANALYSIS

Based on a predicted moderate effect size of $d = 0.5$ [10] and baseline self-esteem measures (Rosenberg Score = 18±4) we determined that the minimum expected changes in self-esteem would require 64 participants at $\beta = 0.8$, $\alpha = 0.05$. To account for drop outs and non-responders we recruited 86 participants. Overall, 75 participants completed all parts of the procedures providing statistical power of $\beta = 0.91$, $\alpha = 0.05$.

We created means and standard deviations for all variables and tested between-sex differences using independent t-tests. Where there were significant differences between variables these were analysed separately in further analyses. To determine the effects of green and control exercise on self-esteem we used two-way repeated measures analysis of variance (rm-ANOVA) for green and control exercise with pre- and post-exercise measurements as factors.

We also used repeated measures t-tests, to examine differences in RPE and enjoyment between exercise and green conditions and stepwise multiple regression to assess the relative impact of physical activity, fitness and condition on enjoyment and RPE. We also used Pearson's product moment correlation to assess the relationship measures of physical activity and fitness had with measures of enjoyment and RPE during both conditions.

4.3 RESULTS

The descriptive characteristics of the sample are shown in Table 1 and show similarities in age and stature of boys and girls. As expected, females were significantly heavier than males at this age due to earlier pubertal development. Females reported significantly lower levels of physical activity in the previous seven days and completed fewer laps during the 20 m shuttle-run test indicating lower cardio respiratory fitness compared with males.

There were no significant order effects for SE, ($t(75) = 0.23$, $p = 0.97$) enjoyment ($t(75) = 0.32$, $p = 0.76$) or RPE ($t(75) = 1.4$, $p = 0.15$). Figure 1 shows the SE values before and after both exercise conditions (means ± SD). As there were no significant differences in SE between boys and girls or between measurements made before either exercise conditions, male and female cases were analysed together. There was a significant main effect for exercise on self-esteem ($F(1,74)$, = 12.2, $p<0.001$), but no main effect for exercise condition ($F(1,74) = 0.02$, $p = 0.898$) and no interaction ($F(1,74)$, = 0.13, $p = 0.72$).

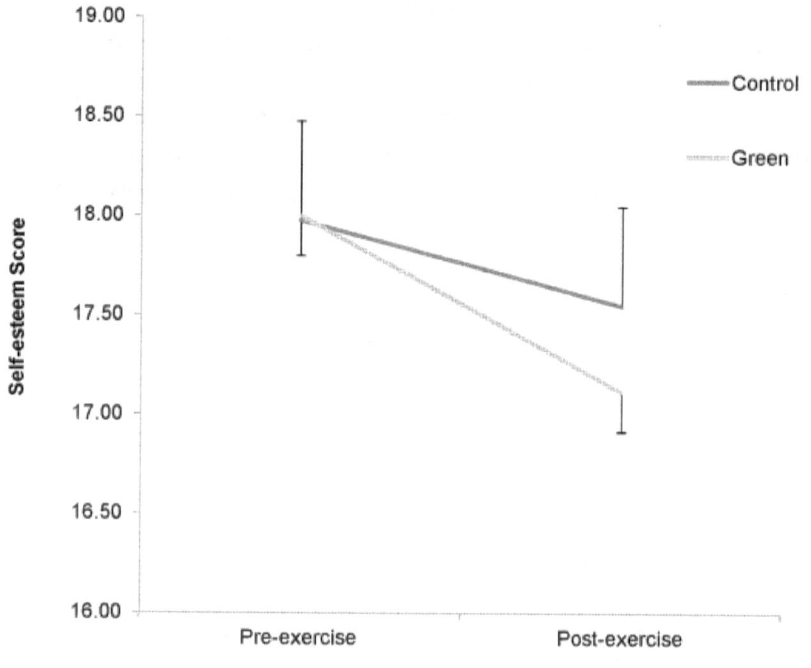

FIGURE 1: Self esteem pre- and post exercise in control and green exercise conditions. Self esteem; measured using the Rosenberg scale (a lower score shows higher self-esteem).

TABLE 1: Descriptive anthropometric, physical activity, fitness and self-esteem scores for sample.

	Males		Females		p-value
	Mean	SD	Mean	SD	
Age (years)	11.4	0.2	11.4	0.3	0.98
Stature (cm)	150.2	7.5	148.4	12.0	0.44
Body mass (kg)	40.3	6.5	44.5	10.1	0.03
PAQ score	2.9	0.7	2.5	0.6	0.004
Shuttle run (laps)	67.2	15.3	45.3	15.8	0.001
Self esteem	17.1	4.0	18.8	4.0	0.09

PAQ-physical activity questionnaire (Kowalski et al. 1997). SE-self esteem; measured using the Rosenberg scale (a lower scale shows higher self-esteem).

TABLE 2: Changes in self-esteem, ratings of perceived exertion and enjoyment in green exercise versus control.

	Control Exercise		Green Exercise		p-value
	Mean	SD	Mean	SD	
ΔSelf Esteem	0.5	4.2	0.9	2.6	0.72
RPE	13.6	3.6	13.5	3.6	0.91
Enjoyment	83.6	34.7	89.2	31.4	0.66

SE-self esteem; measured using the Rosenberg scale (a lower score shows higher self-esteem). ΔScore is pre-test minus post-test value. RPE-Rating of Perceived Exertion; measured using Borg's 6-20 scale. Enjoyment-score out of 120 measured using a visual analogue scale (a higher score shows greater enjoyment).

Values for ΔSE, RPE and enjoyment in both conditions are shown in Table 2. RM t-tests showed there were no significant differences between green and control exercise in terms of enjoyment ($t(75) = 0.43$, $p = 0.66$), RPE ($t(75) = 0.11$, $p = .914$) or change in self-esteem ($t(75) = 0.13$, $p = 0.72$).

Ratings of perceived exertion and fitness showed similar negative correlations in the control and green exercise conditions (Table 3). There was a significant, negative relationship between physical activity and RPE in the control condition but this relationship was not evident when RPE scores from the green exercise condition were correlated with physical activity (Table 3).

TABLE 3: Relationship of fitness and physical activity with ratings of perceived exertion and enjoyment in the green exercise and control conditions.

		RPE			Enjoyment		
		R value	R^2 Value	P value	R value	R^2 value	P value
Fitness	Control	–0.37	0.14	0.001	0.45	0.20	0.000
	Green	–0.36	0.13	0.002	0.41	0.17	0.000
Physical Activity	Control	–0.26	0.07	0.04	0.30	0.09	0.003
	Green	–0.07	0.00	0.551	0.26	0.70	0.022

RPE-Rating of Perceived Exertion; measured using Borg's 6-20 scale. Enjoyment-Score out of 120 measured using a visual analogue scale (a higher score shows greater enjoyment). Fitness-Assessed using the FITNESSGRAM PACER test. Physical Activity-Measured using the PAQ for adolescents.

There was a positive correlation between fitness (measured as shuttle score) and enjoyment in the control and green exercise conditions (Table 3). Self-reported physical activity was positively correlated with enjoyment in the control condition. This relationship was less strong but remained significant in the green exercise condition (Table 3).

Fitness significantly accounted for 11.2% of the variance in RPE ($\beta = -0.37$; $P<0.001$), but neither physical activity ($\beta = 0.001$; $P = 0.987$) or exercise condition ($\beta = -0.007$; $P = 0.927$) made significant contributions. Similarly fitness accounted for a significant (11.7%) proportion of variance in enjoyment scores ($\beta = 0.374$; $P<0.001$), whilst neither physical activity ($\beta = 0.141$; $P = 0.084$) or exercise condition ($\beta = 0.083$; $p = 0.264$) did so.

4.4 DISCUSSION

The aim of this study was to determine if exercising in a natural, "green" environment could have additive effects to the established positive effects that exercise has on children's self-esteem [6]. Despite a reasonable consensus that green exercise can enhance self-esteem in adults [10], [28], this hypothesis has not been examined using rigorous experimental design in children.

The result of our repeated measures experiment showed that green exercise did not create an additional improvement in self-esteem above that observed in the control exercise condition. General physical activity and structured exercise both have positive effects on children's self-esteem [6], [29], however the current findings do not suggest that exposure to nature has a significant additive effect compared to exercise alone. One of the proposed mechanisms for the additive effects of green exercise is the ability of green spaces to provide distraction from daily stresses [11], [13]. Since the current study was performed during a physical education lesson whereby teachers were present and instructing the participants, it is possible that the green run was merely viewed as an extension of school activity. If this was the case, the green run may not have had the same impact as it would have done if it was performed outside of the school day.

The lack of additional impact of green exercise for self-esteem in children might also be due to their low levels of everyday interaction with nature. The current generation of youth spend less time interacting with nature than previous generations [30] due to parental concerns over stranger danger, increasing road traffic [31], [32], the decline in the availability of green space [33], [34] and the attraction of indoor technology [35]. Only 10% of young people have regular contact with nature compared to the 40% of adults who did so 30–40 years ago [35]. Young people are increasingly confined to indoor and urban areas, and may have developed a disconnection from and lack of understanding of the natural world as a consequence [30]. It is proposed that to receive benefits from having contact with nature an individual needs to understand its features and be "connected" to it in some way [36]. Thus it is possible that children are not benefitting from green exercise like adults, because they are not connected to the natural environment in the same way that adults are.

4.4.1 ASSESSMENT OF SECONDARY AIMS

Whilst there was no additional impact of green exercise on self-esteem, there may be other potential benefits to "green exercise" as a means to engage people with exercise and to help adherence to programmes through enjoyment. To assess the other potential benefits of green exercise and to account for individual differences in physical activity and fitness we examined differences in enjoyment and perceived exertion between green and control exercise. We also aimed to explore whether green exercise altered the relationships that measures of physical activity and fitness had with enjoyment and perceived exertion.

There were no significant differences between enjoyment and ratings of perceived exertion in the control and green conditions. While these findings support the null hypothesis this result is noteworthy because the green exercise condition was actually more physically demanding than the control condition, for two reasons. Running over rough terrain requires greater energy expenditure than running on manmade surfaces [37]. The experiment was conducted in the English autumn after heavy rainfall (although conditions were rain-free on all testing days). The children were required to get wet feet, jump large puddles and all finished the course with significant amounts of mud and debris attached to their training shoes. The green condition also had an overall climb (and subsequent descent) of 46 m compared with the completely (±2 m) flat control run. The physical work of carrying body weight means that running uphill requires greater energy expenditure but gradient also negatively affects running economy [38]. Therefore, although we did not measure energy expenditure, we can assume that this was greater in the green condition. The identical RPE and enjoyment scores may give some tentative indication that green exercise feels easier and that natural environments can help more intense exercise to be as enjoyable as less intense exercise in an urban environment. Green exercise may therefore be an important tool for enabling children to achieve activity recommendations and could improve exercise adherence.

We did find significant associations between baseline values for fitness and physical activity and RPE. Unsurprisingly, fitness negatively correlated with RPE; the fitter the child, the easier they perceived the run to be. This was similar in both conditions. Differences in genetic endowment, maturity and sex may all account for differences in fitness. Physical activity is closely related to fitness in children. Unlike fitness, however, it is a modifiable behaviour and a good target for interventions aiming to improve children's health. In the control condition there was a negative association between physical activity and RPE. In common with fitter children, the more active children perceived the control run as easier. This was not the case in the green exercise test. Physical activity was unrelated to perceived exertion meaning that exertion within the green condition was perceived similarly by children with differing levels of habitual physical activity. This may be a potential avenue for future research into green exercise. If less active participants perceive green exercise to be "easier" (due perhaps to distraction) then it may be a means by which to engage those in most need, and with most to potentially gain [39] from exercise.

More active children tend to enjoy formal PE more [16], [17], but it is difficult to determine the direction of this effect. Enjoyment is an important factor mediating engagement in PE [40] and as experience of PE at school can predict adult activity patterns (especially in females) we wanted to know how enjoyment of the two conditions was related to physical activity and aerobic fitness. Unsurprisingly, enjoyment was positively associated with both fitness and physical activity in the control condition. The fitter or more active the child the greater enjoyment rating they gave the control run. There was a similar positive relationship between fitness and enjoyment in the green exercise condition; however the relationship between physical activity and enjoyment was slightly attenuated for the green exercise condition.

Together with the finding from RPE the attenuated association between physical activity and enjoyment during green exercise is encouraging. Compared with a standard 1.5 mile run, the green exercise condition attenuated the well documented association showing that more active children find PE activities less strenuous and was more equally enjoyable for children with a range of activity levels. A study designed with the primary aim of confirming the associations is needed, perhaps also using alternative measures of enjoyment after each exercise condition.

4.4.2 LIMITATIONS AND RECOMMENDATIONS

There are several limitations to the present study. The Rosenberg Self-Esteem Scale is typically used as a trait scale and may have reduced the study's sensitivity. This selection was a deliberate attempt to replicate findings of earlier green exercise studies reviewed [10], many of which have successfully used this tool to show changes in self-esteem. Our aim was to test the green exercise hypothesis using a robust scientific design and analysis. We therefore needed to use the same tools as previous researchers. Future studies would benefit from the use of a state self-esteem questionnaire [41].

The control condition, although typical of a school PE lesson in some respects remained somewhat artificial. The time spent exercising was relatively short and the lesson was contaminated by the presence of external researchers. This was the second lesson the researchers had attended as fitness testing and anthropometry were carried out the previous week but we cannot rule out some reactivity of the children to our presence. The condition was also held outside and although the children were contained within an urban environment, they could occasionally see trees or grassy patches at some points during their run. Furthermore, the differences between the two courses in terms of terrain and elevation makes comparing the energy expenditure and "effort" needed to complete them difficult. This is, however, a common weakness in such natural experiments and was unavoidable in the present protocol. It would however be useful for future research to obtain a measure of energy expenditure so that exercise conditions can be compared. It would also be beneficial to perform a follow-up study incorporating different green exercise modes such as walking and running, in order to determine if the role of the environment in improving self-esteem varies according to exercise intensity. Factors such as relatedness to nature, perceptions and attitudes and perceived level of engagement would also need to be controlled for to develop further insights into the effects of green exercise in children. The school itself was chosen because of its location and was unique of nine potential schools visited in being able to offer both an urban setting and a nearby, wooded, rural area in which to exercise.

The use of retrospective RPE has been mentioned previously and future studies should take such measures during the exercise trails. To further examine the relationships activity and fitness may have with enjoyment and RPE during green exercise a larger sample is needed. This would also allow the observation of between-sex differences. We could not make relevant comparisons here due to sample size but of note, all changes and correlations were similar in magnitude between boys and girls, despite lower fitness and physical activity in the latter.

4.5 CONCLUSIONS

This study assessed the impact of green exercise using a rigorous methodology in children. The effects of green exercise on children's self-esteem were no greater than those of exercise using standard analysis. Despite no evidence for synergy between exercise and nature for increasing self-esteem we did find some promising trends for both enjoyment and ratings of perceived exertion. Though identical between the conditions the increased energy expenditure during the green condition may indicate that natural environments make more intense exercise seem equally as easy and enjoyable as less intense exercise in built environments. Green exercise could therefore be used as a tool for engaging children in more moderate to vigorous physical activity, in line with current recommendations. Also promising was the lack of association between physical activity and perceived exertion and the attenuated association between physical activity and enjoyment in the green condition. We tentatively suggest that green exercise may offer an enjoyable and accessible form of physical activity to less active children who may not typically be well-engaged in physical education.

REFERENCES

1. Green H, McGinnity A, Meltzer H, Ford T, Goodman R (2005) Mental health of children and young people in Great Britain 2004. London: Crown. 388 p.

2. Bagley C (2001) Normative data and mental health constuct validity for the Rosenberg self-esteem scale in British adolescents. Int J of Adolesc Youth 9: 117–126. doi: 10.1080/02673843.2001.9747871
3. Watson AC, Corrigan P, Larson JE, Sells M (2007) Self-stigma in people with mental illness. Schizophr Bull 33: 1312–1318. doi: 10.1093/schbul/sbl076
4. Deslandes A, Moraes H, Ferreira C, Veiga H, Silveira H, et al. (2009) Exercise and mental health: many reasons to move. Neuropsychobiology 59: 191–8. doi: 10.1159/000223730
5. Rees DI, Sabia JJ (2010) Exercise and adolescent mental health: new evidence from longitudinal data. J Ment Health Policy Econ 13: 13–25.
6. Ekeland E, Heian F, Hagen KB, Abbott J, Nordheim L (2004) Exercise to improve self-esteem in children and young people. Cochrane Database Syst Rev 1: CD003683. doi: 10.1002/14651858.cd003683
7. NHS Information Centre (2011) Health survey for England 2010. London: Health and Social Care Information Centre.
8. Wells N (2000) At home with nature- Effects of "greenness" on children's cognitive functioning. Environ Behav 32: 775–795. doi: 10.1177/00139160021972793
9. Wells N, Evans G (2003) Nearby Nature: A buffer of life stress among rural children. Environ Behav 35: 311–330. doi: 10.1177/0013916503035003001
10. Barton J, Pretty J (2010) What is the best dose of nature and green exercise for improving mental health? A multi-study analysis. Environ Sci Technol 44 3947–3955.
11. Pretty J, Peacock J, Sellens M, Griffin M (2005) The mental and physical health outcomes of green exercise. Int J Environ Health Res 15: 319–337. doi: 10.1080/09603120500155963
12. Pretty J, Angus C, Bain M, Barton J, Gladwell V, et al.. (2009) Nature, childhood and life pathways. Colchester: University of Essex. 36 p.
13. Berger BG, Motl RW (2000) Exercise and mood: A selective review and synthesis of research employing the profile of mood states. J Appl Physiol 12: 69–92. doi: 10.1080/10413200008404214
14. LaCaille RA, Masters KS, Heath EM (2004) Effects of cognitive strategy and exercise setting on running performance, perceived exertion, affect and satisfaction. Psychol Sport Exerc 5: 461–476. doi: 10.1016/s1469-0292(03)00039-6
15. Crocker P, Hoar S, McDonough M, Kowalski K, Niefer C (2004) Emotional Experience in Youth Sport. In: Weiss M, editor. Developmental Sport and Exercise Psychology: A lifespan perspective. Morgantown VW: Fitness Information Technology. 197–222.
16. Sallis JF, Prochaska JJ, Taylor WC, Hill JO, Geraci JC (1999) Correlates of physical activity in a national sample of girls and boys in grades 4 through 12. Health Psychol 18: 410–5. doi: 10.1037/0278-6133.18.4.410
17. Sallis JF, Prochaska JJ, Taylor WC (2000) A review of correlates of physical activity of children and adolescents. Med Sci Sports Exerc 32: 963–75. doi: 10.1097/00005768-200005000-00014
18. Kimball J, Jenkins J, Wallhead T (2009) Influence of high school physical education on university students' physical activity. European Physical Education Review 15: 249–269. doi: 10.1177/1356336x09345226

19. Coon JT, Boddy K, Stein K, Whear R, Barton J, et al. (2011) Does participating in physical activity in outdoor natural environments have a greater effect on physical and mental wellbeing than physical activity indoors? A Systematic Review. J Epidemiol Community Health 65: A38–A38. doi: 10.1021/es102947t
20. Kowalski KC, Crocker P, Kowalski NP (1997) Convergent validity of the Physical Activitiy Questionnaire for Adolescents. Ped Exerc Res 9: 342–352.
21. Meredith MD, Welk GJ (2004) Chapter 9. Interpreting Fitnessgram results In: Meredith MD, Welk GJ, Editors. Fitnessgram/Activitygram administration manual. Champaign, IL: Human Kinetics. 59–68.
22. 22. Voss C, Sandercock G (2009) Does the twenty metre shuttle-run test elicit maximal effort in 11 to 16 year olds? Ped Exerc Res 21: 55–62.
23. Rosenberg M (1965) Society and the adolescent self-image. Princeton, NJ: Princeton University Press. 326 p.
24. Borg GAV (1973) Perceived Exertion – Note on History and Methods. Med Sci Sports Exerc 5: 90–93. doi: 10.1249/00005768-197300520-00017
25. Hansen CJ, Stevens LC, Coast JR (2001) Exercise duration and mood state: how much is enough to feel better? Health Psychol 20: 267–75. doi: 10.1037/0278-6133.20.4.267
26. Office for National Statistics (2007) The English Indices of Deprivation 2007 (revised). London: Office of the Deputy Prime Minister. 127 p.
27. Geoconvert website. Available: http://geoconvert.mimas.ac.uk/index.htm Accessed 2008 Jan 1.
28. Bowler DE, Buyung-Ali LM, Knight TM, Pullin AS (2010) A systematic review of evidence for the added benefits to health of exposure to natural environments. BMC Public Health 10: 456. doi: 10.1186/1471-2458-10-456
29. Gruber J (1986) Physical activity and self-esteem development in children: a meta-analysis. In: Stull G, Eckern H, Editors. Effects of physical activity on children. Champaign, IL: Human Kinetics. 330–348.
30. Bird W (2007) Natural Thinking: Investigating the Links between the Natural Environment, Biodiversity and Mental Health. Reading: Royal Society for the Protection of Birds. 113 p.
31. Biddle S, Gorely T, Stensel D (2004) Health-enhancing physical activity and sedentary behaviour in children and adolescents. J Sports Sci 22: 679–701. doi: 10.1080/02640410410001712412
32. Department for Children Schools and Families and Department for Culture Media and Sport (2008) The play strategy. Nottingham: Department for Children Schools and Families. 86 p.
33. Maller C, Townsend M, Pryor A, Brown P, St Leger L (2006) Healthy nature healthy people: 'contact with nature' as an upstream health promotion intervention for populations. Health Promotion Interventions 21: 45–54. doi: 10.1093/heapro/dai032
34. Maas J, Verheij R, Groenewegen P, de Vries S, Spreeuwenberg P (2006) Green space, urbanity, and health: how strong is the relation? J Epidemiol Community Health 60: 587–592. doi: 10.1136/jech.2005.043125
35. Natural England (2009) Childhood and nature: A survey on changing relationships with nature across generations. Cambridgeshire: Natural England. 32 p.

36. Bratman GN, Hamilton JP, Daily GC (2012) The impacts of nature experience on human cognitive function and mental health. Ann N Y Acad Sci 1249: 118–136. doi: 10.1111/j.1749-6632.2011.06400.x
37. Jensen K, Karkkainen LJOP (1999) Economy in track runners and orienteers during path and terrain running. J Sports Sci 17: 945–950. doi: 10.1080/026404199365335
38. Margaria R, Cerretelli P, Aghemo P, Sassi G (1963) Energy cost of running. J Appl Physiol 18: 367–70.
39. Bouchard C, Rankinen T (2001) Individual differences in response to regular physical activity. Med Sci Sports Exerc 33: S446–51. doi: 10.1097/00005768-200106001-00013
40. Wallhead T, Buckworth J (2004) The role of physical education in the promotion of youth physical. QUEST 56: 285–301. doi: 10.1080/00336297.2004.10491827
41. Heatherton TF, Polivy J (1991) Development and validation of a scale for measuring state self-esteem. J Pers Soc Psychol 60: 895–910. doi: 10.1037//0022-3514.60.6.895

CHAPTER 5

LONG-TERM EFFECT OF A SCHOOL-BASED PHYSICAL ACTIVITY PROGRAM (KISS) ON FITNESS AND ADIPOSITY IN CHILDREN: A CLUSTER-RANDOMIZED CONTROLLED TRIAL

URSINA MEYER, CHRISTIAN SCHINDLER, LUKAS ZAHNER, DOMINIQUE ERNST, HELGE HEBESTREIT, WILLEM VAN MECHELEN, HANS-PETER BRUNNER-LA ROCCA, NICOLE PROBST-HENSCH, JARDENA J. PUDER, AND SUSI KRIEMLER

5.1 INTRODUCTION

Clinical markers of chronic disease in adulthood like atherosclerosis, obesity and osteoporosis are due to lifelong processes that originate in childhood with physical inactivity and low aerobic fitness as key players in the high burden of chronic disease.[1] In children, both factors are associated with increasing prevalence of cardiovascular risk factors[2], [3] even independent of body weight.[4] There is strong evidence that high aerobic fitness and physical activity protect adults—with or without increased body fat—from increased morbidity and mortality. [5] Yet, aerobic performance levels in youth have almost globally decreased over the last decades[6] and not even half of the children meet physical activity recommendations. [7]

The importance of primary prevention by promoting physical activity in general[8] as well as in the scope childhood obesity has become indisputable,[9] as most pediatric obesity treatment interventions are marked by small changes in adiposity,[10] a substantial relapse rate and by a strong tracking of overweight into adulthood.[11] School-based intervention studies promoting a healthy lifestyle have shown favourable immediate health effects.[12] However, there is a striking paucity of information on long-term follow-up especially of high-quality randomised, controlled, theory driven trials that had shown efficacy at the end of their interventions.[12], [13] Therefore, we report the 3-year follow-up results of a cluster-randomised, controlled trial ("Kinder- und Jugendsportstudie"; KISS) comparing a school-based stringent physical activity program to traditional physical education during one school-year. This trial has shown beneficial short-term effects on aerobic fitness, physical activity, body fat and a composite cardiovascular risk factor score.[14]

5.2 METHODS

5.2.1 ETHICS STATEMENT

The study was approved by the ethics committees of the University of Basel and the Swiss Federal Institute of Technology Zurich, as well as by the Cantonal Ethical Committee of Aargau, Switzerland. Written informed consent was provided by at least one parent and all children gave their assent for participation to the whole study and specifically for the blood withdrawal. The protocol for this trial and supporting CONSORT checklist are available as supporting information; see Checklist S1 and Protocol S1.

5.2.2 DESIGN AND STUDY POPULATION

The design and the short-term effects have been published previously.[14],[15] Briefly, this cluster randomized controlled trial with a multi-component physical activity intervention was performed between August 2005 and July 2006 in two of 26 provinces of Switzerland comprising 10% of the Swiss population. Of the 95 schools fulfilling our stratification criteria, i.e. rural versus urban localisation, and a prevalence of 10–30% children from other ethnicities as in the Swiss population, and, for practical reasons, the presence of at least one first and fifth grade class per school, we randomly selected 15 schools and assigned them in a 3:2 ratio to an intervention (n = 9 schools) and a control arm (n = 6 schools). Randomization by school was done to avoid a contamination of treatments and was performed based on a computer-generated random-number table which was in the hands of a person not involved in the study. All measurements were performed at school. The younger children, now in fifth grade, were contacted through and tested in their respective schools (June 2009). The former fifth graders now attending different secondary schools/colleges were contacted individually and testing was done in an easily reachable, centrally located school (August to November 2009). For participation in the baseline and post-intervention testing, children received a swim towel with the KISS logo and parents received a written report about individual results of their child. Participants in the follow-up received a small kite (younger children) and a gift voucher (value 30 CHF for younger children or 50 CHF for older children).

5.2.3 INTERVENTION

The intervention was targeted both at the cluster and the individual level and was based on a socio-ecological conceptual model focusing on increasing daily physical activity as previously described.[15] Briefly, children in both groups had three physical education lessons per week (45 minutes each) given by the usual classroom teachers. The intervention group had two additional physical education lessons (45 minutes each) on the remaining school days that were taught by physical education teachers. The curriculum for all physical education lessons for the intervention group was prepared by a team of expert physical education teachers and the same curriculum aiming at increasing quality of physical education and quantity of at least moderately intense physical activity was provided to all intervention classes. In addition, three to five short activity breaks (two to five minutes each) were introduced every day during academic lessons, comprising motor skill tasks such as jumping or balancing on one leg. The children also received daily physical activity homework of about 10 minutes. Children and parents of the control group were not informed about the existence of the intervention program in other schools. The teachers in the control group knew about the intervention arm, but were not informed about its content. After the intervention, none of the schools continued to provide additional physical education.

5.2.4 OUTCOME MEASURES

All measures were taken exactly the same way at baseline, post-intervention and at follow-up.[14], [15] Blinding of the assessors at follow-up was fulfilled, except for waist circumference and skinfold assessment measured by the same persons as before. As in the initial analyses, primary outcome measures included the sum of four skinfolds, aerobic fitness, physical activity and quality of life. Secondary outcome measures included body mass index (BMI) and a cardiovascular risk score comprising all variables of the metabolic syndrome. Overweight was calculated based on WHO criteria.[16] Skinfold thickness was measured in triplicate to the nearest 0.5 mm with Harpenden calipers (HSK-BI, British Indicators, UK). The sum of four sites (triceps, biceps, subscapular and suprailiacal) was calculated.[17] Aerobic fitness was determined using the 20 m shuttle run test.[18] Physical activity was monitored by an accelerometer (MTI/CSA 7164/GT1M, Actigraph, Shalimar, FL, USA) which was worn continuously around the hip for 7 weekdays during each measure period. The sampling epoch was set at one minute. Time periods with over 15 minutes of continuous zero values were omitted. An individual child's physical activity data were included if at least three weekdays of measurements with a minimum of 12 hours and one weekend day of at least 10 hours were recorded.[19] Physical activity was expressed as average counts/min (cpm) and moderate-vigorous physical activity (MVPA) as minutes above 2000 cpm (which is equivalent to walking at about 4 km/h). A physical activity questionnaire was used to assess children's sports club and leisure time sports participation, as well as parental support for and attitude towards physical activity. Quality of life was assessed by the child health questionnaire[20] distributed at school in coded envelopes and completed by the child, if necessary, with the help of the parents. Blood pressure was measured at the right arm five times after a resting period of five minutes using an automated oscillograph (Oscillomatc, CAS Medical Systems, Branford, CT, USA). The mean of the three measurements with the smallest variation was taken and then z-transformed.[21] Blood was drawn in the morning while fasting for measurements of glucose, insulin, and lipids as previously described[15] and a composite cardiovascular risk score[22] was computed by averaging the z-scores of all components of the metabolic syndrome (waist circumference, blood pressure (mean of systolic and diastolic blood pressure z-score), glucose, inverted high density lipoprotein-cholesterol (HDL), and triglycerides). Skewed data were ln-transformed. Z-scores were derived from published age- and gender-specific norm values for BMI[23] and blood pressure.[21] The remaining variables were z-transformed using grade- and gender-specific means and standard deviations derived from the whole sample at each measurement period. Reported time spent in sport clubs (in min/wk), leisure-time physical activity (in min/wk) and parents' support for or attitude towards physical activity in a 5-point Likert scale were assessed by questionnaire.

5.2.5 STATISTICAL ANALYSIS

Children with both, baseline and follow-up data were included in the analysis and defined as "participants". Baseline comparisons were done using a multilevel linear or logistic regression model with school as random effect using participation (1 = participants vs. 0 = non-participants), group (1 = intervention vs. 0 = control group) and the interaction participation

× group as explanatory variables. Analyses of a selection bias for physical activity measures were done using multilevel linear regression models adjusting for sex and grade, comparing children with and without physical activity data for the other primary outcomes. We also used inverse probability weighting based on baseline characteristics (i.e., sex, age, initial fitness, parental education level) and stratifying weight models by group, to assess the direction in which effect estimates might have been biased by differential missing of data (including missing data due to non-participation). For each of the main outcomes, separate weight models were derived. To facilitate interpretation, descriptive results are reported on the original scale according to group and participation status, but all statistical comparisons were done using age and sex-specific z-scores. We used multilevel linear models with z-scores at follow-up as dependent variables, group, gender and grade as fixed factors, the respective baseline z-score as covariate. As BMI and pubertal stage are known to influence aerobic fitness, physical activity and their changes the baseline model was further adjusted by change in BMI z-score and change in Tanner stage. The original school class was the smallest cluster in the sampling design and therefore used as random effect. We did not adjust for multiple comparisons. We did not add a second cluster adjustment for the new class of the older age group since the students were spread into a large number of new classes. We did not include pubertal stage, migrant or socio-economic status, in the final model since their addition to the model did not change the results (data not shown). For each outcome measure, the size of the intervention effect is reported as difference in its average z-scores at follow-up and Cohen effect sizes between the intervention and control group after adjustment for grade, gender, baseline values and clustering within the original school classes. In secondary analyses, potential interactions of the intervention with gender, grade, or baseline BMI, divided into two at the median were assessed and subgroup analyses by gender and grade were performed for the primary outcomes. In an additional step, we also included the group-specific participation propensity scores centered at the respective participation rates to the model in order to adjust for differences in baseline characteristics. According to our original calculation, primarily performed for the outcome of the shuttle run test but equally valid for the other outcomes, a sample size of 360 children at the three year follow-up was sufficient to detect a true mean effect size of half a standard deviation with 79% probability for an intracluster correlation (ICC) within schools of 0.10 and with 90% probability for an ICC of 0.06. A new power calculation, backed up by a Monte Carlo simulation, revealed that our original calculation was too conservative. With 16 intervention and 12 control classes that would each contribute at least 10 children for the 3-year follow-up (n = 280), we would actually already have had a power of 80% to detect a true effect size of 0.5 standard deviations for an ICC of 0.1, and a power of 89% for an ICC of 0.06. The actual ICCs in the follow-up were even lower.

5.3 RESULTS

Figure 1 provides sample size information and Table 1 baseline characteristics stratified by allocation arm and participation at follow-up. Characteristics at follow-up are given in Table 2. Overall participation in the 3-year follow-up assessments was 289 (58%) children of the original baseline sample. Most dropouts at follow-up were caused by non-willingness to participate at the measurements. Participation among groups was not different among the younger and older age group, but non-participation was much more common for the older age group irrespective of group (78% of the intervention group and 66% of the control group of non-participants were from the older age category). There were no major differences in baseline characteristics between participants and non-participants at follow-up except for z-scores of sum of four skinfolds, BMI and waist circumference which were lower in participants than in non-participants. The only significant group × participation interaction existed for BMI z-scores, i.e. with lower values for participants of the intervention compared to controls. Missing values mainly occurred in blood and accelerometer parameters, mainly including invalid accelerometer recordings due to too short wearing time. However, there were no statistically significant differences in any of the primary outcomes between children with and without blood samples and between children with and without valid accelerometer data.

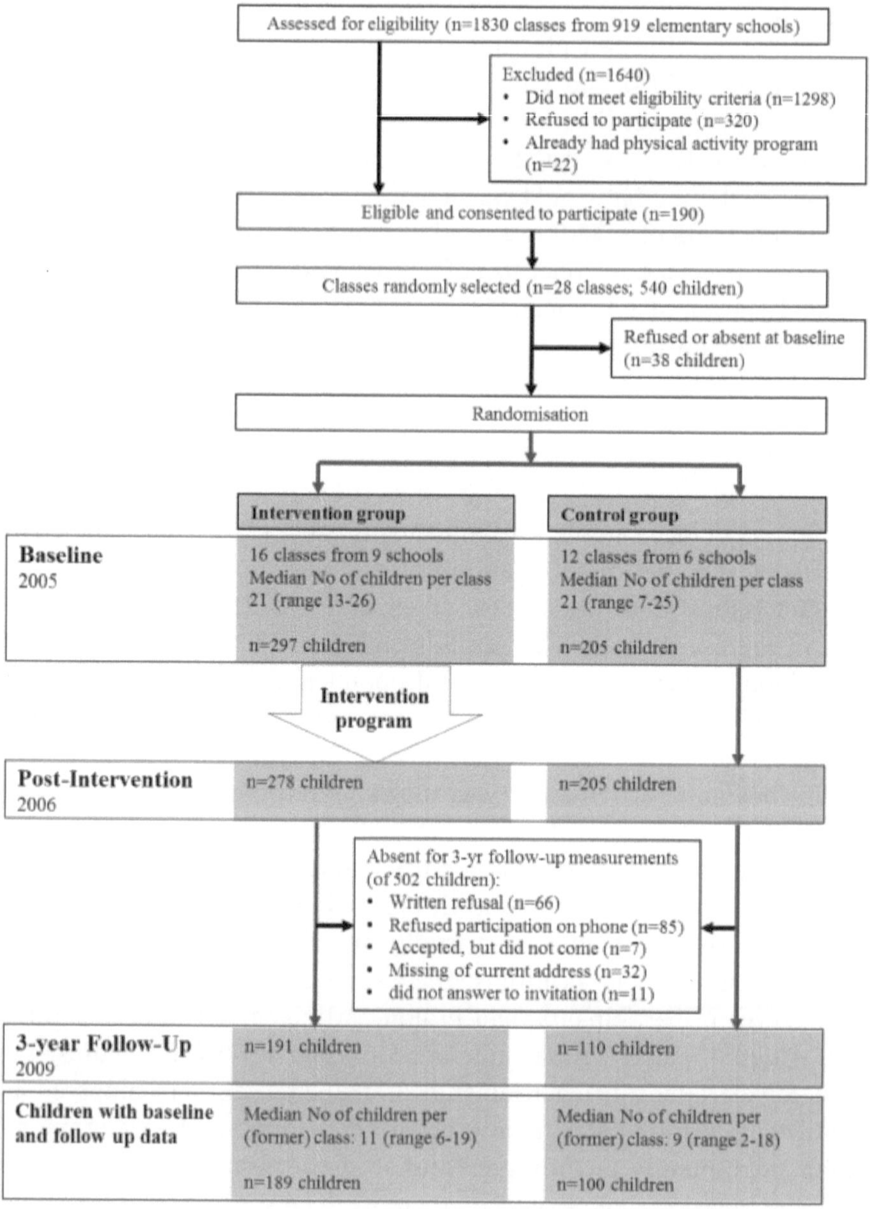

FIGURE 1: Flow of individual participants through study with outcome measures. Post-intervention results have been published elsewhere [14].

TABLE 1: Baseline characteristics of children according to treatment arm and participation at follow-up. Values are means (SD) unless stated otherwise.

		First graders		Fifth graders		Baseline differences between participants and non-participants[a]		
		INT (n = 108)	CON (n = 65)	INT (N = 81)	CON (n = 35)			
		Mean (SD)	Mean (SD)	Mean (SD)	Mean (SD)	p_{part}	p_{group}	$p_{group\ x\ part}$
Age (years)	Participants	6.9 (0.3)	6.9 (0.3)	10.9 (0.5)	11.1 (0.6)	0.07	0.29	0.63
	Non-participants	7 (0.3)	6.9 (0.4)	11.1 (0.6)	11.3 (0.6)			
Height (cm)	Participants	122.5 (5.2)	122.8 (5.6)	144.9 (7.6)	147.2 (7.5)	0.62	0.99	0.34
	Non-participants	124.9 (5.1)	121 (5.2)	145.5 (5.6)	146.7 (7.4)			
Weight (kg)	Participants	24.4 (3.7)	23.6 (4.1)	37.3 (7)	37.4 (7.8)	0.02	0.39	0.33
	Non-participants	25.8 (7.6)	24.8 (4.9)	38.5 (8)	39.9 (8.7)			
Gender, % girls	Participants	51 (47%)	36 (55%)	48 (59%)	23 (66%)	0.04	0.47	0.22
	Non-participants	13 (65%)	19 (79%)	41 (51%)	27 (39%)			
Overweight (5)[b]	Participants	27 (25%)	9 (14%)	15 (19%)	5 (14%)	<0.001	0.1	0.02
	Non-participants	3 (15%)	11 (46%)	20 (25%)	20 (29%)			
Prepubertal/early-pubertal/pubertal[c]	Participants	108/0/0	65/0/0	44/36/1	20/12/3	0.22	0.98	0.68
	Non-participants	24/0/0	36/0/0	36/40/4	33/21/3			
Migrants (5)[d]	Participants	34 (31%)	16 (25%)	16 (20%)	5 (14%)	0.01	0.55	0.13
	Non-participants	10 (50%)	15 (63%)	25 (31%)	20 (29%)			
No formal parental education (%)	Participants	9 (8%)	2 (3%)	2 (2%)	3 (9%)	0.2	0.09	0.31
	Non-participants	3 (15%)	2 (8%)	17 (21%)	8 (12%)			

TABLE 1: *Cont.*

[a]Main effects of group and participation and potential interactions between the two age-group and gender specific z-scores were assessed using mixed linear or logistic regression models including indicator variables for participation (part) and group (intervention (INT) vs. controls (CON)), and an interaction term group x participation as well as a random effect for original school class. [b]Categorization based on WHO z-scores. [c]Pubertal stages are based on Tanner stages: prepubertal (Tanner 1), early pubertal (Tanner 2 and 3), pubertal (Tanner 4 and 5). [d]Both parents from Eastern or Southern European countries, Africa, Asia, Central or South America, or other less developed countries.

TABLE 2: Follow-up characteristics of participating children according to treatment arm. Values are means (SD) unless stated otherwise.

	First graders		Fifth graders	
	INT (n = 108)	CON (n = 65)	INT (n = 81)	CON (n =35)
	Mean (SD)	Mean (SD)	Mean (SD)	Mean (SD)
Age (years)	10.6 (0.3)	10.6 (0.4)	15.0 (0.5)	15.1 (0.6)
Height (cm)	145.0 (7.0)	144.1 (6.9)	167.6 (9.8)	167.3 (7.9)
Weight (kg)	37.7 (7.6)	35.8 (8.6)	58.4 (9.7)	56.9 (11.1)
Gender, n (%) girls	51 (47%)	36 (55%)	48 (59%)	23 (66%)
Overweight (%)[a]	32 (31%)	9 (14%)	16 (20%)	7 (20%)
Pubertal stages[b], n (%)				
Prepubertal	54 (50%)	32 (49%)	1 (1%)	0 (0%)
Early pubertal	51 (47%)	32 (49%)	18 (22%)	9 (26%)
Pubertal	3 (3%)	1 (2%)	62 (77%)	26 (74%)
Migrants, n (%)[c]	34 (31%)	16 (25%)	16 (20%)	5 (14%)
No formal parental education, n (%)	9 (8%)	2 (3%)	2 (2%)	3 (9%)

[a]Categorization based on WHO z-scores. [b]Pubertal stages are based on Tanner stages: prepubertal (Tanner 1), early pubertal (Tanner 2 and 3), pubertal (Tanner 4 and 5). [c]Both parents from Eastern or Southern European countries, Africa, Asia, Central or South America, or other less developed countries.

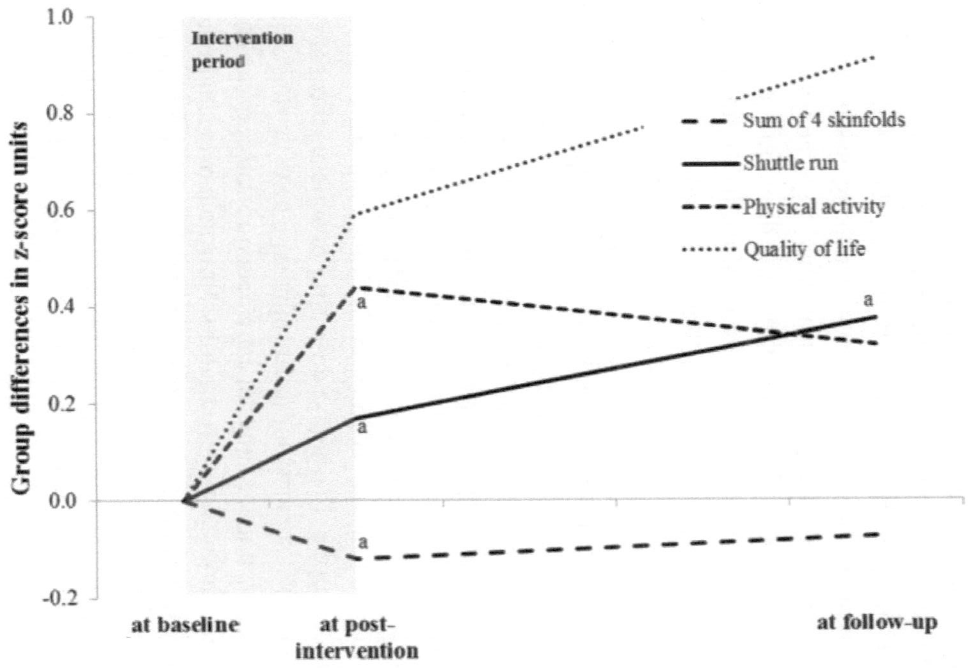

FIGURE 2: Schematic illustration of the differences for the four primary outcomes between the intervention and the control group at baseline, after nine months physical activity intervention, and three years after cessation of the intervention. Post-intervention results derive from previously published results with different sample sizes [14] (for body fat (n = 485 at post-intervention/n = 293 at follow-up); fitness (n = 472/n = 281); physical activity (n = 303/n = 145); quality of life (n = 427/n = 191)). [a]significantly different values in favour of the intervention group compared to the control group.

5.3.1 PRIMARY AND SECONDARY OUTCOMES

Long-term results of the primary and secondary outcomes are presented in Table 3 and Figure 2. Compared to controls, children in the intervention group showed a significant higher aerobic fitness in the shuttle run by 0.373 z-score units (95% CI 0.157 to 0.590), equivalent to a shift from the 50th to the 65th percentile. This effect was found in 1st and 5th graders of both sexes and corresponded to an average difference of improved running distance of about 150 m at the highest speed reached during the test between the two groups. Children of the intervention group continued to increase their fitness from post-intervention to the follow-up while controls lost performance after the intervention had finished. The results were similar, even after adjustment for changes in BMI z-score and Tanner stage from baseline to follow-up (Table 4). Children from the intervention showed a trend towards higher levels of physical activity. Cohen's d effect sizes were 0.35 for total physical activity and 0.65 for aerobic fitness, respectively. Intervention effects on primary outcomes were comparable in children with and without complete physical activity data (all interaction terms $p>0.4$). The remaining primary and secondary outcome variables were not significantly different among groups nor among subgroups by gender or grade. This was also true for the variables that showed beneficial effects in favour of the intervention at the end of the intervention period, including sum of four skinfolds, physical activity and the cardiovascular risk score with one exception. The sum of 4 skinfolds and waist circumference at follow up were significantly lower in the intervention compared to the control group in the 5th graders by 12 and 10%, respectively (both $p<0.03$). The ICCs were ≤ 0.1 indicating a low level of clustering within school classes. Secondary analyses that involved the study of potential effect modifications by gender, grade, or baseline BMI (being dichotomised at the median) did not show any significant result. Inverse probability weighting to adjust for differential missing of data among groups led to slight increases in beneficial effects while non-significant associations showed changes in both directions. The inclusion of the propensity score led to stronger effects for aerobic fitness (β-coef: 0.64 (95%CI: 0.30 to 0.98); $p<0.001$) and significant intervention effects for the sum of four skinfolds (−0.42 (−0.68 to −0.15); $p = 0.002$) and waist circumference

(−0.37 (−0.65 to −0.09); p = 0.009). Reported time spent in sports club was significantly higher in the intervention than the control group (reported difference: 72 min per week (95% confidence interval: 10 to 133; p = 0.022)) while leisure-time physical activity, parents' support for, or attitude towards physical activity did not explain group differences (all p>0.05).

5.4 DISCUSSION

At the current 3-years follow-up of a school-based physical activity intervention over nine months in primary school, aerobic fitness remained significantly higher in favour of the intervention group. The other initially seen beneficial effects on physical activity and a composite cardiovascular risk score were not sustained, except for body fat in the fifth graders that remained lower in the intervention compared to the control group. Reported time spent in sports club during the follow-up period was higher in the intervention group than in controls, while other explanatory factors such as reported leisure-time physical activity and parental attitude towards physical activity were not. This study is one of the few long-term follow-ups of school-based lifestyle interventions to shed light on sustainability of such programs.[12]

The increase in aerobic fitness in favour of the intervention group three years after the end of the intervention, equivalent to a shift from the 50th to the 65th percentile is higher than immediately after the intervention, where it was equivalent to a shift of 5 percentile units. This is due to both a further increase in aerobic fitness in the intervention group and a reduction of aerobic fitness in the control group. Importantly, the differences remained relevant independent of pubertal stage, BMI and their respective changes excluding different developments in body composition or puberty over the study period as confounder. A difference in 150 m of running distance at the highest speed translates into a difference in VO_2max of 5 ml/kg/min or 5%. The decrease in the control group corresponds well to the internationally reported decline of youth fitness by 0.43% per year over the last two decades.[14], [24] Such an improved aerobic fitness is clinically meaningful and from a Public health respect most important, if one considers that an increase of aerobic fitness of 5% in adults translates into 6–7% lower risk for cardiovascular events and mortality.[25]

In the participants of our intervention, some behavioural changes—possibly based on positive experiences by the intervention—occurred. Time spent in sports club during the follow-up was higher in the intervention compared to the control group. Even more importantly, these behavioural changes resulted also in some health enhancing effects such as increased aerobic fitness. Part of the maintained effects may also be related to an increased quality and quantity of the physical education at least in the younger age group. This younger age group attended the same school as during the intervention. Of note, 70% of the teachers and 90% of the children wanted daily physical education to continue after the intervention had stopped.[14]

Children's physical activity levels at follow-up were not different among groups, although there was a trend that pointed towards higher levels in children from the intervention compared to controls. This is consistent with a very similar study,[26] but in contrast to other long-term follow-up studies in which reported leisure-time physical activity was still increased three to 20 years after the intervention.[27]–[30] It is possible that the validity of these studies which were based on activity assessments by questionnaires may have been hampered by factors such as social desirability and reporting or selection bias as these few programs did not measure or show persistent effects on aerobic fitness.[31], [32] The lack of significant physical activity results in our study might reflect insufficient power due to a considerable dropout and non-compliance to wear the accelerometer, even in the children that attended the follow-up assessment. Although our observed intervention effect on physical activity lacks statistical significance, its effect size of $d = 0.35$ would be relevant if it reflected the truth.

Our intervention had initially resulted in an improved body composition with less body fat and lower cardiovascular risk scores that included all components of the metabolic syndrome immediately after the intervention. Unfortunately, this effect was only sustained for the sum of four skinfolds at follow-up for the 5th graders. Only two controlled study in children with a similar follow-up duration and after a one [26] or six [31], [33] year intervention period had reported persistent beneficial effects on blood pressure, [26], [33] blood lipids [31] and glucose metabolism [26] while the few studies that measured long-term effects lost their beneficial effects on adiposity or cardiovascular risk factors. [29], [34], [35] Although one has to be careful with interpreting these data because of methodological limitations and high dropout rates in many of these studies, the maintenance of intervention programs seem necessary over longer time spans, preferably over the whole school period, to have sustained global health effects.

Process evaluation models like the RE-AIM (Reach, Efficacy, Adoption, Implementation and Maintenance of an intervention)[36] that describe the overall health impact of an intervention should always be considered as statistical probabilities or effect sizes on their own do not fully define the real public health impact of an intervention. This important procedure is now taken up by some leading groups in the field, [37], [38] although we were not able to perform it due to financial constraints. In our example with KISS, effect sizes for aerobic fitness and physical activity were relatively large, but its impact is only meaningful if the intervention also reaches a significant part of the population of children and their families. An example in this respect is a small efficacy trial that was performed in a few schools of one province in Canada documenting beneficial effects of a school-based lifestyle intervention.[39] As response to the results the program was then widely implemented throughout the province with the help of the provincial government that mandated 30 minutes of daily physical activity in schools by law. Indeed, the Swiss government has, in part based on results of the KISS study established a National program (Youth and Sport Kids 5–10) that supports schools in establishing additional physical activity programs in primary school by educating classroom teachers to ameliorate quality of physical education teaching and in concert providing financially support. These political steps are promising although their effectiveness has to be proven in the future.

5.4.1 LIMITATIONS AND STRENGTHS

Similarly to every long-term follow-up of school-based intervention studies published so far, the most important limitation of the current study is the considerable dropout rate. It has to be acknowledged that more obese children and those with a migrant background dropped out although other participants' and non-participants' baseline characteristics did not systematically differ. Nevertheless, we cannot rule out the presence of some selection bias. We tried to account for this possible bias by adding a propensity score to our model (to adjust for differential participation) showing that our results remained the same despite adjustment for participation differences. This is especially true for BMI z-scores, for which we had a participation bias in favour of initially leaner children being more prevalent in the intervention than in the control group. Yet, there were no group differences for participation in the other more precise obesity variables such as waist circumference and the sum of the four skin folds and the intervention effects on aerobic fitness remained significant even after adjusting for BMI z-scores (Table 4), and the results did not change with the inclusion of propensity scores for participation. In terms of level of dropout, our study is comparable to other studies of similar length of follow-up, [26], [35] but persistent participation was still much higher than in long-term follow-ups of extended time windows. [30], [31] We did everything to maximize participation: careful update of addresses, offering of multiple test dates, testing during official school time to motivate children, multiple attempts of motivational inputs given by teachers and the KISS staff, and gift vouchers of choice (books, clothes, sport gear, music, jewellery) were provided. Still, these consistently high dropout rates have to be considered when interpreting the results and in future power analyses especially when adolescents with their "unpredictable attitudes" are involved. This may indeed be one or even the major reason explaining the lack of long-term follow-up studies. There is substantial debate whether one should adjust for multiple comparisons in our study. As an intervention like a physical activity program is intended to have simultaneous effects on different health outcomes (like body composition, physical activity, fitness and quality of life) and most of these outcomes are to some extent related. The four primary endpoints mentioned in the protocol represent parallel research questions and not different facets of a global hypothesis. Thus, we have not considered one isolated highly significant intervention effect as proof of success of our intervention, but originally expected a promising public health intervention to have beneficial and relevant effects in most, if not all dimensions. All differences in the main outcome measures were in favour of the intervention group, but only the observed effect on aerobic fitness reached statistical significance. Thus, despite the strong result for aerobic fitnessour expectations were not fully met, possibly due also to a lack of statistical power.

5.5 CONCLUSIONS

After initial beneficial effects in aerobic fitness, physical activity, body fat and a composite cardiovascular risk score were reached by a multicomponent physical activity intervention in school over an academic year, sustained benefits after three years were clearly seen only for aerobic fitness. Although this is highly relevant from a Public Health perspective, longer term interventions throughout the school years are needed to attain persistent beneficial health effects in different relevant dimensions other than fitness.

REFERENCES

1. Beaglehole R, Bonita R, Horton R, Adams C, Alleyne G, et al. (2011) Priority actions for the non-communicable disease crisis. Lancet 377: 1438. doi: 10.1016/s0140-6736(11)60393-0
2. Andersen LB, Riddoch C, Kriemler S, Hills A (2011) Physical activity and cardiovascular risk factors in children. Br J Sports Med 45: 871–876. doi: 10.1136/bjsports-2011-090333
3. Andersen LB, Harro M, Sardinha LB, Froberg K, Ekelund U, et al. (2006) Physical activity and clustered cardiovascular risk in children: a cross-sectional study (The European Youth Heart Study). Lancet 368: 299–304. doi: 10.1016/s0140-6736(06)69075-2
4. Brage S, Wedderkopp N, Ekelund U, Franks PW, Wareham NJ, et al. (2004) Features of the metabolic syndrome are associated with objectively measured physical activity and fitness in Danish children: the European Youth Heart Study (EYHS). Diabetes Care 27: 2141–2148. doi: 10.2337/diacare.27.9.2141
5. Lee DC, Sui X, Church TS, Lavie CJ, Jackson AS, et al. (2012) Changes in fitness and fatness on the development of cardiovascular disease risk factors hypertension, metabolic syndrome, and hypercholesterolemia. J Am Coll Cardiol 59: 665–672. doi: 10.1016/j.jacc.2011.11.013

6. Tomkinson GR, Olds TS (2007) Secular changes in pediatric aerobic fitness test performance: the global picture. Med Sport Sci 50: 46–66. doi: 10.1159/000101075
7. Sisson SB, Katzmarzyk PT (2008) International prevalence of physical activity in youth and adults. Obes Rev 9: 606–614. doi: 10.1111/j.1467-789x.2008.00506.x
8. Ekelund U, Luan J, Sherar LB, Esliger DW, Griew P, et al. (2012) Moderate to vigorous physical activity and sedentary time and cardiometabolic risk factors in children and adolescents. JAMA 307: 704–712. doi: 10.1001/jama.2012.156
9. van Sluijs EM, McMinn A (2010) Preventing obesity in primary schoolchildren. Br Med J 340: c819. doi: 10.1136/bmj.c819
10. Oude Luttikhuis H, Baur L, Jansen H, Shrewsbury VA, O'Malley C, et al. (2009) Interventions for treating obesity in children. Cochrane Database Syst Rev: CD001872.
11. Singh AS, Mulder C, Twisk JW, van Mechelen W, Chinapaw MJ (2008) Tracking of childhood overweight into adulthood: a systematic review of the literature. Obes Rev 9: 474–488. doi: 10.1111/j.1467-789x.2008.00475.x
12. Kriemler S, Meyer U, Martin E, van Sluijs EM, Andersen LB, et al. (2011) Effect of school-based interventions on physical activity and fitness in children and adolescents: a review of reviews and systematic update. Br J Sports Med 45: 923–930. doi: 10.1136/bjsports-2011-090186
13. Dobbins M, De Corby K, Robeson P, Husson H, Tirilis D (2009) School-based physical activity programs for promoting physical activity and fitness in children and adolescents aged 6–18. Cochrane Database Syst Rev: Cd007651.
14. Kriemler S, Zahner L, Schindler C, Meyer U, Hartmann T, et al. (2010) Effect of school based physical activity programme (KISS) on fitness and adiposity in primary schoolchildren: cluster randomised controlled trial. Br Med J 340: c785–c785. doi: 10.1136/bmj.c785
15. Zahner L, Puder JJ, Roth R, Schmid M, Guldimann R, et al. (2006) A school-based physical activity program to improve health and fitness in children aged 6–13 years ("Kinder-Sportstudie KISS"): study design of a randomized controlled trial [ISRCTN15360785]. BMC Public Health 6: 147.
16. de Onis M, Onyango AW, Borghi E, Siyam A, Nishida C, et al. (2007) Development of a WHO growth reference for school-aged children and adolescents. Bull World Health Organ 85: 660–667. doi: 10.2471/blt.07.043497
17. Lohman TG, Roche AF, Martorell R (1988) Anthropometric Standardization Reference Material. Champaign: Human Kinetics.
18. Leger LA, Mercier D, Gadoury C, Lambert J (1988) The multistage 20 metre shuttle run test for aerobic fitness. J Sports Sci 6: 93–101. doi: 10.1080/02640418808729800
19. Freedson P, Pober D, Janz KF (2005) Calibration of accelerometer output for children. Med Sci Sports Exerc 37: S523–S530. doi: 10.1249/01.mss.0000185658.28284.ba
20. Landgraf JM, Maunsell E, Speechley KN, Bullinger M, Campbell S, et al. (1998) Canadian-French, German and UK versions of the Child Health Questionnaire: methodology and preliminary item scaling results. Qual Life Res 7: 433–445. doi: 10.1023/a:1008810004694
21. National High Blood Pressure Education Program Working Group on High Blood Pressure in Children and Adolescents (2004) The fourth report on the diagnosis, evaluation, and treatment of high blood pressure in children and adolescents. Pediatrics 114: 555–576. doi: 10.1542/peds.114.2.s2.555

22. Eisenmann JC (2008) On the use of a continuous metabolic syndrome score in pediatric research. Cardiovasc Diabetol 7: 17. doi: 10.1186/1475-2840-7-17
23. Woringer V, Schutz Y (2003) [Obesity in Switzerland: body mass index (BMI) percentiles of a child and adolescent population born in 1980 in Lausanne and comparison with Swiss norms (1955)]. Soz Praventivmed 48: 121–132.
24. Tomkinson GR, Leger LA, Olds TS, Cazorla G (2003) Secular trends in the performance of children and adolescents (1980–2000): an analysis of 55 studies of the 20 m shuttle run test in 11 countries. Sports Med 33: 285–300. doi: 10.2165/00007256-200333040-00003
25. Kodama S, Saito K, Tanaka S, Maki M, Yachi Y, et al. (2009) Cardiorespiratory fitness as a quantitative predictor of all-cause mortality and cardiovascular events in healthy men and women: a meta-analysis. JAMA 301: 2024–2035. doi: 10.1001/jama.2009.681
26. Bugge A, El-Naaman B, Dencker M, Froberg K, Holme IM, et al. (2012) Effects of a 3-year intervention: The Copenhagen School Child Intervention Study. Med Sci Sports Exerc [Epub ahead of print].
27. Kelder SH, Mitchell PD, McKenzie TL, Derby C, Strikmiller PK, et al. (2003) Long-term implementation of the CATCH physical education program. Health Educ Behav 30: 463–475. doi: 10.1177/1090198103253538
28. Klepp KI, Tell GS, Vellar OD (1993) Ten-year follow-up of the Oslo Youth Study Smoking Prevention Program. Prev Med 22: 453–462. doi: 10.1006/pmed.1993.1037
29. Nader PR, Stone EJ, Lytle LA, Perry CL, Osganian SK, et al. (1999) Three-year maintenance of improved diet and physical activity: the CATCH cohort. Child and Adolescent Trial for Cardiovascular Health. Arch Pediatr Adolesc Med 153: 695–704. doi: 10.1001/archpedi.153.7.695
30. Trudeau F, Laurencelle L, Tremblay J, Rajic M, Shephard RJ (1999) Daily primary school physical education: effects on physical activity during adult life. Med Sci Sports Exerc 31: 111–117. doi: 10.1097/00005768-199901000-00018
31. Manios Y, Kafatos A (2006) Health and nutrition education in primary schools in Crete: 10 years follow-up of serum lipids, physical activity and macronutrient intake. Br J Nutr 95: 568–575. doi: 10.1079/bjn20051666
32. Trudeau F, Espindola R, Laurencelle L, Dulac F, Rajic M, et al. (2000) Follow-up of participants in the Trois-Rivieres Growth and Development Study: Examining their health-related fitness and risk factors as adults. Am J Hum Biol 12: 207–213. doi: 10.1002/(sici)1520-6300(200003/04)12:2<207::aid-ajhb6>3.0.co;2-8
33. Kafatos I, Manios Y, Moschandreas J, Kafatos A (2007) Health and nutrition education program in primary schools of Crete: changes in blood pressure over 10 years. Eur J Clin Nutr 61: 837–845. doi: 10.1038/sj.ejcn.1602584
34. Trudeau F, Laurencelle L, Tremblay J, Rajic M, Shephard RJ (1998) A long-term follow-up of participants in the Trois-Riviäres semi-longitudinal study of growth and development. Pediatr Exerc Sci 10: 366-377.
35. James J, Thomas P, Kerr D (2007) Preventing childhood obesity: two year follow-up results from the Christchurch obesity prevention programme in schools (CHOPPS). Br Med J (Clin Res Ed) 335: 762. doi: 10.1136/bmj.39342.571806.55

36. Glasgow RE, Vogt TM, Boles SM (1999) Evaluating the public health impact of health promotion interventions: the RE-AIM framework. Am J Public Health 89: 1322–1327. doi: 10.2105/ajph.89.9.1322
37. De Meij JS, Chinapaw MJ, Kremers SP, Van der Wal MF, Jurg ME, et al. (2010) Promoting physical activity in children: The stepwise development of the primary school-based JUMP-in intervention applying the RE-AIM evaluation framework. Br J Sports Med 44: 879–887. doi: 10.1136/bjsm.2008.053827
38. Collard DC, Chinapaw MJ, Verhagen EA, van Mechelen W (2010) Process evaluation of a school based physical activity related injury prevention programme using the RE-AIM framework. BMC Pediatr 10: 86. doi: 10.1186/1471-2431-10-86
39. Naylor PJ, Macdonald HM, Warburton DE, Reed KE, McKay HA (2008) An active school model to promote physical activity in elementary schools: action schools! BC. Br J Sports Med 42: 338–343. doi: 10.1136/bjsm.2007.042036

There are two tables and several supplemental files that are not available in this version of the article. To view this additional information, please use the citation on the first page of this chapter.

CHAPTER 6

SCHOOL PROGRAMS AND CHARACTERISTICS AND THEIR INFLUENCE ON STUDENT BMI: FINDINGS FROM HEALTHY PASSAGES

TRACY K. RICHMOND, MARC N. ELLIOTT, LUISA FRANZINI, ICHIRO KAWACHI, MARGARET O. CAUGHY, M. JANICE GILLILAND, COURTNEY E. WALLS, FRANK A. FRANKLIN, RICHARD LOWRY, STEPHEN W. BANSPACH, AND MARK A. SCHUSTER

6.1 BACKGROUND

Numerous interventions aimed at reversing the childhood obesity epidemic have focused on schools. Schools are a logical place to intervene because children and adolescents spend at least one third of their annual waking hours in school, may consume as much as 50% of their daily calories at school, and are potentially exposed to numerous opportunities for physical activity through school [1]–[3]. However, schools do not currently provide students equal opportunities for healthy choices. Schools have rapidly re-segregated since mandatory racial/ethnic desegregation laws were repealed in the early 1990s [4], [5]. This re-segregation likely has health implications as studies have demonstrated poorer nutritional and physical activity offerings in schools with high concentrations of racial/ethnic minority and low-income students [1], [3].

Several studies have demonstrated differences between high schools in average student weight status; in at least two of these studies, between-school differences were not fully explained by the divergent demographics of the student populations [6], [7]. Questions remain, however, whether school-level differences in weight status exist in elementary schools and if physical activity and nutrition programming or demographics can explain these differences in weight status. Additionally, it is unclear whether school characteristics can partially explain racial/ethnic differences in weight status.

Our objectives were to determine if: 1) school characteristics or resources are associated with individual student BMI; 2) school characteristics and resources partially explain racial/ethnic disparities in individual student weight status; and 3) individual student and/or school characteristics can explain between-school differences in student BMI. We hypothesized that students attending a school with higher physical activity and nutrition resources and higher median income would have on average lower BMIs than those students attending schools with lower physical activity and nutrition resources and lower median income and that differential resources could partially explain racial/ethnic and between-school differences in student BMI.

6.2 METHODS

We used data from the Healthy Passages Longitudinal Study of Adolescent Health, a prospective cohort study of 5th grade students in Birmingham, AL, Los Angeles, CA, and Houston, TX [8], [9]. Healthy Passages has a multilevel approach, collecting data from the individual andhis/her parent or caregiver, school, and neighborhood in an effort to understand the complex influences on risk and protective factors, health behaviors, and health outcomes. We used data from the baseline data collection (2004–2006).

6.2.1 PARTICIPANTS

The sample was derived from the study population that included all fifth-grade students enrolled in public schools with an enrollment of ≥25 fifth graders in each of three geographic areas (25 contiguous public school districts in Los Angeles County, CA; 20 contiguous public school districts in and around Birmingham, AL; and the largest public school district in Houston, TX). Healthy Passages used a two-stage probability sampling strategy, described in detail elsewhere [9], to ensure adequate sample sizes of non-Hispanic Blacks, Hispanics, and non-Hispanic Whites. The 5,147 participants were nested in 112 schools within the three survey sites.

Parents provided written consent for their own as well as their child's participation; the child participant provided written assent. The Institutional Review Boards of the sites (RAND/University of California Los Angeles, University of Alabama Birmingham, University of Texas Houston branch) approved the consent process. Computer-assisted Spanish or English interviews were conducted in the participants' homes, at a study center, or another preferred location. Our research team received only de-identified data. Our analyses were approved through a waiver of the Boston Children's Hospital Institutional Review Board.

6.2.2 OUTCOME VARIABLE

6.2.2.1 BODY MASS INDEX (KG/M^2)

Respondents' BMIs were calculated from measured height and weight. Height and weight measurements were performed by trained field interviewers. Height was measured using a portable stadiometer and measurements were recorded to 0.1 cm. Weight was measured using a portable Tanita electronic scale and was recorded to 0.1 kg. Height and weight were measured two times and averaged; if the two differed by more than a pre-specified amount (0.5 cm for height, 0.2 kg for weight), three measurements were performed and the average of the 2 measurements with the smallest difference was taken.

6.2.3 INDIVIDUAL-LEVEL PREDICTOR VARIABLES

6.2.3.1 RACE/ETHNICITY

Our primary predictor variable was student race/ethnicity. Participants and participants' parents were asked whether the student was of Hispanic/ Latino ethnicity and of which racial group they were a member. When available, the participant-response to Hispanic/Latino ethnicity and participant-chosen racial group was used. Where participant-response of either ethnicity or racial group was unavailable, the parental report was used. We used U.S. Census definitions to initially classify the sample into the following mutually exclusive categories: Asian/Pacific Islander; Black; Hispanic; Multi-racial; Native American/Alaskan Native; and White. We classified any individual who checked Hispanic as Hispanic regardless of additional racial/ethnic categories indicated. We categorized anyone not choosing Hispanic but choosing more than one racial category as Multi-racial. Because of small sample sizes in groups other than Blacks, Whites, and Hispanics, we collapsed groups that consisted of Asian/Pacific Islander, Multi-racial, and Native American/Alaskan into a racial category named "Other."

6.2.3.2 SOCIO-ECONOMIC STATUS MEASURES

Healthy Passages attempted to interview a parent/caregiver for all participants and selected the parent/caregiver with the most knowledge about the child's health and education, usually the mother or female guardian. The parent or caregiver was asked to report all household income by choosing one of the following response categories: <$25,000; $25,000–$49,999; $50,000–$99,999; and >$100,000. They were also asked to report the highest educational level achieved by a household member, including that of step- or foster parents, siblings, grandparents, or significant others of caregivers with the following response options: less than high school graduation; high school graduate or GED; some college or 2 year degree; college graduate or beyond.

6.2.3.3 PARENTAL/CAREGIVER WEIGHT STATUS

Objective measurements of the height and weight of the parent/caregiver participating in the interview—typically the mother or female guardian–were taken at the time of the interview. We calculated BMI from height and weight (weight (kg)/height^2(m^2)) and then categorized weight status as low/normal weight v. overweight/obese (BMI$\geq$25 kg/m^2). Where objective heights and/or weights were missing (9.5% of cases), we inserted the mean parental/caregiver BMI of the sample and added an indicator flag to indicate missing data. We constructed models with and without the mean parental/caregiver BMI substituted to assess bias and found no material difference in the findings. Thus, we present only the models with the mean parental BMI substituted for those with missing data to avoid potential bias and inefficiency from deleting participants.

6.2.3.4 ADDITIONAL DEMOGRAPHICS

Age and gender were self-reported by participants.

6.2.4 SCHOOL-LEVEL PREDICTOR VARIABLES

Information regarding school policies and resources was provided by school staff members (typically the school principals or assistant principals—the school nurse or other administrative personnel completed the survey when the principal or assistant principal was unavailable).

6.2.4.1 PHYSICAL ACTIVITY/NUTRITION RESOURCES

We examined a number of variables that described school physical activity and dietary resources (Table 1) individually and as part of a school physical activity/nutrition summary score. The school physical activity/nutrition summary score included the following variables: 1) Physical Education (PE) taught in school 4 or 5 days/week; 2) PE taught in school ≥36 weeks/year; 3) 5th graders have regular recess; 4) physical activity taught in health class; 5) school does not have a pouring contract with a beverage company; 6) nutrition taught in health class; 7) brand name fast food items are not available in the cafeteria. In addition, we explored three additional variables school offers breakfast; an outside food company manages food service; and school participates in the USDA lunch program. We did not include these variables, however, in the summary score as we had no a priori hypothesis regarding the direction of their influence on BMI. Approximately 10% of school personnel surveyed did not answer the question regarding whether or not school nutrition was taught in school. When asked how many weeks/year PE was taught, a number of school personnel survey respondents answered more than 52 weeks, an implausible value. Due to a large degree of missing or implausible data for these two variables (total ~10%) and because neither was associated with the outcome, we constructed the school summary score with and without these variables and found no material differences in the findings. In order to maximize the sample size and avoid bias, this study presents results with the school summary score not including weeks/year of PE and whether nutrition is taught in school. The school physical activity/nutrition summary score represents a count of the positive factors that apply to each school (range: 0–5).

As an additional sensitivity analysis, we conducted a factor analysis of the variables in the physical activity/nutrition summary score. This analysis resulted in three factors, one related to gym and recess, a second related to foods and beverages available in the cafeteria, and a final one related to the number of weeks gym was taught. None of the factors was associated with individual BMI so we present only findings related to the summary score.

6.2.4.2 SCHOOL DEMOGRAPHICS

We controlled for additional school-level demographics, including the school administrator report of the percentage of students who were White and the school median household income aggregated from individual parent/caregiver report of individual household income as described above.

TABLE 1: Bivariate associations between individual and school characteristics and individual race/ethnicity.

Individual Variable	White	Black	Hispanic	Other	p-value
	N = 1256	N = 1755	N = 1813	N = 321	
Age[a]	11.2 (0.03)	11.2 (0.02)	11.1 (0.03)	11.0 (0.03)	0.001
Household income					<0.001
<$25,000	9%	54%	53%	23%	
$25,000–$49,999	16%	27%	32%	27%	
$50,000–$99,999	35%	14%	11%	25%	
≥$100,000	40%	5%	4%	25%	
Highest education level in household					<0.001
Some HS	3%	10%	45%	2%	
HS/GED	9%	31%	24%	10%	
Some college	17%	37%	21%	29%	
College plus	71%	23%	10%	60%	
School-level variables					
Avg proportion of student body that is white	80%	10%	10%	40%	<0.001
Median school household income[a]	$80,427 (5542)	$27,681[b] (1876)	$29,806[b] (2218)	$54,540[b] (4406)	<0.001
Physical education is taught 4 or 5 days/week	75%	56%	30%	49%	<0.001
Physical education is taught ≥36 weeks/year	94%	89%	69%	86%	<0.001
5th graders have regular recess	59%	56%	91%	90%	<0.001
Physical activity and fitness taught in health class	98%	99%	99%	99%	0.22
School participates in USDA school lunch program	69%	93%	93%	93%	0.003
School does not have pouring contract with beverage company	76%	47%	74%	74%	0.002
Nutrition taught in health class	89%	83%	89%	87%	0.54
School serves breakfast	73%	99%	99%	89%	<0.001
Outside food service cooperates food service program	15%	29%	35%	25%	0.01
Brand name fast food items not available	93%	93%	89%	85%	0.42
School physical activity/nutrition resource summary score[a]	4.01 (0.16)	3.16[b] (0.11)	3.87 (0.13)	3.92 (0.18)	0.049

Avg means Average. [a]Values presented as mean (SE). [b]Indicated mean or percent as significantly different from that of the White group, p-values derived from overall F-test.

6.2.4.3 SITE

Finally, we controlled for the survey site: Birmingham, Los Angeles, and Houston.

6.2.5 PROCEDURES/DATA ANALYSIS

We began by examining univariate distributions of the variables of interest. We then examined bivariate associations of our variables of interest with individual race/ethnicity. Because students were nested within schools in the sample we employed multi-level modeling strategies next in order to estimate both random and fixed effects at both the student and school level and to account for the effects of clustering in the data. Using STATA SE 12 [10] and employing weights to account for probabilities of selection and non-response, we constructed a series of three two-level "mixed" (random and fixed effect) linear regression models predicting individual BMI. Early on in our model building strategy we tested for the potential effect modification by gender on associations between race/ethnicity and BMI and found justification for gender-stratified modeling strategies.

We began with a null model with only school-level random effects to assess variation in BMI by school in terms of school-level variance components. In our second model we added student-level fixed effects (e.g., individual race/ethnicity) to allow us to examine the associations of individual characteristics with BMI. In our third model we added specific school-level variables (e.g., school demographics and school physical activity/nutrition resources) to the second model as well as study site fixed effects to examine the associations of school programs and characteristics with BMI (addressing Objective 1). We assessed changes in the parameter estimates for individual race/ethnicity from Model 2 to 3 with the addition of school characteristics (to address Objective 2). In order to better understand the contribution of individual and school-level characteristics to differences in school-level BMI (addressing Objective 3) we compared the change in between-school variance in BMI across Models 1, 2 and 3.

TABLE 2: The association of individual and school factors with female BMI in the Healthy Passages cohort.

	Model 1 (β coefficient)	Model 2 (β coefficient)	Model 3 (β coefficient)
Fixed Effects			
Intercept	20.62 (19.96, 21.29)	6.01 (–0.86, 12.88)	10.79 (4.59, 17.06)
Individual level variables			
Race/ethnicity			
Hispanic		0.41 (–0.34, 1.16)	–0.04 (–0.76, 0.68)
Black		1.40 (0.75, 2.06)	0.77 (0.03, 1.51)
Other		–0.26 (–1.16, 0.646)	–0.38 (–1.30, 0.54)
White [Ref]		0	0
Age		1.06 (0.45, 1.67)	0.76 (0.22, 1.31)
Household income			
<$25,000		1.05 (0.22, 1.89)	0.68 (–0.17, 1.52)
$25,000–$49,9998		1.28 (0.49, 2.07)	0.72 (–0.06, 1.49)
$50,000–$99,999		0.95 (0.30, 1.59)	0.73 (0.08, 1.39)
≥$100,000 [Ref]		0	0
Highest education level in household[a]		–0.07 (–0.34, 0.20)	–0.04 (–0.30, 0.23)
Parent is overweight and obese		2.37 (1.94, 2.81)	2.43 (1.98, 2.87)
Parent is missing weight status flag		1.24 (0.28, 2.20)	1.22 (0.20, 2.25)
School-level variables			
Proportion of student body that is white			–0.60 (–2.01, 0.81)
School income (tens of thousands of dollars)			–0.12 (–0.21, –0.02)
School Nutrition/ Physical Activity Index[b]			–0.10 (–0.38, 0.18)
Site			
Houston	0.77 (–0.10, 1.63)	0.18 (–0.34, 0.71)	0.35 (–0.31, 1.00)
Birmingham	0.54 (–0.38, 1.47)	0.23 (–0.31, 0.77)	0.57 (–0.01, 1.12)
Los Angeles [Ref]	0	0	0
Random Effects			
sigma_u	1.34 (1.01, 1.65)	0	0.27 (0.01, 7.40)
sigma_e e	4.93 (4.66, 5.21)	4.82 (4.56, 5.08)	4.67 (4.42, 4.93)

Ref = reference group; sigma_u is the standard deviation of the school-level random effect; sigma_e is the standard deviation of the individual-level random effect. [a]High school levels categorized into some high school, high school graduate or received GED, some college, and college graduate or beyond. [b]School nutrition/physical activity index is a count of the positive nutrition and physical activity resources/programs reported in the school.

TABLE 3: The association of individual and school factors with male BMI in the Healthy Passages cohort.

	Model 1 (β coefficient)	Model 2 (β coefficient)	Model 3 (β coefficient)
Fixed Effects			
Intercept	21.38 (20.82, 21.93)	9.86 (5.07, 14.64)	9.30 (3.89, 14.71)
Individual level variables			
Race/ethnicity			
Hispanic		1.47 (0.77, 2.17)	1.58 (0.81, 2.35)
Black		0.31 (–0.36, 0.98)	0.44 (–0.40, 1.27)
Other		1.30 (0.23, 2.36)	1.36 (0.26, 2.46)
White [Ref]		0	0
Age		0.79 (0.36, 1.21)	0.78 (0.33, 1.22)
Household income			
<$25,000		0.78 (–0.06, 1.63)	0.82 (–0.04, 1.67)
$25,000–$49,9998		0.72 (–0.14, 1.58)	0.79 (–0.10, 1.68)
$50,000–$99,999		1.01 (0.35, 1.68)	0.97 (0.32, 1.63)
≥$100,000 [Ref]		0	0
Highest education level in household[a]		–0.24 (–0.51, 0.03)	–0.25 (–0.54, 0.04)
Parent is overweight and obese		2.41 (1.92, 2.90)	2.45 (1.94, 2.96)
Parent is missing weight status flag		0.35 (–0.45, 1.14)	0.55 (–0.29, 1.68)
School-level variables			
Proportion of student body that is white			0.54 (–1.03, 2.11)
School income (tens of thousands of dollars)			–0.03 (–0.16, 0.10)
School Nutrition/ Physical Activity Index[b]			0.13 (–0.26, 0.53)
Site			
Houston	0.14 (–0.64, 0.92)	–0.25 (–1.02, 0.52)	0.05 (–0.85, 0.96)
Birmingham	–1.33 (–2.07, –0.58)	–0.32 (–1.18, 0.55)	–0.44 (–1.41, 0.53)
Los Angeles [Ref]	0	0	0
Random Effects			
sigma_u	0.97 (0.71, 1.31))	0.68 (0.41, 1.14)	0.77 (0.49, 1.20)
sigma_e e	4.99 (4.73, 5.26)	4.84 (4.59, 5.11)	4.83 (4.56, 5.11)

Ref = reference group; sigma_u is the standard deviation of the school-level random effect; sigma_e is the standard deviation of the individual-level random effect. [a]*High school levels categorized into some high school, high school graduate or received GED, some college, and college graduate or beyond.* [b]*School nutrition/physical activity index is a count of the positive nutrition and physical activity resources/programs reported in the school.*

6.3 RESULTS

6.3.1 CHARACTERISTICS OF SCHOOLS ATTENDED BY PARTICIPANTS OF DIFFERENT RACES/ETHNICITIES

Table 1 shows the results of the bivariate relationship of the variables of interest and race/ethnicity. Schools attended by Blacks, Whites, and Hispanics differed on numerous school characteristics, including demographics and nutritional and physical activity programs.

6.3.2 MULTIVARIATE ANALYSIS OF INDIVIDUAL- AND SCHOOL-LEVEL VARIABLES AND STUDENT BMI

Tables 2 and 3 report findings from the multilevel models 1–3, stratified by gender.

6.3.2.1 ASSOCIATION OF SCHOOL CHARACTERISTICS WITH INDIVIDUAL STUDENT BMI (ADDRESSING OBJECTIVE 1)

Among females, only the school level household income was inversely associated with individual student BMI ($\beta = -0.12$, CI: −0.21,−0.02). For males and females, neither the percent of the student body reported to be White nor the summary score representing nutrition/physical activity programming was associated with BMI. In males and females, although each of the ten variables describing the school physical activity and nutrition resources was tested individually in addition to testing the summary score itself, no statistically significant associations were found (data not presented for individual components of s ummary score).

6.3.2.2 CHANGE IN PARAMETER ESTIMATES FOR RACE/ETHNICITY WITH THE ADDITION OF SCHOOL CHARACTERISTICS (ADDRESSING OBJECTIVE 2)

The parameter estimates for Hispanic and Black race/ethnicity in Model 2 (without school characteristics) and Model 3 (with school characteristics added) were compared. Among females, the addition of school characteristics reduced the effect size of Black race by nearly half (Model 2: β = 1.40, CI: 0.75, 2.06; Model 3: β = 0.77, CI: 0.03, 1.51). In contrast, among males, Black race was not associated with BMI in any model. Hispanic ethnicity was not associated with BMI among females in either Model 2 or 3, while among males the effect sizes were similar in Models 2 and 3.

6.3.2.3 THE CHANGE IN BETWEEN SCHOOL VARIANCE WITH THE ADDITION OF INDIVIDUAL AND SCHOOL CHARACTERISTICS (ADDRESSING OBJECTIVE 3)

Among females and males, the unconditional model (Model 1) indicated significant variation in BMI between schools, as reflected in the sigma_u values for both models. These values are the square roots of school-level variance components and can be interpreted as school-level standard deviations, so that the amount by which a typical school differs from the overall average BMI is about 1 unit (1.34 units for females, 0.97 units for males). In contrast, the standard deviation at the student level is approximately 5 units for both males and females. In females, after controlling for race/ethnicity, age, household demographics, and parental BMI, the between-school variation in BMI was no longer statistically significant and was estimated at 0 after accounting for chance variation at the student level. In males, the inclusion of individual level characteristics did not fully explain the between school variation in BMI among males, although their inclusion did result in an approximate one-third reduction in between-school variance ($sigma\_u^2$) (see Table 3, Model 2). The addition of school characteristics and programs did not further decrease the between-school variance in BMI.

6.3.2.4 ADDITIONAL FINDINGS.

Black females had BMIs averaging 1.4 kg/m^2 higher than White females. Mean BMI did not significantly differ from Whites for any other female racial/ethnic group. Females with an obese/overweight parent or caregiver had BMIs averaging >2 kg/m^2 higher than those who did not have an obese/overweight parent or caregiver.

Hispanic males averaged nearly 1.5 kg/m^2 higher in BMI than their White peers. Both markers of socioeconomic status—household income and highest educational level achieved in the household—had inverse but non-significant relationships with BMI. Males with an obese or overweight parent or caregiver had BMIs averaging >2 kg/m^2 higher than those who did not have an obese/overweight parent or caregiver.

6.4 DISCUSSION

In our study of a multi-ethnic cohort of 5th graders in Los Angeles, Birmingham, and Houston, we found that females attending higher income schools had lower average BMIs than females attending lower income schools. While there were significant disparities in BMI between White and Black females, this difference was largely explained by school characteristics; the difference in Black and White female BMI was reduced by half with adjustment for school factors. With respect to school-level differences in BMI, individual characteristics (i.e., compositional factors), not school factors (i.e., contextual factors), explained all of the between-school variance in female student weight status and a large portion in males. This study found no associations between school physical activity or nutrition resources/programs and individual BMI in this racially diverse cohort of 5th graders. None of the 10 school-level nutrition and physical activity resources or the summary score was associated with BMI in either males or females.

Our findings are in concert with those of Schuster et al. [8] in which disparities in a number of health behaviors and outcomes were noted to be attenuated by school characteristics. Our findings, however, demonstrate that for obesity it is specific to the disparity in weight status between Black and White females.

Unlike prior studies [6], [7], we were able to explain all of the between-school variation in weight status among females by accounting for the student makeup. Much of the variance in males was similarly explained by compositional factors, not contextual factors. In a prior analysis of the National Longitudinal Study of Adolescent Health (Add Health), a nationally representative school-based study of adolescents, Richmond and Subramanian found a 50% reduction in the between-school variability in student BMI when controlling for student- and school-level demographics; however, significant variation in BMI between schools remained for both males and females.(6) Similarly, O'Malley et al. found persistent between-school variation in weight status in the Monitoring the Future high school cohort.(7) Both Add Health and Monitoring the Future have older cohorts (mostly high school aged) and neither has data regarding the weight status of the parents, which may explain the difference in the results.

Having a parent/caregiver who is overweight/obese was associated with notably higher BMI in both males and females, similar to findings from other studies [11], [12]. Parental/caregiver obesity likely influences the students' weight status through multiple mechanisms including, but not limited to, genetic factors, nutritional patterns and role modeling, and physical activity behaviors. The weight status of the caregiver may also reflect the influences of the neighborhood or home environments, influences not accounted for in this analysis.

The lack of statistical association between school nutrition and physical activity resources/programs is not surprising in this cohort and is consistent with findings from other studies. Because the school-level variability was largely explained by individual factors, there was little between-school variability remaining to be explained by school-level resources or programs. These findings echo those from other studies. Terry-McElrath and colleagues found minimal associations between the school food environment and student BMI [13]; in another study using the same cohort they found little association between participation in PE and/or sports and student weight status [14]. In contrast, Fox et al. found promising results when they looked at serving specific menu items and student BMI [15].

6.4.1 LIMITATIONS

There are limitations to this study that should be noted. First, the findings can only be generalized to similar urban populations attending similar schools. Second, our summary score does not capture how physical activity and nutrition programs were actually implemented and the degree of student participation. It is possible that schools that scored similarly on the physical activity/nutritional resources summary score could differ considerably in the quality and participation levels in their programs. Finally, given the cross-sectional nature of the study, no causal inference can be made regarding the findings.

6.4.2 CONCLUSIONS

We find that school characteristics and programs largely explain Black/White disparities in female weight status and that school SES is inversely related to female weight status. However, school nutrition and physical activity programming were not associated with individual weight status in males or females. This study is unable to compare the effects of any school programs vs. none but instead demonstrates that there is no differential impact on BMI when programs in one school are compared with another, even in schools of different incomes and racial/ethnic makeup. The study highlights the need to understand how school programs such as the school lunch program and/or PE are actually implemented and utilized by students. This may allow future researchers to shed light on the influence of different types or intensities of programs and thus identify programs with the greatest promise of impacting student BMI. In the meantime, schools should be viewed as a potential venue in which to intervene on the commonly seen disparities in female BMI.

6.4.3 HUMANS SUBJECT APPROVAL STATEMENT

All analyses were approved by the Boston Children's Hospital Institutional Review Board.

REFERENCES

1. Story M, Kaphingst K, French S (2006) The role of schools in obesity prevention. Future Child 16 (1) 109–142. doi: 10.1353/foc.2006.0007
2. Gleason P, Suitor C (2001) U. S. Food and Nutrition Service. Children's Diets in the Mid-1990s: Dietary intake and its relationship with school meal participation. Alexandria, VA: U.S. Dept. of Agriculture, Food and Nutrition Service.
3. Johnson LD, Delva J, O'Malley PM (2007) Sports participation and physical education in American secondary schools: current levels and racial/ethnic and socioeconomic disparities. Am J Prev Med 33 (6) S195–208.
4. Frankenberg E, Lee C (2002) Race in American schools: rapidly resegregating school districts. Available: http://www.civilrightsproject.harvard.edu/research/deseg/reseg_schools02.php#fullreport. Accessed 2012 Sep 4.
5. Diversitydata.org, Common Core of Data. Available: http://diversitydata.sph.harvard.edu/. Accessed 2012 Sep 12
6. Richmond TK, Subramanian SV (2008) School level contextual factors are associated with the weight status of adolescent males and females. Obesity 16 (6) 1324–1330. doi: 10.1038/oby.2008.48
7. O'Malley P, Johnston L, Delva J, Bachman J, Schulenberg J (2007) Variation in obesity among American secondary school students by school and school characteristics. Am J Prev Med 33: S187–194. doi: 10.1016/j.amepre.2007.07.001
8. Shuster MA, Elliott M Kanouse DE, et al. (2012) Racial and ethnic health disparities among fifth-graders in three cities. N Engl J Med 367: 735–44. doi: 10.1056/nejmsa1114353
9. Windle M, Grunbaum JA, Elliott M, Tortolero SR, Berry S, et al. (2004) Healthy Passages: A multi-level, multi-method longitudinal study of adolescent health. Am J Prev Med 27 (2) 164–172.
10. StataCorp (2011) Stata Statistical Software: Release 12. College Station, TX: StataCorp LP.
11. Whitaker RC, Wright JA, Pepe MS, Seidel KD, Dietz WH (1997) Predicting obesity in young adulthood from childhood and parental obesity. N Engl J Med 337 (13) 869–73. doi: 10.1056/nejm199709253371301
12. Whitaker RC (2010) The infancy of obesity prevention. Arch Pediatr Adolesc Med 164 (12) 1167–1169. doi: 10.1001/archpediatrics.2010.218
13. Terry-McElrath YM, O'Malley PM, Delva J, Johnson LD (2009) The school food environment and student body mass index and food consumption: 2004–2007 national data. J Adolesc Health 45 (3 Suppl) S45–56. doi: 10.1016/j.jadohealth.2009.04.007
14. O'Malley PM, Johnston LD, Delva J, Terry-McElrath YM (2009) School physical activity environment related to student obesity and activity: a national study of schools and students. J Adolesc Health 45 (3 Suppl) S71–81. doi: 10.1016/j.jadohealth.2009.04.008
15. Fox MK, Dodd AH, Wilson A, Gleason PM (2009) Association between school food environment and practices and body mass index of US public school children. J Am Diet Assoc 109 (2 Suppl) S108–117. doi: 10.1016/j.jada.2008.10.065

CHAPTER 7

MODERATING INFLUENCES OF BASELINE ACTIVITY LEVELS IN SCHOOL PHYSICAL ACTIVITY PROGRAMMING FOR CHILDREN: THE READY FOR RECESS PROJECT

PEDRO F. SAINT-MAURICE, GREGORY J. WELK, DANIEL W. RUSSELL, AND JENNIFER HUBERTY

7.1 BACKGROUND

There is considerable public health interest in developing and testing strategies to help youth be more physically active [1]. School-based interventions are a common target due to the opportunity to reach large numbers of youth and the availability of staff and resources [2], but unfortunately, the success of school-based programming is limited [1,3].

A limitation of traditional analyses of school-based interventions is that the focus is on evaluating only the overall group-level effects. This provides a limited perspective of the outcomes since it is possible for interventions to have differential effects within the sample population. An intervention, for example, might have benefits for inactive youth but not for others. It is therefore important to conduct follow-up evaluations of the data collected to examine possible moderating influences.

Members of our team recently reported on the outcomes from a recess-based intervention, the Ready-for-Recess (R4R) project, a controlled trial evaluating environmental modifications to promote physical activity during recess [4]. Recess plays a critical role in children's development and well being [5,6] and recess time has also been shown to make important contributions to children's school and total daily activity [7-10]. Ridgers et al., 2012, recently conducted a systematic review to examine activity levels during recess. The review emphasized the need to explore different activity promotion strategies and how these can impact the behaviors of important subgroups (e.g. boys vs. girls) [11]. Other recess-based studies have examined the benefits of adult supervision [12], and equipment availability during recess [13], but a unique aspect of R4R was that it evaluated the independent and combined effects of adult supervision and equipment on physical activity during recess. Schools in the R4R study (n=12) were randomly assigned to one of four conditions: control group, staff supervision, provision of equipment, and the combination of staff supervision and equipment. The combination of staff supervision and equipment availability led to a significant increase of moderate-to-vigorous physical activity (MVPA) in boys (+14.1%) [4]. These findings suggest that recess interventions can be successful when promoting active behaviors among groups of children.

As with most clinical trials [14], the success of R4R was examined using group-level comparisons with the rate of change across time being defined as a fixed effect. This approach assumes that the amount of change across individuals is the same. While this fixed effects approach is appropriate for the overall evaluation, further work is required so that the assumption of homogeneity across individuals can be examined and to avoid what is defined as the "ecological fallacy" [15,16].

The inter-individual variability in the context of a PA intervention can be examined by allowing the impact of the interventions to be defined as random in the regression model. A test of homogeneity is used to determine if the rate of change across time is consistent across individuals. If there is variability between individuals one can try to explain this variability and thereby better understand individual determinants of PA. This approach can be undertaken using latent growth curve analysis, which is similar to the classic fixed effects model but with the advantage that researchers can specify predictors in the model as random factors [16]. This approach makes it possible to systematically evaluate factors influencing the consistency of change across individuals.

The purpose of this study was to examine if baseline levels of moderate-to-vigorous physical activity (MVPA) moderated the effects from the various R4R treatments.

7.2 METHODS

7.2.1 INTERVENTION DESIGN

The R4R (August 2009-September 2010) project evaluated the independent and combined effects of staff training and equipment on children's participation in MVPA during daily recess. Twelve schools were randomly assigned to one of four conditions: Staff Training (ST), Equipment (EQ), Staff Training+Equipment (STEQ) or a control condition. We have published a main outcome paper that provides additional details about the R4R intervention [4].

7.2.2 PARTICIPANTS

Elementary children (3rd-6th grades, 8–11 years of age) from 12 participating schools were recruited to participate in the evaluation of the R4R intervention. Demographic information obtained from the school included: age, gender, birth date, race, and free and reduced lunch status. The Ready for Recess intervention study was approved by the Institutional Review Board at University of Nebraska at Omaha. Children that returned signed consent forms were enrolled in the study.

7.2.3 ANTHROPOMETRIC MEASURES

Height and weight data on participants were obtained by the research team using standard field based techniques. However, we had to minimize the disruption of the school schedule at some of the schools and therefore were not able collect this information on the entire sample involved in the study.

7.2.4 PHYSICAL ACTIVITY: ACCELEROMETER MEASURE

Physical Activity was assessed with the GT1M Actigraph Accelerometers (Actigraph, Pensacola, FL). Students were asked to wear the activity monitors during the school day (approximately 8:00 AM – 3:00 PM), for 4–5 consecutive days. Members of the research team put the monitors on the children each morning and took them off at the end of the school day to ensure compliance. Teachers provided logs of student attendance and a daily schedule to record time periods for recess, lunch, and physical education.

The data from the Actigraphs were recorded in 5 second epochs and processed using Freedson et al. (2005) age-specific cutpoints (METs = 2.757 + (0.0015 · counts · min-1) – (0.08957 · age [yr]) – (0.000038 · counts · min-1 · age [yr]) [17]. Each epoch during recess was classified as light (1.5 - 3.9 METs), moderate (MPA; 4.0 - 6.0 METs) or vigorous (VPA; > 6.0 METs) and the data were then aggregated to determine time spent in LPA, MPA, VPA and MVPA (MPA + VPA). Participants were included in the final analyses if they were at school (and had data) on at least 3 of the 5 days. Since the activity monitors were only used during school time it was assumed that students wore the monitors during all time unless indicated otherwise by school teachers. Activity outcomes were computed as an average of the valid data extracted from recess periods. The major computed outcome measure was the percent time allocated to MVPA in order to standardize for different lengths of recess.

7.2.5 DATA ANALYSIS

Latent Growth Curve (LGC) models were used to account for the longitudinal nature of the data (repeated-measures) and potential individual differences (nested within schools) when exposed to the different treatments. The variable Trial (coded as 0=trial 1, 1=trial 2) was defined as a level-1 predictor (growth factor), characteristics of the children as level-2 predictors, and schools as level-3 predictors. Post-intervention average percent time in MVPA during recess (activity obtained from valid recess segments) was defined as the main outcome of interest (dependent variable). Level-2 covariates included grade (coded with 0=3rd grade, 1=4th grade, 2=5th grade, and 3=6th grade), gender (coded 0=male and 1=female), average recess duration (in minutes), and baseline (trial 1) percent time in MVPA during recess. The three treatments were used as level-3 predictors and coded using dummy coding (variable Staff coded 0=No Staff, 1=Staff; variable Equipment coded 0=No equipment, 1=Equipment; and variable Staff+Equipment coded 0=No Staff+Equipment, and 1=Staff+Equipment). Other demographic characteristics of the children such as BMI, race, or social economic status were not included since this information was not available for the entire sample. Only individuals with complete activity data at each assessment (Trial) were included in the analysis.

To examine the direction, magnitude and consistency of the moderation of baseline MVPA on each intervention, least-square means comparing each treatment to the control group were computed (using the final LGC model) at three fixed values based on baseline MVPA scores: Mean - 1 standard deviation, Mean, and Mean+1 standard deviation (see magnitude and direction of moderation effect). These three categories were operationalized as Low Active, Moderate Active, and High Active, respectively. These comparisons were performed to examine the overall trend over time (across treatments and control group) and also separately for each activity group. A total of 12 least-square means tests with their respective mean difference (Mean diff), standard errors and p-values are reported.

Results from the nested models (test of model fit for level-1 and level-2 predictors) and moderation effects were computed with 95% confidence intervals ($p < .05$). To account for the increased type I error associated with multiple statistical tests when comparing subgroups of activity, statistical analysis associated with least-square means were performed with a 99% confidence interval and therefore defined as significant if p-value<.01. In addition, mean differences for these analyses were considered borderline significant if p-value was between .01 and .05. Statistical procedures as described above were performed using SAS v9.2 (Cary, North Carolina).

7.3 RESULTS

From the total sample of 667 participants, there were 393 participants (181 boys and 212 girls) who had three days of activity monitor data on both trials. The sample size differs from the main outcome results previously reported by Huberty et al., 2013, since it was important to have robust estimates of individual variability patterns across time. The distribution of participants across gender, grade and intervention is provided in Table 1.

TABLE 1: Distribution (N) of gender and grade per intervention group

	Gender		Grade				
	Boys	Girls	3rd	4th	5th	6th	Total
Control	47	45	20	27	24	21	92
ST	39	69	32	19	34	23	108
EQ	59	51	23	27	38	22	110
STEQ	36	47	8	22	23	30	83
Total	181	212	83	95	119	96	393

ST=Staff treatment; EQ=Equipment treatment; STEQ=Staff+Equipment treatment.

7.3.1 INTER-INDIVIDUAL VARIABILITY AND TEST OF COVARIATES

Preliminary analyses were conducted to test assumptions needed for the use of LGC. We examined the variability in the MVPA scores across time to ensure that there was sufficient variability in the data. The intraclass correlation for individuals was equal to .08, while for schools it was equal to .07 and the covariance parameters indicated that intercept scores for time spent in MVPA were significantly different between individuals (see Figure 1) and schools (see Figure 2) ($p<.05$). Additional testing with level-1 and level-2 predictors revealed significant improvements in the fit of the model (indicated by a significant ($p<.05$) change in the (LLR) value). The results supported the clustered nature of the data and differences on baseline activity levels between individuals and schools. These findings support the planned model used to examine the moderator effect of baseline activity on change in MVPA levels associated with each condition.

7.3.2 THE LATENT GROWTH CURVE MODEL

Interpretation of the latent growth curve model b-weights (Table 2) revealed that change in MVPA from trial 1 to trial 2 in the control group (holding all the other predictors in the model constant) could be explained by initial MVPA scores. Per each unit increase in baseline MVPA score, there was a reduction of 0.76% on MVPA scores change from trial 1 to trial 2 (e.g., children in the control group with lower baseline MVPA scores had greater positive changes in MVPA from trial 1 to trial 2 while the opposite was true for children with higher baseline MVPA scores). Similar trial X baseline MVPA interactions with each condition revealed that this trend was attenuated by ST ($\beta=0.29\pm0.12$, $p=.02$) but not EQ ($p=.35$) or STEQ ($p=.74$). In other words, youth in the Staff condition that were less active at baseline had greater MVPA differences (from their respective control group) in MVPA at trial 2 when compared to their more active peers. Per each unit increase in percent MVPA at baseline, there was an attenuation of the ST effect by 0.47% in MVPA levels at trial 2.

7.3.3 MAGNITUDE AND DIRECTION OF THE MODERATION EFFECT

The overall mean score (across treatments and control group) for percent of time spent in MVPA at baseline was 27.5%. Predicted values were estimated by fixing baseline activity values in the final model as 27.5%, 12.5% (−1SD), and 42.4% (+1SD). These predicted activity scores represented Moderate, Low, and High Active groups, respectively. There were significant changes over time for the three groups but the patterns were very different. The Low Active group had a significant increase in MVPA from trial 1 to trial 2 ($Mean_{diff}=6.3\pm0.9\%$; $t(11)=6.7$; $p<.001$), while the Moderate ($Mean_{diff}=-4.5\pm0.7\%$; $t(11)=-6.8$; $p<.001$) and High active group ($Mean_{diff}=-15.3\pm0.9\%$; $t(11)=-16.2$; $p<.001$) decreased their MVPA levels ($p<.001$).

Further evaluation, however, shows that the response varies depending on the treatment group. When stratified by treatment group, the mean baseline MVPA values (Medium) for the ST, EQ and STEQ treatments were 27.7%, 26.1%, and 27.1%, respectively. The corresponding values for Low Active (−1SD) were equal to, 12.2%, 11.0%, and 13.3% while values for High Active (+1SD) were 43.2%, 41.3%, and 40.8%. The values for Low Active were all similar at baseline (Trial 1) but the levels of MVPA at trial 2 in the ST schools were significantly lower than the respective Low Active control group ($Mean_{diff}=-10.8\pm2.9\%$; $t(10)=-3.6$; $p=.005$). There were also differences in MVPA for the Low Active EQ when compared with the control group but the effect was not significant ($Mean_{diff}=-5.9\pm3.0\%$; $t(10)=-2.0$; $p=.079$). Interestingly, the effect of the STEQ treatment in the Low Active was opposite to the effects for ST and EQ with increases in MVPA occurring when compared to the Low Active control group ($Mean_{diff}=6.6\pm3.0\%$; $t(10)=2.2$; $p=.055$). Results for Moderate active subgroups in the ST and also in the EQ groups were similar to the results for less active individuals (in the same treatment group). MVPA differences from their respective control group had the same direction but a lower magnitude. Results for the ST and EQ treatments were borderline significant (ST: $Mean_{diff}=-7.4\pm2.6\%$; $t(10)=-2.8$; $p=.018$; EQ: $Mean_{diff}=-7.7\pm2.6\%$; $t(10)=-2.9$; $p=.015$). MVPA difference at trial 2 for individuals in the STEQ treatment had the same direction as their less active peers (exposed to the same treatment) but a lower magnitude. MVPA differences were non-significant ($Mean_{diff}=5.5\pm2.7\%$; $t(10)=2.1$; $p=.066$). These trends reflected some variability around the pooled effect of the Ready for Recess (Figure 3).

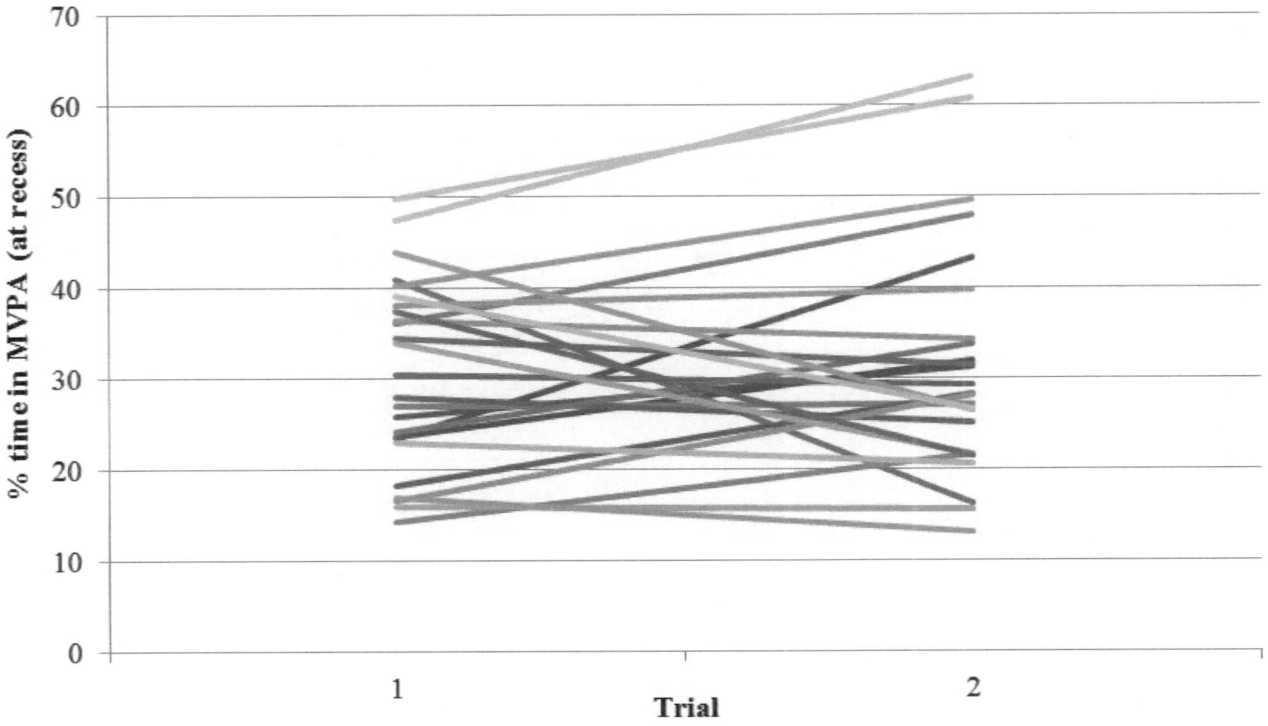

FIGURE 1: Percent time spent in MVPA at recess for a (randomly selected) subgroup of 25 individuals. Each line represents an individual. This figure illustrates a high degree of variability in individual's baseline scores (intercept) and change over time (slopes). This justifies the need for a random intercept term at level-2 (individual).

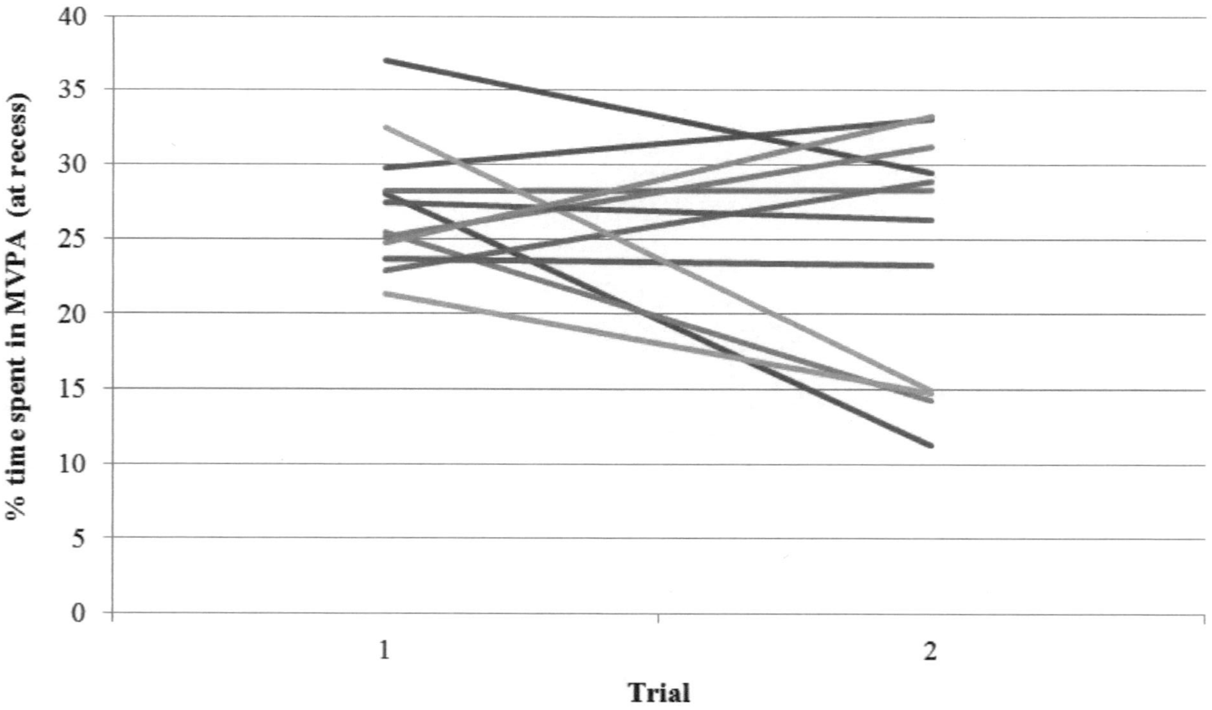

Figure 2: Percent time spent in MVPA at recess for the 12 schools. Each line represents a school. Similarly to Figure 1, there was a significant difference in baseline scores for school clusters, and therefore, justifying the need for random intercepts at this level.

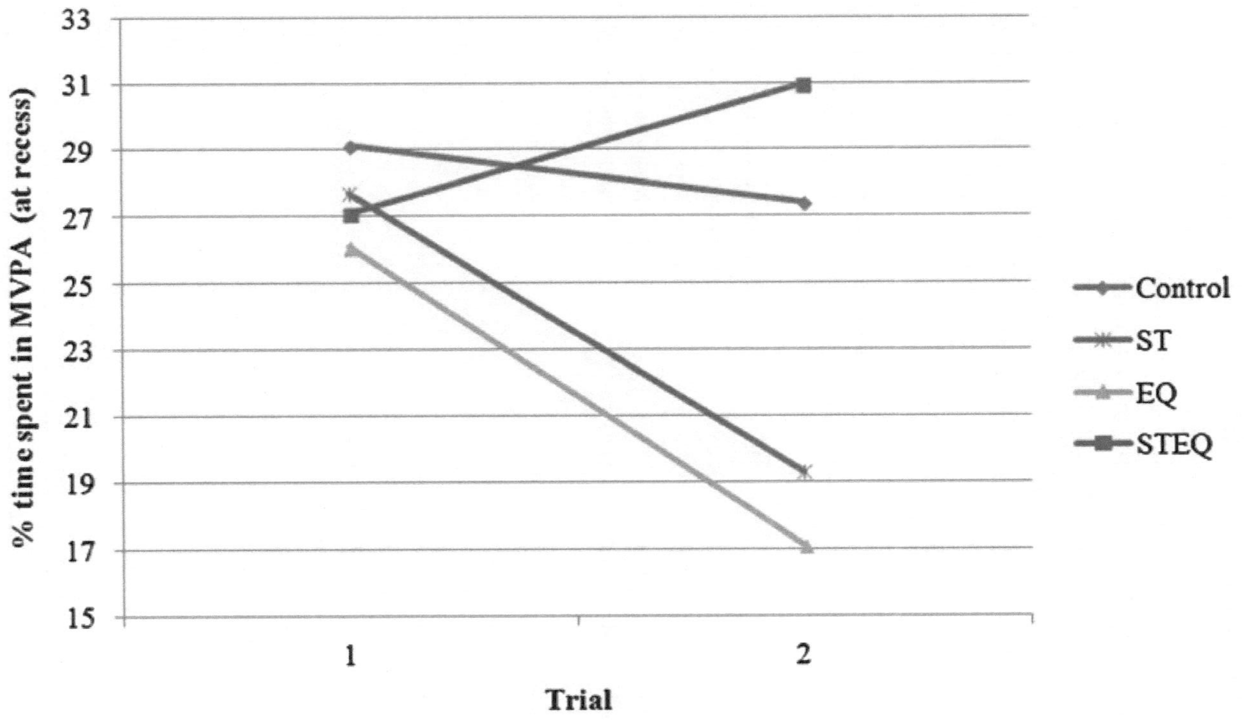

FIGURE 3: Average MVPA scores for the control and each treatment group. Both the Staff (ST) and the Equipment (EQ) treatments had a negative effect on individuals' MVPA. The Staff+Equipment (STEQ) treatment effect was positive.

TABLE 2: Regression coefficients for the final latent growth curve model

	Estimate	SE	df	t-value	p-value
Intercept	−6.73	5.62	8	−1.20	0.27
b-weights					
Trial	20.35	3.00	759	6.78	<.001
Baseline MVPA	1.72	0.15	759	11.72	<.001
Gender	−2.39	0.73	759	−3.26	0.001
Grade	−2.32	0.35	759	−6.69	<.001
Recess duration	0.06	0.07	759	0.84	0.4
ST	17.90	6.71	8	2.67	0.03
EQ	8.41	6.60	8	1.27	0.24
STEQ	−3.07	7.36	8	−0.42	0.69
Trial X ST	−15.73	3.96	759	−3.97	<.001
Trial X EQ	−6.49	3.90	759	−1.66	0.1
Trial X STEQ	5.39	4.39	759	1.23	0.22
Trail X baseline MVPA	−0.76	0.09	759	−8.32	<.001
ST X baseline MVPA	−0.36	0.2	759	−1.85	0.06
EQ X baseline MVPA	0.11	0.20	759	0.57	0.57
(STEQ) X baseline MVPA	0.01	0.20	759	0.05	0.96
Trial X ST X baseline MVPA	0.29	0.12	759	2.39	0.02
Trial X EQ X baseline MVPA	−0.12	0.12	759	−0.94	0.35
Trial X (STEQ) X baseline MVPA	−0.05	0.14	759	−0.34	0.74

SE = standard error; df = degrees of freedom. ST = Staff treatment; EQ = Equipment treatment; STEQ = Staff + Equipment treatment.

The most active individuals in the ST (and the STEQ) treatment had the lowest MVPA differences from their respective control group (Staff: $\text{Mean}_{\text{diff}} = -3.9 \pm 2.9\%$; $t(10) = -1.3$; $p = .215$; STEQ: $\text{Mean}_{\text{diff}} = 4.4 \pm 3.0\%$; $t(10) = 1.5$; $p = .172$). The High Active group in the EQ treatment had the highest MVPA difference from their control group. MVPA levels in this subgroup were significantly lower than the control group ($\text{Mean}_{\text{diff}} = -9.5 \pm 2.9\%$; $t(10) = -3.3$; $p = .009$). A summary of the differences between each treatment group and respective control at trial 2 is available in Figure 4.

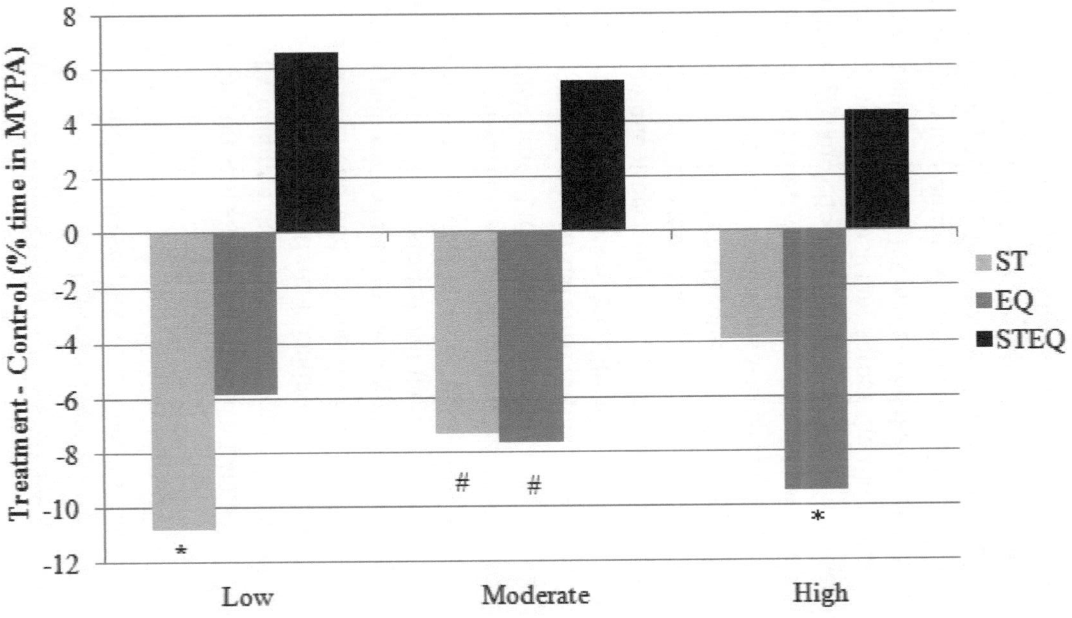

Figure 4: Average % MVPA difference among Low, Moderate, and High active groups, per treatment group. Each activity level subgroup was compared with their respective control group (e.g. % MVPA Difference Low Staff="Low Staff"- "Low Control" at trial 2, holding constant all the remaining variables in the full model). There was a reduced effect trend (from Low to High active individuals) for the Staff (ST), and the Staff+Equipment (STEQ) treatment groups. This trend was reversed in the Equipment (EQ) group (the effect was higher for High active individuals and decreased among Moderate, and Low active subgroups). *Significantly different than respective control group at trial 2 ($p<.01$). #Borderline significantly different than respective control group at trial 2 ($.01<p<.05$).

7.4 DISCUSSION

The present study provides new insights about the outcomes from the R4R project. The main outcome paper from the study [4] reported an overall positive effect of STEQ on boy's MVPA (+14.1%). Interestingly, there was a decrease on MVPA associated with the ST (boys: -13.5% and girls: -11.4%) and similar results were found for the EQ condition. These results were somewhat surprising since positive effects were expected for both of these independent conditions.

In the present study, we utilized a Latent Growth Curve model to more directly examine the consistency of both individual and subgroup change as a result of the different conditions. In this model, time is defined as a level-1 predictor and the mean (pooled) effects essentially replicate the group patterns evident in the original outcome paper (See Figure 3). Initial analyses demonstrated that there was significant variability around the mean trajectories over time so the nested models focused on predicting individual variation around each of the treatment effects. Baseline levels of MVPA proved to be an important source of variability. These findings were supported as initial MVPA was a significant predictor of MVPA at trial 2 (after 6 months of baseline assessment).

A unique aspect of the present analyses is that we used a similar approach to explore the consistency of this effect for the three primary treatment conditions. The direction of this moderation effect across the three different treatment conditions was specifically examined via higher-order interaction terms (i.e., trial by treatment condition by baseline MVPA). Interestingly, the effect of baseline MVPA on subsequent levels of physical activity was not consistent across the three treatments. The results indicated that initial MVPA moderated the effect of ST, but not EQ and STEQ. In our previous study, we found that ST and EQ were both associated with a pooled negative effect. Participants belonging to schools in these conditions decreased their activity levels after 6 months of intervention [4].

The examination of high-order interactions indicated that change in MVPA levels for children in the ST condition were significantly affected by their baseline MVPA levels. Per each unit increase in baseline MVPA scores, there was a 0.47% attenuation on the differential effect of Staff on

MVPA score changes from trial 1 to trial 2. The attenuation means that less active participants were more negatively affected by the presence of trained staff than their more active peers. Surprisingly, the trend was reversed for participants in the EQ condition. The effect was negative but the magnitude of the effect was greater in High Active participants. Nevertheless, the moderation effect of baseline MVPA in this condition was non-significant ($p>.05$). Less active participants in the STEQ condition reacted more positively to this intervention however, the moderation effect for STEQ was also not significant (possibly due to lack of statistical power).

While the moderation effect was not significant for all treatments, it is noteworthy that the less active children (i.e., those who spent approximately 12% of their recess time in MVPA) were shown to be more responsive to the ST and STEQ conditions. Low active children had declines in time spent in MVPA (~11%) when exposed to staff supervision but increases in MVPA (~6%) when staff utilized recreational equipment and implemented games. Interestingly, similarly to the ST findings, the effect of equipment was also negative but reversed, meaning, those who were more active had greater declines in MVPA. In conclusion, staff training reduced physical activity levels, in low and medium active children.

The examination of these relationships has great value to public health researchers, particularly those interested in promotion strategies for physical activity in elementary children. Many school based interventions have been conducted to promote physical activity behavior in youth. Studies have examined interventions during PE class, in class time, during recess and after school. The common form of analyses conducted in these trials has focused on mean responses of groups of children. The results of the present study provide important insights because it suggests that interventions may have varying effects on different segments of the population. A previous analysis [10] revealed some important differences by gender with regard to physical activity during recess. A recent meta-analysis also suggested that age, and both duration and type of intervention can moderate the effect of PA promotion initiatives during recess [18]. As illustrated by this review, there is a lack of research on the moderation effect of typical activity levels. The present analyses reveal moderation of intervention effects by baseline levels of MVPA. Individuals conducting school-based projects should consider the possible differential effects of programming on different segments of the population. Ideally, interventions should be set up to enhance physical activity opportunities for low active youth [19] without detracting from physical activity opportunities in already active youth.

The results of this study suggest that low active youth are more responsive to changes in the environment of school recess programming, but the effects depend on the nature of the intervention. Staff training sites had staff trained to increase physical activity during recess time. This strategy affected the expected trend in activity from trial 1 to trial 2 (illustrated by the control group) and led to a decrease in activity levels in low active groups. This may be because the structure allowed more active and skilled youth to dominate games. Interestingly, low active individuals' activity was not negatively affected by the presence of equipment alone. This may be because the equipment gets claimed by more active (and perhaps more dominant) youth in a recess environment. In contrast, activity patterns of low active youth were significantly increased when staff training and equipment were provided (STEQ).

Activity levels of highly active individuals seem to be unaltered when exposed to staff supervision or a combination of both staff and equipment. However, the presence of equipment tended to cause decreases in levels of MVPA. This may be because the equipment became more interesting than the active games that children play when equipment is not provided.

Some limitations of this study should be considered when interpreting the results. As described in the main outcome paper [4], there was no fidelity testing, so it is not possible to quantify the degree of staff involvement and or the compliance with the training provided. This could influence the results and conclusions regarding this condition. Another possible concern is a possible 'regression to the mean' effect [20] that can be present when baseline measures of the outcome variable are used to predict change over time [21]. Our results indicated that the magnitude of individual MVPA changes over time differed between two conditions (Staff and Equipment) even though group slopes were similar (see Figure 3). Moreover, these changes did not follow similar regression to the mean trends evidenced by the control group. The individual effects were statistically significant for less active individuals in the ST condition but not in the EQ condition. The opposite was found for more active individuals. More active individuals in the EQ condition were significantly affected but similarly active individuals in the ST condition were not significantly affected. Thus, these findings support the idea that differential changes over time in subgroups of individuals could be explained by the R4R intervention and not regression to the mean. Finally, the inclusion of BMI and additional individual-level predictors such as race and/or socio-economical status, in our models could have explained additional variability in the effects of the ready for recess. However these predictors are known to be related with PA and therefore their inclusion might have resulted in over adjustment of our model.

7.5 CONCLUSIONS

The findings from this study provide an important contribution to the field of physical activity and public health. Understanding the differential reactivity effect when children are exposed to different PA promotion strategies can help researchers and policy makers choose appropriate intervention designs based on population needs. For example, less active individuals will benefit more from interventions involving supervised staff combined with equipment availability. Children with higher activity levels seem to benefit to a lesser extent. The results from this study could not confirm the broader benefit from this strategy.

This study complements findings from a previous Ready for Recess study [4]. The potential of different strategies to increase active behaviors should be further examined taking into consideration typical activity levels. The detailed and comprehensive examination of the MVPA outcome did not allow a parallel comparison with sedentary behavior. However, this outcome also has important implications for children's health and therefore should be examined separately.

REFERENCES

1. Metcalf B, Henley W, Wilkin T: Effectiveness of intervention on physical activity of children: systematic review and meta-analysis of controlled trials with objectively measured outcomes (EarlyBird 54). BMJ 2012, 345:e5888.

2. Centers for Disease Control and Prevention: School health guidelines to promote healthy eating and physical activity. MMRW, Volume 60 (RR- 5) 2011, 1-76.
3. Kriemler S, Meyer U, Martin E, van Sluijs EM, Andersen LB, Martin BW: Effect of school-based interventions on physical activity and fitness in children and adolescents: a review of reviews and systematic update. Br J Sports Med 2011, 45:923-930.
4. Huberty JL, Beets MW, Beighle A, Saint-Maurice PF, Welk G: Effects of ready for recess, an environmental intervention, on physical activity in 3rd - 6th grade children. J Phys Act Health 2013. in press
5. Ramstetter CL, Murray R, Garner AS: The crucial role of recess in schools. J Sch Health 2010, 80:517-526.
6. Pellegrini A, Smith P: School recess: implications for education and development. Review of Educational Research 1993, 63:51-67.
7. Erwin H, Abel M, Beighle A, Noland MP, Worley B, Riggs R: The contribution of recess to children's school-day physical activity. J Phys Act Health 2012, 9:442-448.
8. Ridgers ND, Saint-Maurice PF, Welk GJ, Siahpush M, Huberty J: Differences in physical activity during school recess. J Sch Health 2011, 81:545-551.
9. Ridgers ND, Timperio A, Crawford D, Salmon J: Five-year changes in school recess and lunchtime and the contribution to children's daily physical activity. Br J Sports Med 2012, 46:741-746.
10. Saint-Maurice PF, Welk GJ, Silva P, Siahpush M, Huberty J: Assessing children's physical activity behaviors at recess: a multi-method approach. Pediatr Exerc Sci 2011, 23:585-599.
11. Ridgers ND, Salmon J, Parrish AM, Stanley RM, Okely AD: Physical activity during school recess: a systematic review. Am J Prev Med 2012, 43:320-328.
12. Connolly P, TL M: Effects of a game intervention on the physical activity levels of children at recess. Res Q Exerc Sport 1995, 66:A66.
13. Verstraete SJ, Cardon GM, De Clercq DL, De Bourdeaudhuij IM: Increasing children's physical activity levels during recess periods in elementary schools: the effects of providing game equipment. Eur J Public Health 2006, 16:415-419.
14. Parrish AM, Okely AD, Stanley RM, Ridgers ND: The effect of school recess interventions on physical activity: a systematic review. Sports Med 2013, 43:287-299.
15. Bryk SA, Raudenbush SW: Hierarchical Linear Models - Applications and Data Analysis Methods. 2nd edition. Thousand Oaks, CA: Sage Publications; 1992.
16. Preacher KJ, Wichman AL, MacCallum RC, Briggs NE: Latent Growth Curve Modeling. Thousands Oaks, CA: Sage Publications; 2008.
17. Freedson P, Pober D, Janz KF: Calibration of accelerometer output for children. Med Sci Sports Exerc 2005, 37:S523-S530.
18. Erwin HE, Ickes M, Ahn S, Fedewa A: Impact of recess interventions on children's physical activity-a meta-analysis. Am J Health Promot 2014, 28:159-167.
19. Fairclough SJ, Beighle A, Erwin H, Ridgers ND: School day segmented physical activity patterns of high and low active children. BMC Public Health 2012, 12:406.
20. Bland JM, Altman DG: Regression towards the mean. BMJ 1994, 308:1499.
21. Vickers AJ, Altman DG: Statistics notes: analysing controlled trials with baseline and follow up measurements. BMJ 2001, 323:1123-1124.

CHAPTER 8

SCHOOL-BASED PROGRAMS: LESSONS LEARNED FROM CATCH, PLANET HEALTH, AND NOT-ON-TOBACCO

ADELE L. FRANKS, STEVEN H. KELDER, GERI A. DINO, KIMBERLY A. HORN, STEVEN L. GORTMAKER, JEAN L. WIECHA, AND EDUARDO J. SIMOES

8.1 INTRODUCTION

Schools can play a crucial role in improving the health of children and, thus, the adults they will become. Children and adolescents generally attend school 5 days per week throughout most of the calendar year. Schools in the United States are located in communities of every socioeconomic, racial, and ethnic group. In addition to academic skills, students also learn cultural expectations and social norms that strongly influence health behaviors (1).

During childhood and adolescence, habits emerge that influence and reinforce physical activity, eating, and tobacco-use behaviors. These health

---

Franks AL, Kelder SH, Dino GA, Horn KA, Gortmaker SL, Wiecha JL, and Simoes EJ. School-based Programs: Lessons Learned from CATCH, Planet Health, and Not-On-Tobacco. Preventing Chronic Disease, *4,2 (2007). Originally published by the Centers for Disease Control and Prevention.*

behaviors can affect development of cardiovascular disease, cancer, and diabetes, which are now the major causes of premature death and disability in the United States and the Western world (2). Public health professionals are interested in school-based programs that can provide a foundation for lifelong healthy behaviors and thereby significantly reduce the burden of preventable chronic diseases for both individuals and society.

Although more than 80% of U.S. school districts require health education to be taught in their elementary, middle, and high schools, less than half provide a curriculum for teachers (3). Furthermore, available curricula have rarely undergone rigorous evaluation to demonstrate their effectiveness, and they are often out-of-date when compared with current practice standards (4). Thus, there is a largely unmet need for effective school-based programs that promote healthy behaviors among youth. For public health officials who have embraced the concept of evidence-based practice (5), it is imperative that programs be rigorously evaluated. Collaboration between the public health and education sectors is essential to ensure that effective programs are available and meet the needs of youths, teachers, and school administrators.

Creating public health partnerships with schools is challenging for many reasons, including the numerous academic and nonacademic demands placed on schools. In addition, school programs often lack sufficient funds, are subject to political vicissitudes, exist in complex bureaucracies that foster fragmentation, and vary across localities (6). Despite these problems public health and education sectors have worked together successfully on programs that can serve as examples to guide and encourage future collaborative efforts.

The Division of Adolescent and School Health at Centers for Disease Control and Prevention (CDC) funds collaborations between state education and health agencies to promote coordination of school health programs. CDC's Prevention Research Centers (PRCs) engage public health organizations, academic institutions, and communities in partnerships to develop, test, and disseminate programs to improve health outcomes. To be considered effective, these programs must undergo systematic measurement and analysis using solid research methods and study designs. In some cases a PRC participates in the development and testing of new programs; in other cases a PRC participates by studying how to disseminate programs already shown to be effective. This paper explores three effective school-based programs promoted by PRCs and highlights common features and lessons learned for public health practitioners and researchers who wish to partner with schools. Two of these programs promote physical activity and healthy eating among school children—Coordinated Approach to Child Health (CATCH) and Planet Health—and one promotes smoking cessation among adolescents—Not-On-Tobacco (N-O-T).

8.2 COORDINATED APPROACH TO CHILD HEALTH (CATCH)

CATCH is an elementary school program focused on supporting positive environmental influences to increase physical activity and improve healthy eating. CATCH involves classroom and physical education teachers, school food service personnel, and families of students. Input from school administrators, teachers, food service employees, and parents played an important role in program development to ensure the program would be compatible with the needs of the people who would implement it. From 1991 through 1994, researchers funded by the National Heart, Lung, and Blood Institute conducted a 3-year randomized controlled trial evaluating the program in California, Louisiana, Minnesota, and Texas. The evaluation involved ethnically and racially diverse groups of students from 96 elementary schools (7).

The CATCH program is focused on changing the behavior of elementary school students—both in and out of school. Classroom teachers use a prepared, age-appropriate curriculum to teach about physical activity and healthy eating. Students in regular classes practice new skills designed to improve their physical activity and eating behaviors. In physical education classes, teachers encourage students to actively participate in physical activity that is fun. School cafeterias serve healthy, low-fat foods that have been tested for their appeal to elementary students. Study results showed that as a result of the CATCH program, students in the intervention schools significantly increased time spent in moderate to vigorous physical activity within physical education classes (from 40% to 50%) and considerably decreased their consumption of fat in school meals (from 39% to 32%) (7).

A 3-year follow-up study between 1995 and 1998 assessed diet, physical activity, and related health indicators among 3714 (73%) of the initial CATCH participants. Students receiving the CATCH intervention in grades three through five maintained a diet considerably lower in total fat and saturated fat and participated in more vigorous physical activities in grades six through eight than did students in control groups (8). These findings reinforced the expectation that participation in the CATCH program could contribute to better cardiovascular health as students mature.

A recent replication study of CATCH in a Hispanic community on the U.S.–Mexico border in El Paso, Tex, showed that participation in the CATCH program stemmed the rate of increase in overweight among both girls and boys in grades three through five. Without the CATCH intervention, overweight increased among students in these grades from 26% to 39% among girls and from 40% to 49% among boys (9). These figures can be compared with 30% to 32% for girls and 40% to 41% for boys who participated in CATCH. Thus, participation in the CATCH program appears to help address the obesity epidemic affecting children today, and researchers using the results of the El Paso study found CATCH to be cost-effective (S. Brown, oral communication, June 2005).

Since completion of these two studies, the CATCH program 1) has expanded its curricula to include kindergarten, first, and second grades; 2) has developed and evaluated an after-school program for kindergarten through fifth grade (10); and 3) has created a physical education module for grades six through eight.

In 1996, with support from the Texas Department of State Health Services, local Texas foundations, and the CDC PRC program, a dissemination team consisting of Texas faculty investigators and field staff responsible for the randomized controlled trial was formed to translate CATCH research into practice. The models eventually selected for dissemination were based on elements from Rogers' diffusion theory (11), social cognitive theory (12), and social marketing (13) as described by Hoelscher et al (14). Factors that influenced the extent of dissemination and adoption included the attributes of the interventions, characteristics of the adopter, types of decisions required to implement the program, channels of communication, social context of the system into which the innovation is introduced, and the efforts of change agents.

The CATCH dissemination team developed strategies to reach the maximum number of school opinion leaders, teachers, and administrators in Texas. By mid-2006, more than 2000 elementary schools in Texas had purchased the CATCH program, and more than 900,000 students had potentially been exposed to the program. Results of mailed surveys to these schools indicated a high level of program implementation and fidelity (15). A recent study showed that training of school staff is important and influences whether or not schools continue to use the CATCH program (16).

8.2.1 LESSONS LEARNED FROM THE CATCH PROGRAM

1. During development of the CATCH program, those who were going to use the program (e.g., teachers, food service employees, administrative staff, students, parents) were included in the planning and design. Their inclusion was essential to ensure program acceptability.
2. Successful diffusion requires program staff who can contact decision makers, answer questions, present the program at professional meetings, conduct training, and ensure quality control.
3. The supportive involvement of a school principal or other administrator is crucial.
4. Effective training of interdisciplinary teams (i.e., classroom and physical education teachers and food service staff) to implement the CATCH program curriculum is important for program success.
5. To gain the support and enthusiastic participation of teachers, prepared lessons aligned with state education standards should be provided along with sufficient training and flexibility in delivering materials.

8.3 PLANET HEALTH

Planet Health was developed by researchers at Harvard University in collaboration with teachers and principals (17) for public middle schools. The focus of this interdisciplinary curriculum is to improve cardiovascular health and lower the prevalence of obesity among sixth- through eighth-grade students. The curriculum was designed 1) to fit easily into existing language, mathematics, science, social studies, and physical education classes; 2) to foster basic educational competencies required by the state; and 3) to provide teaching materials that are easy to use. Planet Health's goals for youths are based on evidence that healthy eating and physical activity are important and emphasize increasing consumption of fruits and vegetables and decreasing consumption of high-fat foods.

One Planet Health innovation is promoting child health by stressing the importance of decreasing television viewing. This intervention goal was based on recent evidence that television viewing contributes to obesity through both the sedentary act of television watching and exposure of viewers to relentless broadcast encouragement to consume high-calorie, high-fat, nutrient-poor foods (18,19).

A 21-month randomized controlled study of Planet Health between 1995 and 1997 was funded by the National Institute of Child Health and Human Development in 10 public middle schools. This study showed 1) a reduction in television watching for both girls and boys enrolled in Planet Health compared with controls, 2) a significant decrease in prevalence of obesity among girls in the study, 3) an increase in fruit and vegetable consumption among girl participants, and 4) less of an increase in daily calories consumed by girls enrolled in Planet Health (20). Additional analyses of the data funded by CDC showed that girls participating in Planet Health were less likely to report weight control behavior disorders (21) or early menarche (22).

CDC researchers conducted an independent economic analysis of Planet Health based on estimated program costs of $14 per student per year and found the program to be highly cost-effective: for every dollar spent on middle school Planet Health programs, researchers projected a savings of $1.20 in medical costs and lost wages by the time students reach middle age (40 to 65 years of age) (23).

Boston Public Schools (BPS) expressed interest in the Planet Health program after they heard about its success from Harvard PRC researchers. A partnership was formed between BPS and the Harvard PRC that included the original Planet Health researchers. This team planned a pilot test of the Planet Health curriculum in BPS public school settings to determine the feasibility and sustainability of the Planet Health program in settings where resources are severely limited.

A BPS and Harvard PRC advisory board provided guidance by using a model of community-based participatory research. BPS selected a sample of six inner-city middle schools to participate, and the PRC provided copies of the Planet Health curriculum, training workshops for teachers, small stipends for teacher coordinators, and evaluation and research expertise. This study was funded by CDC and demonstrated that 90% of the teachers found the curriculum effective and believed it made a positive contribution to their classes (24).

BPS has endeavored to sustain and expand use of the Planet Health curriculum through independent funding. BPS first secured funding from the U.S. Department of Education's Physical Education for Progress grant program for pilot expansion to 12 schools during 2002 through 2003. BPS later received financial support for further expansion from the Boston Public Health Commission under the auspices of the Steps to a HealthierUS (STEPS) project sponsored by the U.S. Department of Health and Human Services. In 2004, BlueCross BlueShield of Massachusetts announced a 4-year, $3-million program of grants to Massachusetts middle schools to implement Planet Health and offer after-school programs. Hundreds of Massachusetts middle school teachers and school administrators have adopted Planet Health, and efforts to disseminate and evaluate the Planet Health curriculum in additional state school systems are under way.

More than 4000 copies of the Planet Health curriculum have been purchased in 48 states and 20 countries. The program has the potential to benefit thousands of children, has demonstrated that it is effective, feasible, and sustainable in a public school environment, and has shown that it is accepted by participants and teachers. In the long term, the program is cost effective and is projected to save society money.

8.3.1 LESSONS LEARNED FROM PLANET HEALTH

1. Honoring the scientific evidence that television viewing has a major influence on obesity in children was worthwhile. Planet Health included limitation of television viewing among its targets for be-

havioral change, achieved a considerable reduction, and found this reduction to be beneficial.

2. By working closely with teachers and principals, holding focus groups with students and parents, and working with project advisory boards, Planet Health developed materials that resonated well with the interests and resources of the stakeholders. Participation of all parties was crucial to developing materials that were liked by everyone. For example, researchers would not have known in advance that teachers preferred development of a textbook for their use rather than Web-based materials.
3. From the beginning, researchers looked to the work of Rogers (11) when planning both the diffusion and sustainability of the intervention materials. Researchers were well aware that school systems throughout the United States were reducing their focus on health education and physical education because of financial constraints and the rising importance of high-stakes testing. This understanding led them to develop a low-cost interdisciplinary curriculum that used existing teachers and stressed literacy across the curriculum. These curriculum characteristics tended to increase the perceived relative advantage of the intervention.

8.4 NOT-ON-TOBACCO (N-O-T)

West Virginia led the nation in teenage smoking during the mid–1990s, and as a result, the West Virginia University PRC partnered with West Virginia's Bureau for Public Health, Department of Education, and other members of the state's public health community to strengthen school-based tobacco control initiatives. West Virginia needed an effective, user–friendly teenage smoking cessation program that could be adopted statewide and that would support a newly developed state tobacco-free school policy emphasizing prevention and cessation support rather than punitive action (25,26).

Later inclusion of the American Lung Association (ALA) into the partnership brought a national scope to the West Virginia teenage smoking cessation efforts. The partnership identified local and national needs and took on the shared goal of developing a theoretically based, scientifically tested teenage smoking cessation intervention (26). With funding from CDC and other organizations, the West Virginia University PRC launched a smoking cessation project that was committed to community-based participatory research methods and included the following contributions: 1) teachers, students, and school health professionals provided input for program development; 2) the ALA provided program expertise, funding, and a means for disseminating programs; and 3) PRC researchers provided a scientific framework to evaluate the effectiveness of programs and a commitment to program dissemination.

The partnership decided the intervention should be initially developed for use in schools because schools can promote tobacco-free environments through policy, can offer services for students and staff who want to quit smoking, and can reach youth efficiently (27). Program goals were to create a smoking cessation program that could 1) enhance adolescent health, 2) fulfill the needs of students who want to quit smoking, 3) reduce school tobacco policy violations, and 4) provide an educational alternative to punitive measures for violating school tobacco policy.

Through an iterative, collaborative process, the partnership developed a smoking cessation program designed for 14- to 19-year–old daily smokers (27). The program was given the youth-approved name, Not-On-Tobacco. In addition to smoking cessation, other N-O-T goals include reducing smoking; increasing healthy lifestyle behaviors (e.g., physical activity, healthy eating); and improving stress management, decision making, coping ability, and social support skills. Students participate in the program on a voluntary basis, and the program includes 10 hour-long weekly sessions and 4 booster sessions in same-sex groups with same-sex facilitators (e.g., teachers, school nurses, counselors, volunteers).

Facilitators are trained by the ALA and may lead sessions in both schools and other community settings. They assist participants with 1) identifying reasons for smoking and excuses for not quitting, beliefs and behaviors that reinforce smoking and self-defeating behaviors, triggers for smoking, and other barriers to the quitting process; 2) recognizing and understanding the process of nicotine addiction, advertising ploys to encourage youth smoking, and situations that may spark relapse; and 3) developing skills in cognitive restructuring, coping with stress and peer pressure, identifying and maintaining social supports, goal setting, and assertiveness and other behavior changes (27,28).

After the N-O-T program was developed, partners collaborated to implement the program and assess its efficacy and acceptability in school settings (29-32). Because the need for a youth smoking cessation program was so great, ALA field workers were anxious to use N-O-T even before effectiveness studies were complete. As a result, while the N-O-T demonstration studies in West Virginia and several other states were under way, other local uses of the program were allowed if results were carefully monitored (26).

Over a 7–year period the N-O-T program went through several iterations, testing, refinement, and retesting. Demonstration studies were conducted in West Virginia, North Carolina, Florida, New Jersey, Illinois, Wisconsin, and Washington by the West Virginia team and independent investigators. Studies have consistently shown that adolescents enrolled in N-O-T programs have significantly greater quit and reduction rates than adolescents in more conventional smoking cessation programs. A recent review of N-O-T program outcomes in different locations included more than 6000 youths in 489 schools and showed that after 3 months, adolescents enrolled in N-O-T programs were twice as likely to have quit smoking than adolescents in conventional smoking cessation programs (33). The N-O-T program has been designated a model program by the federal Substance Abuse and Mental Health Services Administration and the federal Office of Juvenile Justice and Delinquency Prevention and is considered a research tested intervention program by the National Cancer Institute.

PRC researchers and the ALA developed a national training prototype by using the tested curriculum and scientific study results and initiated a N-O-T media campaign in 2000. The ultimate success of an evidence-based program is reflected in its widespread dissemination and adoption (34), and as of 2005, N-O-T trainings have occurred in 47 states and in Europe and Canada. It is estimated that since 1998, at least 100,000 adolescents have participated in N-O-T programs in the United States (American Lung Association, 2005). N-O-T program leaders estimate conservatively that one in five participants quits smoking (33); this rate suggests that N-O-T programs have helped up to 20,000 U.S. adolescents quit smoking. In

West Virginia, there are trained N-O-T facilitators in 75% of high schools, and program dissemination is supported by the Bureau for Public Health, the Department of Education, and the American Lung Association's West Virginia chapter.

N–O–T programs are supported in Canada and a number of U.S. states. Some states, including Virginia, Vermont, Wisconsin, Delaware, and Rhode Island, incorporate the N-O-T program into their state tobacco control plans.

8.4.1 LESSONS LEARNED FROM THE N-O-T PROGRAM

1. Involvement of multiple stakeholders, including school personnel and students, in the N-O-T program design resulted in a program that is feasible and effective and that attracts local champions to spearhead implementation in multiple locales.
2. Dissemination of the N-O-T program was a goal from its beginning, and this aim was a valuable guide to keep the program practitioner-friendly, consistent with local policies, and appealing to local funding agencies.
3. Having a partner with experience in national dissemination (the ALA) provided the capacity for widespread diffusion and adoption of the N-O-T program.

8.5 DISCUSSION

The lessons learned in the course of developing and disseminating these three school-based programs—CATCH, Planet Health, and N-O-T—are remarkably similar. Each program included multiple stakeholders to plan, implement, evaluate, and disseminate interventions. Although stakeholder groups varied in some ways, school administrators and teachers were included in all three programs. PRC researchers became familiar with the culture of schools and learned that a school-based intervention must be easy and inexpensive to implement, needs to allow flexibility for local adaptation, and should be aligned with current political constraints and academic mandates to be successful. All three programs provided teacher-friendly, inexpensive prepared curricula that appealed to students. Training was crucial to all three programs but was not burdensome in terms of time commitment or budget. Planning for dissemination from the start helped maintain a focus on feasibility and acceptability.

All three programs used the work of Rogers (11) as a foundation for design and dissemination efforts. His diffusion theory posits that adoption is more likely when innovations are perceived to have 1) relative advantage (the innovation is better than the status quo), 2) compatibility (the innovation is consistent with current values), 3) low complexity (the innovation is not difficult to understand and use), 4) observability (results of the innovation are noticeable to others), and 5) trialability (the innovation can be tried out on a partial or temporary basis). Other factors that encourage adoption, use, and maintenance of programs are involvement of advocates and adequate training to enhance user competency.

Another characteristic common to these programs was that each was shown to be effective through sound research studies. There is no substitute for demonstrating through methodologically sound science that an intervention leads to desirable behavior change (when compared with the status quo) in real-world settings. Such evidence of effectiveness also helps promote sustainable support since external agencies that fund school health programs are likely to favor those that are shown to be effective. Each of these programs has found strong local interest and financial support.

PRC involvement is an important feature shared by these three successful school-based programs. The CDC-administered PRC program is intended to build durable partnerships between public health professionals and organizations, academia, schools, community organizations, and community members to foster development and dissemination of programs that improve community health. Improving and maintaining community health requires a stable infrastructure that allows cultivation and maintenance of complex partnerships. PRC funding helps create this necessary infrastructure by supporting staff dedicated to improving health in underserved communities and by providing scientific research and evaluation expertise. PRCs help hold partnerships together and make it possible for local institutions to seek sustainable funding for effective health programs and polices.

The lessons learned from these three programs should encourage public health practitioners to consider schools as a potential venue for public health improvement. Public health practitioners who wish to work with schools, whether to implement programs or conduct research, need to develop an understanding of the school environment and how educational bureaucracy is structured (35). Schools are best approached through appropriate channels, such as a Coordinated School Health Program, a state or district coordinator, or an individual school health coordinator. These sources understand the current school policy environment in the state and can provide pertinent information, advice, and routes of communication.

Public health professionals can engage schools on their own ground to demonstrate the value of public health to school personnel. By attending local school board or district school health council meetings, public health professionals can offer valuable information to develop policies to promote high-quality health education and physical education courses, high-quality school food services, and a healthy school environment. Public health practitioners can also work with state coalitions for healthy schools or participate in professional organizations with a mission to support school health programs. Resources to build school health programs, such as promising practices for state leaders, funding opportunities, evidence-based guidelines, key strategies, and physical education curriculum analysis tools are available at www.cdc.gov/healthyyouth.

The School Health Index (SHI) is a CDC resource that can assist public health partnerships with schools through a structured process that helps schools assess their competencies in components of a coordinated school health program. The SHI requires interdisciplinary involvement from school personnel, promotes a collaborative culture within participating schools, and raises awareness of needs for health-related curricula, services, and policies. Schools that have used SHI programs are primed to improve their overall school health program, to welcome the involvement of public health experts who offer to test new health promotion programs, and to consider implementation of programs shown to be effective elsewhere.

Although challenges to working with schools are substantial, experience shows that success is possible. Understanding the school milieu, ensuring participation of relevant stakeholders (e.g., teachers, administrators, students, parents) in all stages, keeping potential dissemination in mind in all stages, and providing ample training and easy-to-use prepared curricula are features of the successful school-based interventions promoted by the PRC program.

APPENDIX

The following Web sites are for organization and agency information used in research for this article.

- Action for Healthy Kids: http://www.actionforhealthykids.org/
- American Lung Association Not On Tobacco Program: http://www.lungusa.org/site/pp.asp?c=dvLUK9O0E&b=39866
- American School Health Association: http://www.ashaweb.org/
- CATCH Texas: http://www.sph.uth.tmc.edu/catch/
- CDC Healthy Youth Program School Health Index: http://apps.nccd.cdc.gov/shi/default.aspx
- Harvard Prevention Research Center on Nutrition and Physical Activity, Planet Health: http://www.hsph.harvard.edu/prc/proj_planet.html
- National Association of State Boards of Education (NASBE) Center for Safe and Healthy Schools: http://www.nasbe.org/healthy_schools/intro.htm
- National Cancer Institute Research–tested Intervention Programs: http://rtips.cancer.gov/rtips/index.do
- Office of Juvenile Justice and Delinquency Prevention, U.S. Department of Justice: http://www.ojjdp.ncjrs.org/programs/mpg.html
- Substance Abuse and Mental Health Services Administration (SAMHSA) Model Programs: http://www.modelprograms.samhsa.gov/template_cf.cfm?page=model&pkProgramID=521
- Rhode Island Tobacco Control Program School Tobacco Cessation: http://www.health.state.ri.us/disease/tobacco/school-cessation.php

REFERENCES

1. Perry CL, Kelder SH, Komro K. The social world of adolescents: family, peers, schools, and community. In: Millstein SG, Peterson AC, Nightengale EO, editors. Promoting the health of adolescents: new directions for the twenty-first century. Oxford University Press; New York (NY): 1992.
2. U.S. Department of Health and Human Services. Health: United States, 2004. With chartbook on trends in the health of Americans. Hyattsville (MD): National Center for Health Statistics; 2004.

3. Kann L, Brener ND, Allensworth DD. Health education: results from the School Health Policies and Programs Study 2000. J Sch Health. 2001;71(7):266–278.
4. Marx E, Wooley S, Northrop D, editors. Health is academic: a guide to coordinated school health programs. New York (NY): Teachers College Press; 1998.
5. Brownson RC, Baker EA, Leet TL, Gillespie KN. Evidence-based public health. New York (NY): Oxford University Press; 2003.
6. Kolbe L. Education reform and the goals of modern school health programs. State Educ Standard 2002;3(4):4–11.
7. Luepker RV, Perry CL, McKinlay SM, Nader PR, Parcel GS, Stone EJ, et al. Outcomes of a field trial to improve children's dietary patterns and physical activity. The Child and Adolescent Trial for Cardiovascular Health. CATCH collaborative group. JAMA. 1996;275(10):768–776.
8. Nader PR, Stone EJ, Lytle LA, Perry CL, Osganian SK, Kelder S, et al. Three-year maintenance of improved diet and physical activity: the CATCH cohort. Child and Adolescent Trial for Cardiovascular Health. Arch Pediatr Adolesc Med. 1999;153(7):695–704.
9. Coleman KJ, Tiller CL, Sanchez J, Heath EM, Sy O, Milliken G, et al. Prevention of the epidemic increase in child risk of overweight in low-income schools: the El Paso coordinated approach to child health. Arch Pediatr Adolesc Med. 2005;159(3):217–224.
10. Kelder S, Hoelscher DM, Barroso CS, Walker JL, Cribb P, Hu S. The CATCH Kids Club: a pilot after-school study for improving elementary students' nutrition and physical activity. Public Health Nutr. 2005;8(2):133–140.
11. Rogers EM. Diffusion of innovations. 5th ed. The Free Pres; New York (NY): 2003.
12. Bandura A. Social foundations of thought and action: a social cognitive theory. Prentice Hall; Englewood Cliffs (NJ): 1986.
13. Siegel M, Doner L. Marketing public health: strategies to promote social change. Gaithersburg (MD): Aspen Publishers, Inc.; 1998. Applying marketing principles to public health.
14. Hoelscher DM, Kelder SH, Murray N, Cribb P, Conroy J, Parcel P. Dissemination and adoption of the child and adolescent trial for cardiovascular health (CATCH): A case study in Texas. J Public Health Manag Pract. 2001;7(2):90–100.
15. Owens N, Glanz K, Sallis J, Kelder S. Evidence-based approaches to dissemination and diffusion of physical activity interventions. Am J Prev Med. 2006 Oct;31(4 Suppl):S35–S44.
16. Hoelscher DM, Feldman HA, Johnson CC, Lytle L, Osganian SK, Kelder SH, et al. School-based health education programs can be maintained over time: results from the CATCH institutionalization study. Prev Med. 2004;38(5):594–606.
17. Carter J, Wiecha J, Peterson KE, Gortmaker SL. Planet Health. Champaign (IL): Human Kinetics Press; 2001.
18. Dietz WH, Gortmaker SL. Do we fatten our children at the TV set? Obesity and television viewing in children and adolescents. Pediatr 1985;75(5):807–812.
19. Epstein LH, Paluch RA, Consalvi A, Riordan K, Scholl T. Effects of manipulating sedentary behavior on physical activity and food intake. J Pediatr. 2002;140(3):334–339.

20. Gortmaker SL, Peterson K, Wiecha J, Sobol AM, Dixit S, Fox MK, Laird N. 15341999. 409–418.418Reducing obesity via a school-based interdisciplinary intervention among youth: Planet Health Arch Pediatr Adolesc Med
21. Austin SB, Field AE, Wiecha J, Peterson KE, Gortmaker SL. The impact of a school-based obesity prevention trial on disordered weight-control behaviors in early adolescent girls. Arch Pediatr Adolesc Med. 2005;159(3):225–230.
22. Chavarro JE, Peterson KE, Sobol AM, Wiecha JL, Gortmaker SL. Effects of a school-based obesity-prevention intervention on menarche (United States) Cancer Causes Control. 2005;16(10):1245–1252.
23. Wang LY, Yang Q, Lowry R, Wechsler H. Economic analysis of a school-based obesity prevention program. Obes Res. 2003;11(11):1313–1324.
24. Wiecha JL, El Ayadi AM, Fuemmeler BF, Carter JE, Handler S, Johnson S, et al. Diffusion of an integrated health education program in an urban school system: Planet Health. J Pediatr Psychol. 2004;29(6):467–474.
25. Tompkins NO, Dino GA, Zedosky LK, Harman M, Schaler G. A collaborative partnership to enhance school-based tobacco control policies in West Virginia. Amer J Prev Med 1999;16(Suppl 3):S29–S34.
26. Dino GA, Horn KA, Goldcamp J, Kemp-Rye L, Westrate S, Monaco K. Teen smoking cessation: making it work through school and community partnerships. J Pub Health Manag Pract. 2001;7(2):71–80.
27. Dino G, Horn K, Zedosky L, Monaco K. A positive response to teen smoking: Why N-O-T? NASSP Bull 1998;82:46–58.
28. Horn K, Dino G, Gao X, Momani A. Feasibility evaluation of Not On Tobacco: the American Lung Association's new stop smoking program for adolescents. Health Educ 1999;99(5):192–206.
29. Dino GA, Horn KA, Goldcamp J, Massey CJ, Maniar SD, Fernandes A. A statewide demonstration of Not On Tobacco: a gender-sensitive teen smoking cessation program. J Sch Nurs. 2001;17(2):90–97.
30. Dino GA, Horn KA, Goldcamp J, Fernandes A, Kalsekar I, Massey CJ. A 2-year efficacy study of Not On Tobacco in Florida: An overview of program successes in changing teen smoking behavior. Prev Med. 2001;33(6):600–605.
31. Horn K, Dino G, Kalsekar I, Massey CJ, Manzo-Tennant K, McGloin T. Exploring the relationship between mental health and smoking cessation: a study of rural teens. Prev Sci. 2004;5(2):113–126.
32. Horn K, Dino G, Kalsekar I, Fernandes AW. Appalachian teen smokers: Not On Tobacco 15 months later. Am J Public Health. 2004;94(2):181–184.]
33. Horn K, Dino G, Kalsekar I, Mody R. The impact of Not on Tobacco on teen smoking cessation: end-of-program evaluation results, 1998 to 2003. J Adolescent Res 2005;20(6):640–661.
34. Glasgow RE, Lichenstein E, Marcus AC. Why don't we see more translation of health promotion research to practice? Rethinking the efficacy-to-effectiveness transition. Am J Public Health. 2003;93(8):1261–1267.
35. How schools work & how to work with schools: a primer for professionals who serve children and youth. National Association of State Boards of Education; Alexandria (VA): 2003.

CHAPTER 9

ASSOCIATIONS BETWEEN EATING FREQUENCY, ADIPOSITY, DIET, AND ACTIVITY IN 9–10-YEAR-OLD HEALTHY-WEIGHT AND CENTRALLY OBESE CHILDREN

AMY JENNINGS, AEDHN CASSIDY, ESTHER M. F. VAN SLUIJS, SIMON J. GRIFFIN, AND AILSA A. WELCH

9.1 INTRODUCTION

Worldwide childhood obesity rates are reaching epidemic proportions with established health consequences that include both the presence of cardiovascular risk factors and strong links to adult morbidity and mortality (1). The distribution of body fat is also thought to predict cardiovascular disease risk with central (abdominal) obesity being more strongly related than total adiposity (2). Evidence also suggests that measures of central obesity, in particular waist-to-height ratio, predict adverse health outcomes including cardiovascular disease independently of BMI. Waist-to-height ratio is also associated with percentage body fat in children (3). Poor diet, next to lack of physical activity, has been implicated as a key

Printed with permission from Jennings A, Cassidy A, van Sluijs EMF, Griffin SJ and Welch AA. Associations Between Eating Frequency, Adiposity, Diet, and Activity in 9–10 year old Healthy-Weight and Centrally Obese Children. Obesity **20**,7 *(2012), DOI: 10.1038/oby.2012.72.*

determinant of obesity (1); however, it is not clear which specific aspects of dietary behavior, such as eating frequency (EF), should be targeted to reduce obesity (4,5). In order to develop effective strategies for obesity prevention, it is critical to determine how different aspects of children's diet relate to body composition and body fat distribution to enable more specific guidance and intervention strategies in the future.

EF (number of eating occasions/meals per day) is one aspect of the diet that is thought to be associated with both weight status and with risk factors associated with chronic diseases (6). Studies in adults have shown that increased EF is associated with improved weight status, although the evidence is equivocal (7,8,9,10,11) perhaps due to the use of different methodologies (12), different definitions of intake occasions (12), underreporting (13), or limited data on energy expenditure (7). The evidence in children is more consistent with four previous studies showing that EF is associated with reduced obesity status (14,15,16,17). These studies, however, have only used questionnaires to examine EF and physical activity meaning they have been unable to concurrently examine distribution and content of meals and snacks and objectively measured physical activity throughout the course of the day. These data would allow us to examine whether the mechanisms proposed to explain the association between increased EF and improved weight status in adults, including elevated physical activity levels (7), and better adjustment of energy intake (EI) in response to preceding eating occasions (7,14,18) also act in children. To date, it has been suggested that the specific distribution of meals and snacks may be important in the maintenance of body weight in children with data showing that increased snacking and breakfast consumption are associated with reduced risk of overweight and obesity (19,20). However, studies have not investigated the composition of foods within eating occasions.

The aims of the current cross-sectional study were as follows: first, to assess whether, in a well-characterized population-based sample of children aged 9–10 years, EF was associated with objectively measured parameters of adiposity when children were stratified by central obesity status. Second, to examine whether any observed associations might be attributable to differences in the composition of the diet or physical activity levels in an attempt to elucidate the potential mediating mechanisms whereby EF might influence bodyweight. Because breakfast consumption and snacking have been highlighted as key meals in terms of weight control and energy regulation, we chose to focus specifically on dietary intake at these meals (19,20,21). It was hypothesized that the children who ate more frequently would have more favorable adiposity status, dietary behaviors, and physical activity levels as compared with children who ate less frequently.

9.2 METHODS AND PROCEDURE

9.2.1 PARTICIPANTS

A total of 92 schools in the county of Norfolk, UK, agreed to take part in the SPEEDY study (Sport, Physical activity and Eating behaviour: Environmental Determinants in Young people), which was designed to quantify dietary habits, physical activity, and their correlates in a population-based sample of 9- to 10-year-old children. A total of 2,064 children participated and detailed descriptions of the sampling strategy, participation rates, and measurement procedures have been previously reported (22). Briefly, children aged 9–10 years were recruited from schools during the 12-week summer term of 2007 (April to July). Trained researchers took anthropometric measurements, and instructed children on how to complete questionnaires and diaries, and how to use an accelerometer. The University of East Anglia local research ethics committee approved the study protocol and the written consent of all participating children and their parents was obtained.

9.2.2 PROCEDURE

Assessment of dietary intake. Dietary intake was recorded using a 4-day food and drink diary where children, with assistance from their parents, were asked to record everything they ate and drank over a 4-day period (including two weekend days). This method has previously been used and validated with children aged 9–10 years (23). Estimated weights of portions were then calculated using published values, including those specific to children (24,25), and mean nutrient intakes estimated using the WISP nutritional analysis software, version 3.0 (Tinuviel Software, Warrington, UK) using nutrient values from McCance and Widdowson's the Composition of Foods (26).

Children were asked to record their food and drink consumption in predefined time periods (6–9 am, 9 am–12 pm, 12–2 pm, 2–5 pm, 5–8 pm, 8–10 pm, 10 pm–6 am). Daily EF was defined as the number of time periods in which children reported consuming any food or drink. Breakfast was defined as consuming any food or drink during the first eating period (between 6 am and 9 am), a mid-day meal as any food or drink consumed in the third eating period (between 12 pm and 2 pm) and an evening meal as food and drink consumed in the fifth eating period (between 5 pm and 8 pm). A snack was defined as food or drink consumed at any other time.

Underreporting of EI was assessed by calculating the ratio of reported EI to estimated energy requirements (EERs), which were estimated using equations from the Food and Agriculture Organization/World Health Organization/United Nations University Expert Consultation Report on Human Energy Requirements (27). A 95% confidence interval for the accuracy of EI:EER was calculated by taking into account the amount of variation inherent in the methods used to estimate EI and EER (28). For the SPEEDY data, the 95% confidence interval for EI:EER was 0.71–1.30 and, therefore, reports of EI within 71–130% of EER were considered to be in the range of normal measurement. As excluding children who underreport can distort dietary intake data, energy reporting quality (ratio of EI:EER) was examined as a continuous variable in all statistical models (29).

Assessment of anthropometry variables. Portable Leicester height measures (Seca, Hamburg, Germany) were used to assess height to the nearest millimeter. A nonsegmental bioimpedance scale (type TBF-300A; Tanita, Tokyo, Japan) was used to measure weight (to the nearest 0.1 kg) and impedance. Previously validated and published equations were used to calculate percentage body fat (30). BMI was calculated as weight in kilograms divided by height in meters squared and transformed to standardized z-scores using the least mean square method and the 1990 British Growth Reference data (31). Waist circumference was measured twice to the nearest millimeter (or three times if a discrepancy of more than 3 cm was observed) at the midpoint between the lower costal margin and the level of the anterior superior iliac crests, using a calibrated measuring tape (Seca, Birmingham, UK), a 0.5-cm correction was applied to account for clothing. Waist-to-height ratio was calculated as waist (cm) divided by height (cm) and used to classify children as centrally obese (>0.46 boys and >0.45 girls) or healthy weight (≤0.46 boys and ≤0.45 girls) using recently developed age-appropriate cutoffs to define central obesity (3). We chose to use waist-to-height ratio as the measurement to define obesity in this study for a number of reasons. First, there is substantial evidence that abdominal obesity is a better predictor of cardiovascular risk than BMI in children (2,32,33). Second, waist-to-height ratio has benefits over waist circumference when defining central obesity as it is known that height influences the observations of fat accumulation and distribution. Third, the use of waist-to-height ratio has also been highlighted as a useful public health tool in that very similar cutoff values can be used in different age, gender, and ethnic groups (34). A greater interest in and advocacy for the use of waist-to-height ratio to define obesity has, therefore, been observed in recent years (34).

Assessment of confounding variables. Information on highest parental education (in categories) was obtained from parental self-report. Free-living physical activity was assessed over 1 week with the ActiGraph activity monitor (GTIM; ActiGraph, Pensacola, FL) using a recording epoch of 5 s. Children were fitted with the monitor on the measurement day at school and received both verbal and written instructions regarding its use. They were instructed to wear the monitor during all waking hours, except while engaged in water-based activities. A special written program (MAHUffe; www.mrc epid.cam.ac.uk) was used for data cleaning, reduction, and further analyzes. Zero activity periods of 10 min or longer were interpreted as "not worn time" and these periods were removed from the summation of activity in line with previous research (35). Participants who did not manage to record valid data for at least 500 min per day for at least 3 days were excluded from further analyses. Physical activity was defined as mean daily activity counts per minute, an indicator of overall energy expenditure, and minutes in activity of moderate (2,000–3,999 counts/min) and vigorous activity (>4,000 counts/min).

TABLE 1: Characteristics of 1,700 healthy-weight and centrally obese children aged 9–10 years from the SPEEDY study

	All children (n = 1,700)	Healthy-weight children (n = 1,034)	Centrally obese children (n = 666)
Gender (% girls)	56	53	62[a]
Age (years)	10.3 (0.3)	10.3 (0.3)	10.2 (0.3)
Parental education (%)			
None or school leaving certificate	7	5	9
GCSE (exams usually taken at age 16 years)	51	49	55
A-level (exams usually taken at age 18 years)	25	28	21
University	17	18	15[a]
Height (cm)	141 (6.6)	140 (6.3)	142 (6.9)
Weight (kg)	36.6 (8.3)	32.7 (4.9)	42.7 (8.9)[a]
BMI (kg/m^2)	18.2 (3.1)	16.5 (1.4)	21.0 (3.1)[a]
BMI (z-score)	0.4 (1.1)	–0.3 (0.8)	1.4 (0.8)[a]
Waist (cm)	64.1 (8.1)	59.4 (3.6)	71.5 (7.7)[a]
Waist:height (cm)	0.454 (0.051)	0.422 (0.109)	0.504 (0.044)[a]
Body fat (%)	30.6 (7.9)	26.1 (4.9)	37.7 (6.1)[a]
Eating occasions			
Eating frequency (occasions/day)	4.3 (0.8)	4.4 (0.7)	4.3 (0.7)
Snacking frequency (occasions/day)	1.57 (0.68)	1.58 (0.68)	1.56 (0.69)
Breakfast frequency (% days)	89.2 (18.0)	89.8 (17.6)	88.3 (18.7)
Composition of the diet			
Energy density (kcal/g)	1.97 (0.31)	1.98 (0.31)	1.97 (0.32)
Total fat (% energy/day)	37.0 (4.6)	36.9 (4.4)	37.2 (4.7)
Carbohydrate (% energy/day)	48.6 (5.1)	48.9 (5.0)	48.3 (5.1)[a]
Protein (% energy/day)	14.3 (2.3)	14.2 (2.3)	14.5 (2.3)[a]
Fiber (g/day)	9.7 (3.4)	9.7 (3.4)	9.7 (3.4)
Fruit and vegetable (g/day)	196 (115)	198 (115)	192 (115)
Physical activity			
Moderate activity (min/day)	48.3 (14.3)	49.2 (14.5)	47.0 (13.9)[a]
Vigorous activity (min/day)	25.0 (13.2)	26.9 (13.9)	22.0 (11.5)[a]
Total activity (counts/min)	668 (218)	691 (227)	631 (197)[a]

Values are mean (SD) or %, n = 1,700. GCSE, General Certificate of Secondary Education; SPEEDY, Sport, Physical activity and Eating behavior: Environmental Determinants in Young People. [a]Significant difference between healthy-weight and overweight children ($P<0.05$; independent sample t-test or χ^2 test for categorical data).

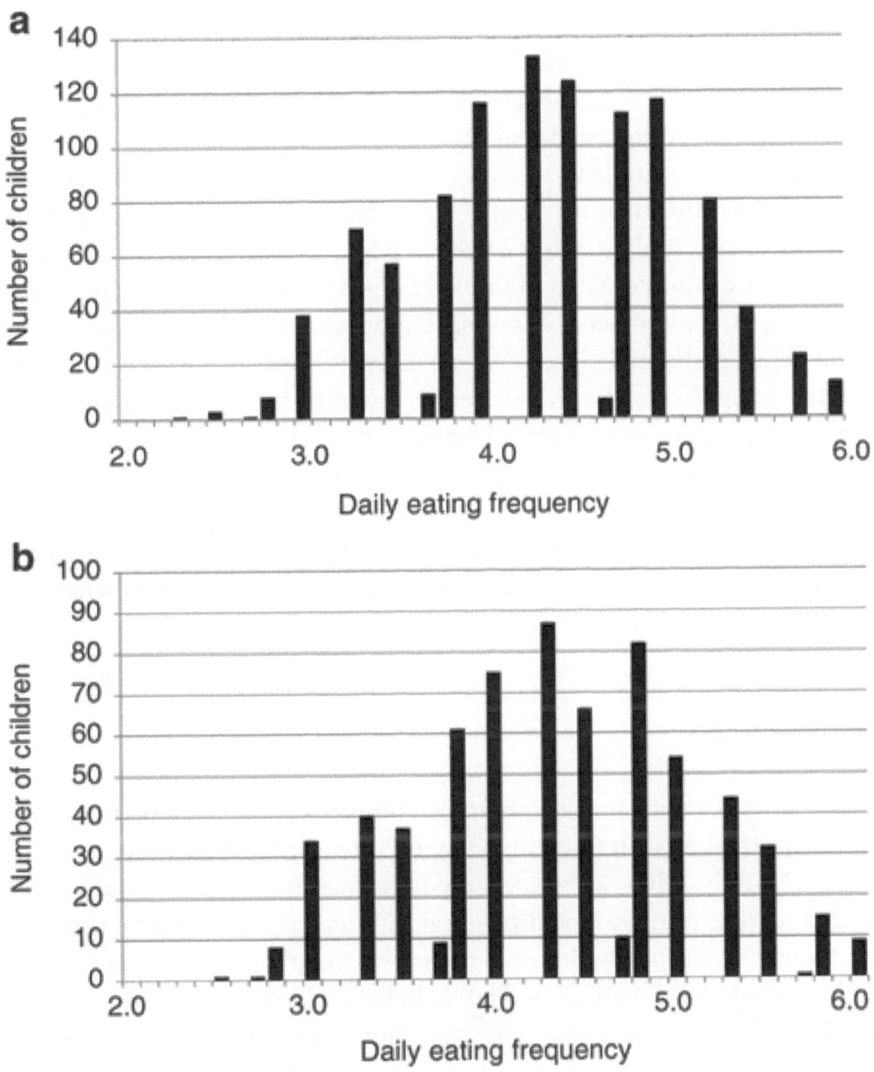

FIGURE 1: Distribution of eating frequency in 1,700 children aged 9–10 years. (a) Healthy-weight children (n = 1,034). (b) Centrally obese children (n = 666).

9.2.3 STATISTICAL ANALYSIS

As overweight children have been shown to have different dietary and physical activity patterns to healthy-weight children (36), and differences in meal frequencies have been shown between obese and healthy-weight adults (37), we examined the relationships between EF and adiposity separately in healthy-weight and centrally obese children using stratified analyses. Independent sample t-tests and χ^2 test for categorical data were used to examine the differences between characteristics of the healthy-weight and centrally obese children. Associations between EF and children's adiposity status were evaluated using multiple regression analysis after adjustment for relevant confounders. The distribution and nutritional composition of breakfast and snacks, and physical activity levels, were determined in quartile categories of EF. Mean percentage differences, adjusted for relevant confounders, are presented between the highest and lowest quartile (Q4–Q1), with statistical comparisons made using analysis of covariance. Potential confounders included gender, parental educational attainment, underreporting (EI:EER), EI (kcal), and physical activity (counts/min). Statistical analyses were performed using SPSS, version 16.0 for windows (SPSS, Chicago, IL).

9.3 RESULTS

Descriptive statistics for demographic and physical characteristics of the children are shown in Table 1. Of the 2,064 children recruited for the SPEEDY study 1,700 (82%) had adiposity measurements taken, completed diet diaries, provided valid physical activity data, and data on relevant confounders. All the children were aged between 9 and 10 years (10.3 ± 0.3 years) and 56% were girls. The included children did not differ in age to those who were excluded, although there were differences by gender (56% girls included sample v 50% girls excluded sample; $\chi^2 = 4.71$; $P = 0.030$). Centrally obese children were more likely to be girls ($\chi^2 = 12.6$; $P < 0.001$) and have parents with lower levels of education ($\chi^2 = 22.1$; $P = 0.001$). As expected, the healthy-weight children had significantly lower anthropometric measures (all $P < 0.05$) and higher physical activity levels (t = 6.05; P < 0.001) than the centrally obese children. There were no clear differences in the nutrient intake of the two groups although the healthy-weight children consumed more energy from carbohydrate (t = 2.42; P = 0.015) and less energy from protein (t = −2.31; P = 0.021), as compared with the centrally obese children.

TABLE 2: Association between daily eating frequency and adiposity in 1,700 healthy-weight and centrally obese children aged 9–10 years

	All children (n = 1,700)			Healthy-weight children (n = 1,034)			Centrally obese children (n = 666)		
	β	SE	P value	β	SE	P value	β	SE	P value
Weight (kg)	−0.02	0.31	0.479	−0.78	0.24	0.001	0.64	0.52	0.220
BMI (kg/m²)	0.02	0.12	0.867	−0.17	0.07	0.020	0.30	0.18	0.088
BMI (z-score)	−0.03	0.04	0.556	−0.10	0.04	0.014	0.09	0.05	0.047
Waist circumference (cm)	0.41	0.31	0.893	−0.38	0.17	0.031	0.71	0.45	0.118
Waist:height (cm)	0.002	0.002	0.313	0.000	0.001	0.849	0.005	0.003	0.036
Body fat (%)	−0.03	0.27	0.992	−0.20	0.21	0.347	0.40	0.33	0.226

Values are β coefficients and SE for a one unit increase in eating frequency, multivariate linear regression adjusted for gender, parental education, underreporting, energy intake, and physical activity.

Mean EF was 4.3 eating occasions/day (SD 0.8, range 2.3–6.0). There was no significant difference in reported frequency of meals and snacks between the healthy-weight and centrally obese children (4.4 eating occasions/day, SD 0.7, range 2.3–6.0 vs. 4.3 eating occasions/day SD 0.7, range 2.5–6.0; t = −0.31; P = 0.308), and the distribution of EF in each subgroup was similar (Figure 1). The mean number of snacks reported was 1.6/day in this sample (SD 0.68, range 0.0–3.0). The observed relationship between EF and adiposity differed between the healthy-weight children and the centrally obese children (Table 2). In healthy-weight children, increased EF was associated favorably with adiposity; each unit increase in EF was inversely associated with weight (β = −0.78 kg; P = 0.001), BMI (β

= −0.17 kg/ m²; $P = 0.020$), BMI z-score ($\beta = -0.10$; $P = 0.014$), and waist circumference ($\beta = -0.38$ cm; $P = 0.031$). In centrally obese children, each increase in eating occasion was positively associated with BMI z-score ($\beta = 0.09$; $P = 0.047$) and waist-to-height ratio ($\beta = 0.005$ cm; $P = 0.036$).

EF was significantly associated with both the number of snacks consumed and the nutritional composition of the snacks. As compared with the least-frequent eaters, the most-frequent eaters consumed more snacks (healthy-weight children 188% Q4–Q1, $P < 0.001$; centrally obese children 200% Q4–Q1, $P < 0.001$). Moreover, their snacks were lower in energy density (healthy-weight children −35% Q4–Q1, $P < 0.001$; centrally obese children −33% Q4–Q1, $P < 0.001$) and higher in carbohydrate (healthy-weight children 10% Q4–Q1, $P < 0.001$; centrally obese children 15% Q4–Q1, $P < 0.001$), fiber (healthy-weight children 57% Q4–Q1, $P < 0.001$; centrally obese 62% Q4–Q1, $P < 0.001$), and fruit and vegetables (healthy-weight children 201% Q4–Q1, $P < 0.001$; centrally obese children 209% Q4–Q1, $P < 0.001$; Figure 2).

Breakfast consumption was reported on an average of 89.2% of days (SD 18.0, range 0–100%). EF was associated with the number of days that breakfast consumption was reported with children in the highest quartile of EF reporting breakfast consumption most frequently (healthy-weight children 10% Q4–Q1, $P < 0.001$; centrally obese children 9% Q4–Q1, $P < 0.001$). The nutritional composition of food and drinks reported at breakfast time also differed by EF. As compared with the least-frequent eaters (quartile 1) the most-frequent eaters (quartile 5) reported lower EI (healthy-weight children −14% Q4–Q1, $P < 0.001$; centrally obese children −10% Q4–Q1, $P = 0.044$), lower total fat intake (healthy-weight children −18% Q4–Q1, $P < 0.001$; centrally obese children −18% Q4–Q1, $P < 0.001$), and higher carbohydrate intake at breakfast (healthy-weight children 9% Q4–Q1, $P < 0.001$; centrally obese children 10% Q4–Q1, $P = 0.001$; Figure 2).

The percentage differences in EI between extreme EF quartiles were similar for both healthy-weight (1.5% Q4–Q1, $P < 0.001$) and centrally obese children (1.1% Q4–Q1, $P = 0.035$), as were differences in activity of moderate intensity (healthy-weight children 6% Q4–Q1, $P = 0.040$ and overweight children 6% Q4–Q1, $P = 0.104$). The direction of differences in high-intensity activity differed between the two groups, however, with the healthy-weight children who ate most frequently reporting significantly higher levels of vigorous activity than the children who ate least frequently (4% Q4–Q1, P = 0.033), with the converse observed for overweight children, although this did not reach statistical significance (−2% Q4–Q1, P = 0.801; Figure 2).

9.4 DISCUSSION

Using a large population-based sample of 9- to 10-year-old children, we observed that increased EF was associated with improved body weight, BMI, and waist circumference in healthy-weight children with relative mean differences of −2.4% for body weight, −1.0% for BMI, −33% for BMI z-score, and −0.6% for waist circumference detected. Conversely, increased EF was associated with a higher BMI z-score and waist-to-height ratio in centrally obese children, with relative mean differences of 6% and 1%, respectively. Increased EF was also associated with the more favorable nutritional composition of breakfast and snacks in both groups, with children in the highest quartiles of EF reporting improved fruit and vegetable, fat, fiber, and carbohydrate intakes at these meals, as compared with the children in the lowest quartiles. Finally, an inverse association between high-intensity physical activity and EF was seen for the healthy-weight, but not the centrally obese children. These findings were all independent of covariates known to be associated with obesity including gender, EI, physical activity, parental education, and underreporting.

Despite the large amount of work examining the associations between dietary intake and weight status in children, it is not entirely clear how different eating behaviors relate to measures of adiposity in children, or the mechanisms behind these associations. To our knowledge, this is the first time a study has examined the behaviors that may be associated with EF in a large cohort of children using food diaries and objectively measured physical activity. Previous studies in children have shown daily meal frequency to be associated with a lower prevalence of obesity in German children aged 5–6 years (14), lower BMI z-score in German children aged 7–14 years (15), and with lower BMI in Portuguese girls aged 13–17 years (16). Furthermore snacking frequency has shown to be associated with overweight status in the National Health and Nutrition Examination Survey (NHANES) study (19). The current study builds on the results of this previous work by showing EF to be differentially associated with adiposity in healthy-weight and centrally obese children. The magnitude of our findings may have potential clinical relevance as reductions in BMI z-score similar to those observed in the current study have previously been associated with reductions in cardiometabolic risk factors in children of a similar age. Specifically, a decrease in BMI z-score of 0.1 has been associated with significantly lower insulin (−19 pmol/l), and total (−0.1 mmol/l) and low-density lipoprotein cholesterol levels (−0.12 mmol/l; ref. 38).

Our data also suggest that there may be a favorable impact of increased EF on fruit and vegetable, fat, fiber, and carbohydrate intake at the specific meal times examined in this study. These food groups and nutrients are known to be important in terms of weight control in children and are the dietary components forming the basis of public health policy relating to the prevention and treatment of childhood obesity (39). We have also shown that intake of these foods and nutrients are improved at specific meals that have been highlighted as important in terms of reducing obesity in children (19,20).

The positive relationship observed between EF and adiposity in centrally obese children does not appear to have been reported previously in the literature. It is possible that the differences observed in the associations between EF and adiposity between healthy-weight and obese children were linked to disparities in how the children were compensating EI and energy expenditure as our data show no association between physical activity and EF in centrally obese children. This could indicate that centrally obese children who were eating more frequently were, unlike the healthy-weight children, not compensating for their increased EI by being physically active. Previous studies have shown that children are generally good energy compensators, although this ability declines with age, and there is some evidence that overweight children compensate less well than healthy-weight children (40). A further possibility is that some of the centrally obese children were eating fewer meals as a strategy for weight loss, which could make it appear that there were positive associations between frequency of eating and adiposity in this group.

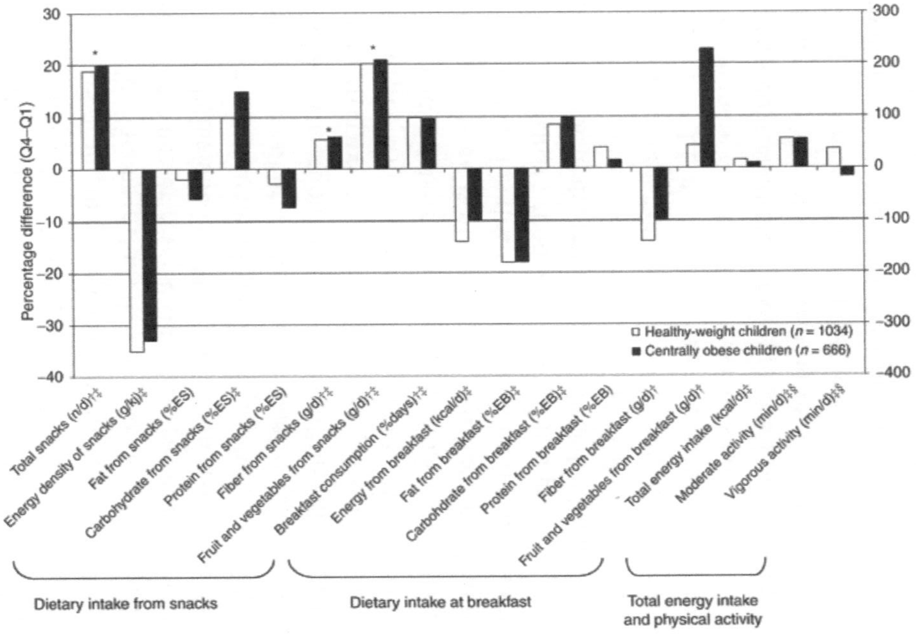

FIGURE 2: Mean percentage differences in dietary intake at specified meals and physical activity by eating frequency. Comparisons were made between the 4th and 1st quartile (healthy-weight children: n = 269 for Q1 and 273 for Q4; centrally obese children: n = 191 for Q1 and 155 for Q4). Values were adjusted for gender, parental education, underreporting, physical activity, and energy intake. %EB, percentage of total energy from breakfast; %ES, percentage of total energy from snacks. *Categories were plotted on the secondary axis. †Values adjusted for energy intake. ‡The difference between the 4th and 1st quartile was significantly different P <0.05 (analysis of covariance) in healthy weight and centrally obese children, or in §healthy-weight children only.

Strengths of this study are robust methodologies that allowed us to collect data on EF, the composition of the diet, and objectively measured physical activity concurrently. Unlike previous studies that have investigated EF, we were able to examine the composition of foods and nutrients within eating occasions. There was also a large sample recruited using a population-based sampling strategy. Underreporting is common in nutritional studies, especially among those who are overweight or obese (29), by using underreporting as a covariate we were able to control for the effect misreporting may have had on any reported associations.

The limitations include the cross-sectional design that means we cannot determine whether reverse causality was a factor. Furthermore, although our sample included children from a diverse range of urban and rural environments and areas of varying deprivation, Norfolk does not have large cities, and is culturally less varied than some parts of the country, as there are a low proportion of families from different ethnic backgrounds. Lower rates of overweight and obesity were also found in the current sample as compared with national averages (22). We acknowledge that our findings would not be generalizable to more ethnically diverse populations and further work is needed to see whether these findings are replicated in other samples. Finally, although food diaries have been shown to provide a valid measure of food intake in this age group (23), underreporting was accounted for in the present analysis and substantial assistance from parents was requested, we cannot entirely eliminate measurement error or the possibility of reporting bias by the children or parents. Furthermore, our definition of EF was restrictive (to a maximum of six eating occasions), although more detailed than previous studies, and it is possible that some children consumed more than one meal or snack in the time periods we considered. This misclassification may have underestimated the magnitude of associations between EF, measures of adiposity, diet, and physical activity in this sample. If EF was more precisely defined, the associations observed may have been of an even greater magnitude.

In conclusion, we found that increased EF was favorably associated with body weight and adiposity measures in healthy-weight children but not centrally obese children. The healthy-weight children who ate most frequently reported significantly higher physical activity levels and improved composition of snacks and breakfast in terms of fruit and vegetables, fat, fiber, and carbohydrates, as compared with the children who ate least frequently. In contrast, our data show no association between objectively measured physical activity and EF in centrally obese children. It is, therefore, important that public health messages supporting increased EF in children, such as those that promote breakfast or snacking consumption, should focus on promoting dietary quality and the importance of physical activity in balancing EI. The findings of this study suggest that future obesity interventions should consider the mediating role of physical activity and diet quality in the relationship between EF and in children, however, further evidence from prospective studies is needed to confirm the findings of this study.

REFERENCES

1. World Health Organization. Obesity: Preventing and Managing the Global Epidemic. Report of a WHO Consultation. World Health Organization: Geneva, 2000.
2. Mokha JS, Srinivasan SR, Dasmahapatra P et al. Utility of waist-to-height ratio in assessing the status of central obesity and related cardiometabolic risk profile among normal weight and overweight/obese children: the Bogalusa Heart Study. BMC Pediatr 2010;10:73.
3. Nambiar S, Hughes I, Davies PS. Developing waist-to-height ratio cut-offs to define overweight and obesity in children and adolescents. Public Health Nutr 2010;13:1566–1574.
4. National Institute for Health and Clinical Excellence. Obesity: Guidance on the Prevention, Identification, Assessment and Management of Overweight and Obesity in Adults and Children. London, 2006.
5. Scottish Intercollegiate Guidelines Network. Management of Obesity. A National Clinical Guideline. Scottish Intercollegiate Guidelines Network: Edinburgh, UK, 2010.
6. Titan SM, Bingham S, Welch A et al. Frequency of eating and concentrations of serum cholesterol in the Norfolk population of the European prospective investigation into cancer (EPIC-Norfolk): cross sectional study. BMJ 2001;323:1286–1288.
7. Duval K, Strychar I, Cyr MJ et al. Physical activity is a confounding factor of the relation between eating frequency and body composition. Am J Clin Nutr 2008;88:1200–1205.
8. Drummond SE, Crombie NE, Cursiter MC, Kirk TR. Evidence that eating frequency is inversely related to body weight status in male, but not female, non-obese adults reporting valid dietary intakes. Int J Obes Relat Metab Disord 1998;22:105–112.
9. Yannakoulia M, Melistas L, Solomou E, Yiannakouris N. Association of eating frequency with body fatness in pre- and postmenopausal women. Obesity (Silver Spring) 2007;15:100–106.

10. Ma Y, Bertone ER, Stanek EJ 3rd et al. Association between eating patterns and obesity in a free-living US adult population. Am J Epidemiol 2003;158:85–92.
11. Ruidavets JB, Bongard V, Bataille V, Gourdy P, Ferrières J. Eating frequency and body fatness in middle-aged men. Int J Obes Relat Metab Disord 2002;26:1476–1483.
12. Bertéus Forslund H, Lindroos AK, Sjöström L, Lissner L. Meal patterns and obesity in Swedish women-a simple instrument describing usual meal types, frequency and temporal distribution. Eur J Clin Nutr 2002;56:740–747.
13. Summerbell CD, Moody RC, Shanks J, Stock MJ, Geissler C. Relationship between feeding pattern and body mass index in 220 free-living people in four age groups. Eur J Clin Nutr 1996;50:513–519.
14. Toschke AM, Küchenhoff H, Koletzko B, von Kries R. Meal frequency and childhood obesity. Obes Res 2005;13:1932–1938.
15. Würbach A, Zellner K, Kromeyer-Hauschild K. Meal patterns among children and adolescents and their associations with weight status and parental characteristics. Public Health Nutr 2009;12:1115–1121.
16. Mota J, Fidalgo F, Silva R et al. Relationships between physical activity, obesity and meal frequency in adolescents. Ann Hum Biol 2008;35:1–10.
17. Nicklas TA, Morales M, Linares A et al. Children's meal patterns have changed over a 21-year period: the Bogalusa Heart Study. J Am Diet Assoc 2004;104:753–761.
18. Bellisle F. Impact of the daily meal pattern on energy balance. Scand J Nutr 2004;48:114–118.
19. Keast DR, Nicklas TA, O'Neil CE. Snacking is associated with reduced risk of overweight and reduced abdominal obesity in adolescents: National Health and Nutrition Examination Survey (NHANES) 1999–2004. Am J Clin Nutr 2010;92:428–435.
20. Rampersaud GC, Pereira MA, Girard BL, Adams J, Metzl JD. Breakfast habits, nutritional status, body weight, and academic performance in children and adolescents. J Am Diet Assoc 2005;105:743–60; quiz 761.
21. McCrory MA, Campbell WW. Effects of eating frequency, snacking, and breakfast skipping on energy regulation: symposium overview. J Nutr 2011;141:144–147.
22. van Sluijs EM, Skidmore PM, Mwanza K et al. Physical activity and dietary behaviour in a population-based sample of British 10-year old children: the SPEEDY study (Sport, Physical activity and Eating behaviour: environmental Determinants in Young people). BMC Public Health 2008;8:388.
23. Crawford PB, Obarzanek E, Morrison J, Sabry ZI. Comparative advantage of 3-day food records over 24-hour recall and 5-day food frequency validated by observation of 9- and 10-year-old girls. J Am Diet Assoc 1994;94:626–630.
24. Crawley H. Food Portion Sizes. H.M. Stationary Office: London, 2002.
25. Wrieden WL, Longbottom PJ, Adamson AJ et al. Estimation of typical food portion sizes for children of different ages in Great Britain. Br J Nutr 2008;99:1344–1353.
26. Food Standards Agency. McCance and Widdowsons's the Composition of Foods, 6th edn. Royal Society of Chemistry: Cambridge, 2002.
27. Torun B. Energy requirements of children and adolescents. Public Health Nutr 2005;8:968–993.

28. Black AE, Cole TJ. Within- and between-subject variation in energy expenditure measured by the doubly-labelled water technique: implications for validating reported dietary energy intake. Eur J Clin Nutr 2000;54:386–394.
29. Rennie KL, Coward A, Jebb SA. Estimating under-reporting of energy intake in dietary surveys using an individualised method. Br J Nutr 2007;97:1169–1176.
30. Tyrrell VJ, Richards G, Hofman P et al. Foot-to-foot bioelectrical impedance analysis: a valuable tool for the measurement of body composition in children. Int J Obes Relat Metab Disord 2001;25:273–278.
31. Cole TJ, Freeman JV, Preece MA. British 1990 growth reference centiles for weight, height, body mass index and head circumference fitted by maximum penalized likelihood. Stat Med 1998;17:407–429.
32. Kahn HS, Imperatore G, Cheng YJ. A population-based comparison of BMI percentiles and waist-to-height ratio for identifying cardiovascular risk in youth. J Pediatr 2005;146:482–488.
33. Savva SC, Tornaritis M, Savva ME et al. Waist circumference and waist-to-height ratio are better predictors of cardiovascular disease risk factors in children than body mass index. Int J Obes Relat Metab Disord 2000;24:1453–1458.
34. Browning LM, Hsieh SD, Ashwell M. A systematic review of waist-to-height ratio as a screening tool for the prediction of cardiovascular disease and diabetes: 0·5 could be a suitable global boundary value. Nutr Res Rev 2010;23:247–269.
35. Riddoch CJ, Bo-Andersen L, Wedderkopp N et al. Physical activity levels and patterns of 9- and 15-yr-old European children. Med Sci Sports Exerc 2004;36:86–92.
36. Oellingrath IM, Svendsen MV, Brantsaeter AL. Eating patterns and overweight in 9- to 10-year-old children in Telemark County, Norway: a cross-sectional study. Eur J Clin Nutr 2010;64:1272–1279.
37. Bertéus Forslund H, Torgerson JS, Sjöström L, Lindroos AK. Snacking frequency in relation to energy intake and food choices in obese men and women compared to a reference population. Int J Obes (Lond) 2005;29:711–719.
38. Kolsgaard ML, Joner G, Brunborg C et al. Reduction in BMI z-score and improvement in cardiometabolic risk factors in obese children and adolescents. The Oslo Adiposity Intervention Study — a hospital/public health nurse combined treatment. BMC Pediatr 2011;11:47.
39. Parliamentary Office of Science and Technology. Childhood obesity. Postnote 2003;205. <http:www.parliament.ukdocumentspostpn205.pdf>.
40. Cecil JE, Palmer CN, Wrieden W et al. Energy intakes of children after preloads: adjustment, not compensation. Am J Clin Nutr 2005;82:302–308.

PART III

RECOMMENDATIONS FOR THE FUTURE

CHAPTER 10

SYSTEMATIC REVIEW OF THE HEALTH BENEFITS OF PHYSICAL ACTIVITY AND FITNESS IN SCHOOL-AGED CHILDREN AND YOUTH

IAN JANSSEN AND ALLANA G. LEBLANC

10.1 BACKGROUND

Canada's first set of physical activity guidelines for children and youth were introduced in 2002 [1,2]. The basic recommendation within these guidelines was that children and youth, independent of their current physical activity level, should increase the time they spend on moderate-to-vigorous intensity physical activity by 30 minutes per day, and over a 5 month period progress to adding an additional 90 minutes of daily physical activity. Recently, a narrative literature review was conduced to provide an update on the evidence related to the biological and psycho-social health benefits of physical activity in school-aged children and youth which has accumulated since the publication of Canada's guidelines [3]. This narrative review explored whether Canada's physical activity guidelines for children and youth are appropriate, and made recommendations as to how the guidelines could be modified to reflect current knowledge.

Several other narrative reviews have examined the relation between physical activity and health in school aged children, a small sample of which are referenced here [4-8]. Although informative, narrative reviews have severe limitations. First and foremost, it is uncertain as to whether all of the relevant scientific evidence has been examined. The authors of a narrative review may be exclusive with the materials they review, and these materials may have been selected and interpreted in a biased manner. Thus, the reader is faced with uncertainty and doubt when interpreting a narrative review. The reader may be better served when the choices made in the review are explicit, transparent, clearly stated, and reproducible. This can be achieved through a systematic review. Systematic reviews attempt to reduce reviewer bias through the use of objective, reproducible criteria to select relevant publications, to synthesize and critically appraise the findings from these publications, and to employ defined evidence-based criteria when formulating recommendations [9].

The purpose of this report was to: 1) perform a systematic review of the evidence informing the relation between physical activity and health in school-aged children and youth, defined here as those aged 5-17 years; and 2) make recommendations on the appropriate volume, intensity, and type of physical activity for minimal and optimal health benefits in school-aged children and youth. A previously developed evaluation system was used to set the level of evidence and grade for the recommendations. This report was part of a much larger project around Canada's physical activity guidelines, and comparable systematic reviews for adults [10] and older adults [11] have also been published in the journal. Additional details on the scope and purpose of the larger project [12] and the interpretation of the recommendations from an independent expert panel [13] can also be found elsewhere in the journal.

10.1.1 OVERVIEW OF EXISTING PHYSICAL ACTIVITY GUIDELINES FOR CHILDREN AND YOUTH

Before conducting the systematic review, this paper provides a brief overview on existing physical activity guidelines for school-aged children, as well as an explanation of the scientific evidence that informed the guideline development process.

The publication of Canada's physical activity guidelines for children and youth in 2002 represented a joint effort of the Canadian Society for Exercise Physiology and Health Canada. Two sets of guidelines were published, one for children aged 6 to 9 years [2] and a second for youth aged 10 to14 years [1]. In addition to the physical activity guides, which highlighted the recommended physical activity levels for these two age groups, a number of other promotional and educational packages were developed, including family booklets [14,15], teacher booklets [16,17], as well as physical activity magazines for children [18] and youth [19].

The key recommendations within Canada's child and youth physical activity guides are:

1. Increase the time currently spent on physical activity by 30 minutes per day, and progress over approximately 5 months to 90 minutes more per day.
2. Physical activity can be accumulated throughout the day in periods of at least 5 to 10 minutes.
3. The 90 minute increase in physical activity should include 60 minutes of moderate activity (e.g., brisk walking, skating, bicycle riding) and 30 minutes of vigorous activity (e.g., running, basketball, soccer).
4. Participate in different types of physical activities—endurance, flexibility, and strength—to achieve the best health results.
5. Reduce non-active time spent on watching television and videos, playing computer games, and surfing the Internet. Start with 30 minutes less of such activities per day and progress over the course of approximately 5 months to 90 minutes less per day.

Many other countries and organizations have developed physical activity recommendations for school-aged children and youth, as recently summarized [3]. With few exceptions, these countries and organizations recommend that children and youth participate in at least 60 minutes of moderate-to-vigorous intensity physical activity on a daily basis. One of these recommendations was published in 2005 as part of a systematic review that linked physical activity to several health and behavioural outcomes in school-aged children and youth [20]. This systematic review was sponsored by the U.S. Centers for Disease Control and Prevention (CDC) and was developed by a multidisciplinary expert panel. The expert panel considered over 850 articles published in 2004 or earlier, identified by computerized database searches and by searching the bibliographies of the panellists' own libraries [20]. Based on conceptual definitions and inclusion and exclusion criteria developed by the panel, participants systematically evaluated relevant articles (primarily intervention studies) for each of the 14 health and behavioural outcomes considered. On the basis of their reviews, the panel provided a summary of the evidence for strength (strong, >60% of studies reviewed; moderate, 30-59% of studies reviewed; and weak, <30% of studies reviewed) and the direction (positive, null, or negative) of the effects of physical activity on each of the health and behavioural outcomes. The strength of evidence was judged from the statistical significance of the outcomes; it did not include other factors usually considered in systematic review, such as the effect sizes of physical activity and the quality and types of studies.

The expert panel reached the following conclusions: (i) Evidence-based data are strong to conclude that physical activity has beneficial effects on adiposity (within overweight and obese youth), musculoskeletal health and fitness, and several components of cardiovascular health. (ii) Evidence-based data are adequate to conclude that physical activity has beneficial effects on adiposity levels in those with a normal body weight, on blood pressure in normotensive youth, on plasma lipid and lipoproteins levels, on non-traditional cardiovascular risk factors (inflammatory markers, endothelial function and heart rate variability), and on several components of mental health (self-concept, anxiety and depression) [20]. A summary of evidence concerning the health outcomes examined by the expert panel is shown in Table 1 [Additional file 1]. The amount, intensity, and type of physical activity required to achieve the result, when clear, is also shown in the table.

In 2008 a second systematic review of literature examining the relation between physical activity and key fitness and health outcomes within school-aged children and youth was published. This systematic review was part of the "Physical Activity Guidelines for Americans" project that was undertaken by the Unites States Department of Health and Human Services [21]. Unlike the 2005 CDC sponsored systematic review that focused on intervention studies, the 2008 review considered both observational and experimental studies. The 2008 systematic review concluded that few studies have provided data on the dose-response relation between physical activity and various health and fitness outcomes in children and youth. However, substantial data indicate that health and fitness benefits will occur in most children and youth who participate in 60 or more minutes of moderate-to-vigorous physical activity on a daily basis. For children and youth to gain comprehensive health benefits they need to participate in the following types of physical activity on 3 or more days per week: vigorous aerobic exercise, resistance exercise, and weight-loading activities.

Although informative, the recommendations made within the 2005 and 2008 systematic reviews did not include a level of evidence or grade, which are now becoming a routine part of evidence based reviews. The level of evidence helps inform the reader about the strength of evidence that informed the recommendation. The grade considers the harms and benefits of implementing the intervention, and informs the reader about whether an intervention should be implemented.

10.1.2 QUESTIONS ADDRESSED IN SYSTEMATIC REVIEW

The following questions were addressed in this systematic review:

1. *How much (volume) physical activity is needed for minimal and optimal health benefits in school-aged children and youth?* To address this question careful consideration was given to whether dose-response relations existed between physical activity and fitness with the various health outcomes, and if so, the pattern of these relations (e.g., linear, or curvilinear relations with large improvements in health occurring with limited increases in physical activity at the low end of the physical activity scale, or curvilinear relations with small improvements in health occurring with increases in physical activity at the low end of the physical activity scale).

2. *What types of activity are needed to produce health benefits?* Specific consideration was given to what types of activity (aerobic, resistance, etc.) influenced the different health outcomes, and whether more than one type of activity would be needed for overall health and well-being.
3. *What is the appropriate physical activity intensity?* Attention was given to the intensity of physical activity measured (observational studies) or prescribed (experimental studies). An underlying assumption was that children and youth would prefer lower intensity activities over higher intensity activities. Therefore, for higher intensity activities to be recommended over lower intensity activities there would need to be either: i) no evidence that low intensity activities were beneficial for health and evidence that higher intensity activities impacted health in a favorable manner, or ii) clear evidence that higher intensity activities impacted the health outcomes to a greater extent than lower intensity activities.
4. *Do the effects of physical activity on health in school-aged children and youth vary by sex and/or age?* Results were examined to see if: i) the moderating effects of sex and/or age on the relations between physical activity and health were explored, and if not, iii) whether there were consistent patterns across studies (either statistically or in order of magnitude) that were suggestive of sex or age differences.

10.2 METHODS

10.2.1 ELIGIBILITY CRITERIA

This systematic review was limited to key indicators of different health outcomes known to be related to physical activity in school-aged children and youth. Decisions on what health outcomes to include in the systematic review were made by examining what outcomes were studied in previously conducted reviews of this nature [20,21] and in consultation with the Steering Committee for the Canadian Physical Activity Guidelines project. These key indicators consisted of:

1. High blood cholesterol, high blood pressure, and markers of the metabolic syndrome as a measure of cardiometabolic risk
2. Overweight/obesity as a measure of adiposity
3. Low bone density as a measure of skeletal health
4. Depression as a measure of mental health
5. Injuries as a negative health outcome of physical activity

We recognized that although cardiorespiratory and musculoskeletal fitness are partially genetic in origin, they are in large measure a reflection of physical activity participation in recent weeks and months [22]. Therefore, the systematic review also included studies that examined the relation between fitness and health. For our purposes, fitness was assumed to be a proxy measure of physical activity. Any studies evaluating the relationship between physical activity or fitness and one or more of the key health outcomes listed above within school-aged children and youth were eligible for inclusion.

In consultation with the Steering Committee of the Canadian Physical Activity Guidelines and Measurement Project and the authors who were completing the adult and older adult systematic reviews, a decision was made to limit the pediatric systematic review to: 1) studies examining the key health indicators above, and 2) for observational studies, the outcomes must have been measured in a dichotomous (yes or no) manner and presented as prevalences or ratio scores (odds ratio, relative risk, hazard ratio). This decision was made for three reasons: (i) to help ensure that the systematic review would be manageable in size and scope for a single research team to complete in a timely manner, (ii) to eliminate many of the observational studies with small sample sizes, and (iii) to ensure that the health outcomes, at least for the observational studies, were presented in a reasonably consistent pattern from study to study. This helped us to make comparisons between studies and to characterize the magnitude of effect for physical activity.

To further illustrate why the aforementioned limitations were put in place, consider the following. Within children and youth physical activity has been related to over two dozen different health outcomes. For adiposity alone, several adiposity measures have been considered including body weight, BMI, several skinfold and circumference measures, total body fat, and several specific body fat depots. Preliminary literature searches on adiposity—as measured using both continuous (e.g., body weight, BMI, visceral fat, skinfolds) and categorical (overweight/obese vs. normal weight) outcomes to capture the measures indicated above, revealed over 15,000 published papers. The results from these papers were presented in several formats including comparison of group means for continuous adiposity measures according to physical activity level, relations between continuous adiposity and physical activity measures which were presented in a variety of ways (e.g., r values, regression coefficients); comparison of group means for physical activity according to adiposity status; ratio scores (odds ratios, relative risks, hazard ratios) for the prediction of obesity status according to physical activity level; comparison of the prevalence of obesity according to physical activity level; etc. Without employing some criteria to limit the types of measures and outcomes, it would have been virtually impossible to synthesize the results from these studies.

Cross-sectional studies, case-control studies, cohort studies (prospective and retrospective) and intervention studies (including randomized and quasi experimental designs) were eligible for inclusion in the systematic review. Only published, English language studies including human participants were included. To be included studies had to be limited to school-aged children and youth between 5-17 years of age, or present data specifically for a subgroup of participants within this age range.

For the observational studies, there were no limitations placed on the form of physical activity (e.g., questionnaire, activity diary, pedometer, accelerometer) or fitness (cardiorespiratory or musculoskeletal fitness) measurements. For intervention studies, all cardiorespriatory and/or musculoskeletal based interventions were eligible for inclusion. Intervention studies were excluded if they included a dietary (e.g., caloric restriction) or other behavioral risk factor component (e.g., smoking cessation) that may have independently affected the health outcomes and subsequently made it impossible to distinguish the independent effect of the physical activity portion of the intervention.

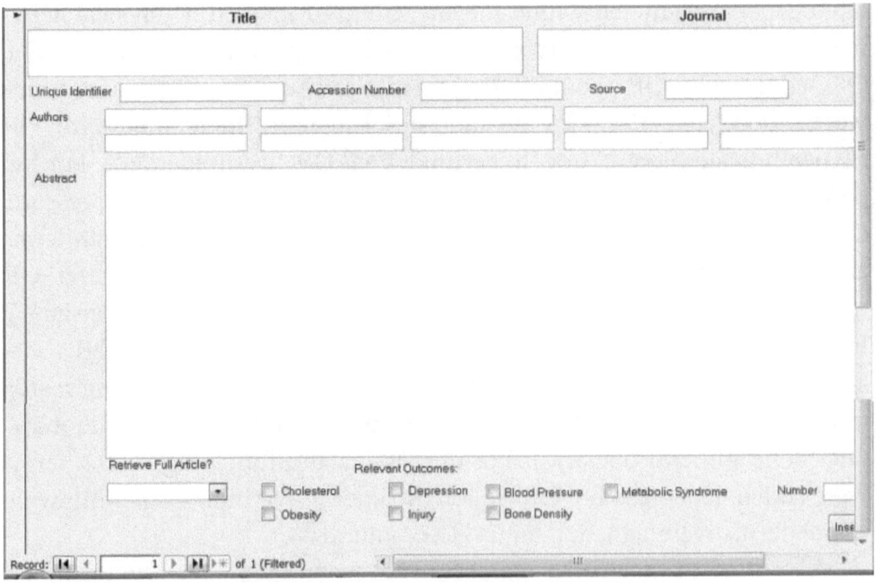

FIGURE 1: Copy of electronic abstract review form.

10.2.2 SEARCH STRATEGY

Literature searches were conducted in MEDLINE (1950-January 2008, OVID Interface), EMBASE (1980-January 2008, OVID Interface), CINAHL (1982-January 2008, OVID Interface), PsycINFO (1967-January 2008, OVID Interface), all Evidence-Based Medicine Reviews (1991-January 2008, OVID Interface), and SPORTDiscus (up to January 2008, EBSCO Interface).

The electronic search strategies were executed by a single researcher (AB) under direction of the primary author (IJ). They were not restricted by publication type or study design; however, they were limited to human participants and English language. The following string of search terms were used for each of the study outcomes to identify physical activity related papers conducted within the age group of interest: ('physical activity' OR 'fitness' OR 'exercise' OR 'energy expenditure') AND ('child' OR 'adolescent' OR 'youth' OR 'juvenile'). The following search terms were added (e.g., AND) for the cholesterol search: ('high cholesterol' OR 'hypercholesterolemia' OR 'hyperlipidemia' OR 'dyslipidemia'). For hypertension the following search terms were added: ('high blood pressure' OR 'hypertension'). For metabolic syndrome the following search terms added: ('metabolic syndrome' OR 'syndrome X' OR 'deadly quartet' OR 'plurimetabolic syndrome' OR 'insulin resistance' OR 'insulin resistant'). For obesity the following search terms were added: ('obese' OR 'obesity' OR 'overweight'). For low bone mineral density the following search terms were added: ('bone density' OR 'bone strength' OR 'bone mass' OR 'bone mineral density'). For depression the following search terms were added: ('depression' OR 'mood disorder'). For injuries the following search terms were added: ('injury' OR 'injuries').

A total of 42 electronic searches were performed (7 health outcomes × 6 search engines) and the information from each search was saved as a text file that included all of the retrieved citations. Using SAS software version 9 (SAS Institute, Carry, NC), the text files were separated back into individual citations and exported into a Microsoft Access database. The database included the following information for each citation: unique identifier for the database, paper title, authors, journal name, volume and issue number, page numbers, and the abstract. See Figure 1 for an illustration of the Microsoft Access database form. Within the Microsoft Access database, duplicate citations—those citations that were identified in more than one of the search engines and/or for more than one of the health outcomes—were identified by a match of the title and were removed using automated procedures.

10.2.3 SCREENING OF CITATIONS

After duplicate citations were removed from the Access database, the abstract of each citation was reviewed by a single reviewer to determine if it should be included within the systematic review. The full-text articles of all potentially relevant citations were obtained, and saved as Adobe-PDF files that were linked to the Access database. Whenever it was uncertain as to whether a citation was appropriate, the full-text copy was obtained. After the first reviewer screened the database, the citations that were deemed ineligible were reviewed by a second reviewer to determine if any potentially relevant citations were missed, and full-text copies of these citations were also obtained. Copies of all of the full-text articles were then reviewed by the two reviewers for inclusion criteria; if uncertain as whether or not to include an article, the article in question was reviewed again until a final decision was made.

10.2.4 DATA ABSTRACTION

A single reviewer (AL) abstracted data from all eligible full-text citations using an electronic data abstraction form. Refer to Figure 2 for an illustration of electronic data abstraction form. The data abstraction was completed in a second Microsoft Access Database, which was linked to the first Microsoft Access Database using a unique identifier. The abstracted data included information on the study design, participants, details of the physical activity (or fitness) measures or interventions, and key findings. After data abstraction was completed, the information was checked by a second reviewer (IJ) and corrected when necessary.

10.2.5 ASSIGNING LEVELS OF EVIDENCE AND FORMULATION OF RECOMMENDATIONS

The goal was to use a rigorous, evidence-based approach to develop levels of evidence on the relation between physical activity and health in school-aged children that could be used to formulate recommendations for the specific volume, intensity, and type of physical activity needed. At present there is no universally accepted method for formulating evidence-based recommendations. In consultation with the Steering Committee for this project and the authors performing the systematic reviews in adults and older adults, we chose to use the process that was recently employed for the development of Canada's obesity prevention and management guidelines [23]. Within this system, the level of evidence for a recommendation is based on an objective appraisal of the literature according to a pre-specified scale as reflected by the study designs and quality. As shown in Table 2 [Additional file 2], the level of evidence can range from 1 (highest) to 4 (lowest). The grade for a recommendation reflects the level of evidence and several additional features, including: benefits and risks of physical activity participation, magnitude of the effects, cost of the intervention, and value of an intervention to an individual or population. As indicated in Table 3 [Additional file 3], the grade for the recommendation may be an A, B, or C. Note that while the level of evidence assigned is not necessarily linked to the corresponding grade, a high grade is less likely in the setting of low-quality of evidence.

Note that the level of evidence in the aforementioned grading system is based in part on the quality of the studies. This grading was particularly relevant for experimental studies wherein the level of evidence would change from Level 1 to Level 2 based on whether or not the randomized controlled trials (RCTs) have important limitations. A single investigator (IJ) assessed the quality of the RCTs included in this systematic review using the validated checklist developed by Downs and Black [24]. This 27-item checklist assess the quality of reporting (e.g., are the interventions of interest clearly described, have all the adverse events that may be a consequence of the intervention been reported), external validity (e.g., were the subjects representative of the population), internal validity (e.g., was an attempt made to blind those measuring the outcome, were the outcome measures accurate), selection bias (e.g., were the study subjects randomized, was randomization assignment concealed until recruitment was complete), and statistical power.

To evaluate the magnitude of effect of physical activity on the various health outcomes examined, in addition to statistical significance, the following criteria were applied to evaluate the strength of the ratio scores (odds ratio, relative risk, hazard ratio) for the observational studies. For positive associations 1.01-1.50 = weak association, 1.51-3.00 = moderate association, and 3.01 or higher = strong association. For negative associations: 0.71-0.99 = weak association, 0.41-0.70 = moderate association, 0.00-0.40 = strong association [25]. For the experimental studies, measures of effect were calculated based on Cohen's d, which was calculated as the difference between the pre- and post-treatment mean within a given treatment group divided by the average of the standard deviation of the pre- and post-treatment means [26]. Cohen's d effect measures $\geq$ 0.49 were considered to be weak, values ranging from 0.50-0.79 were considered to be moderate, and values $\geq$ 0.80 were considered to be strong [26]. Note that several experimental studies did not report the information required to calculate Cohen's d, and for these studies effect measures have not been presented.

When possible (e.g., at least 4 studies) we performed meta-analyses to calculate summary odds ratio and Cohen's d effect size measures for the observational and experimental studies, respectively [27]. These summary estimates represent a weighted average of the estimates provided in the various studies included in the meta-analysis. These meta-analyses were performed separately for each health outcomes, separately for observational and experimental studies, and separately based on type of physical activity measurement or exercise modality prescribed.

10.3 RESULTS

10.3.1 LITERATURE REVIEW

The flow of citations through the systematic review process is shown in Figure 3. For each of the 7 health outcomes, several citations were retrieved in more than one of the 6 search engines. After removing duplicates, a total of 437 citations were identified for cholesterol, 1151 for depression, 2505 for injury, 1181 for bone density, 1677 for blood pressure, 5824 for obesity, and 1677 for the metabolic syndrome. Thus, the grand total was 13174. Many of these 13174 citations were retrieved for 2 or more health outcomes, and after removing these duplicates there was a total of 11,088 unique citations. After the titles and abstracts of these 11,088 citations were reviewed, full-text copies of 454 potentially relevant citations were obtained and reviewed. Of these 454 citations, 86 unique citations passed the eligibility criteria and were included in the systematic review. Several of these 86 citations included results for 2 or more of the 7 relevant health outcomes.

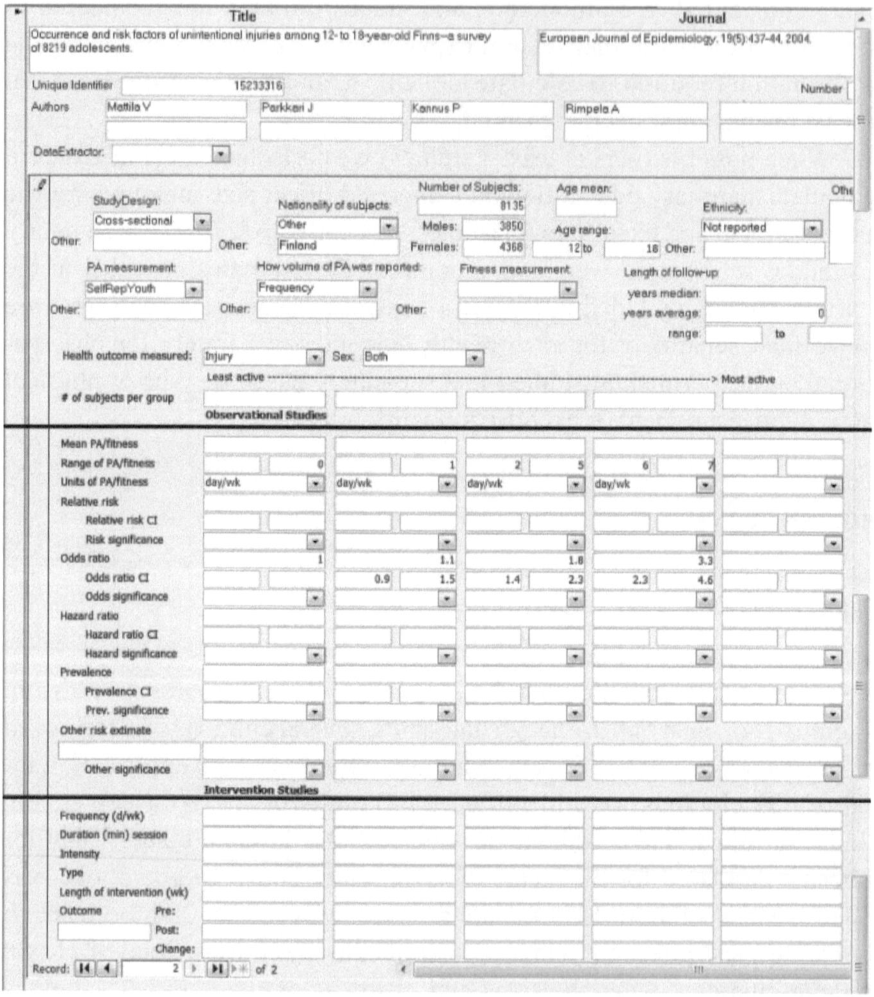

Title: Occurrence and risk factors of unintentional injuries among 12- to 18-year-old Finns—a survey of 8219 adolescents.

Journal: European Journal of Epidemiology, 19(5):437–44, 2004.

Unique Identifier: 15233316

Number:

Authors: Mattila V | Parkkari J | Kannus P | Rimpela A

DataExtractor:

StudyDesign: Cross-sectional

Other:

Nationality of subjects: Other

Other: Finland

Number of Subjects: 8135

Males: 3850

Females: 4368

Age mean:

Age range: 12 to 18

Ethnicity: Not reported

Other:

PA measurement: SelfRepYouth

Other:

How volume of PA was reported: Frequency

Other:

Fitness measurement:

Other:

Length of follow-up

years median:

years average: 0

range: to

Health outcome measured: Injury

Sex: Both

Least active ---> Most active

# of subjects per group					
Observational Studies					
Mean PA/fitness					
Range of PA/fitness	0	1	2 5	6 7	
Units of PA/fitness	day/wk	day/wk	day/wk	day/wk	
Relative risk					
Relative risk CI					
Risk significance					
Odds ratio	1	1.1	1.8	3.3	
Odds ratio CI		0.9 1.5	1.4 2.3	2.3 4.6	
Odds significance					
Hazard ratio					
Hazard ratio CI					
Hazard significance					
Prevalence					
Prevalence CI					
Prev. significance					
Other risk estimate					
Other significance					
Intervention Studies					
Frequency (d/wk)					
Duration (min) session					
Intensity					
Type					
Length of intervention (wk)					
Outcome Pre:					
Post:					
Change:					

Record: 2 of 2

FIGURE 2: Copy of electronic database abstraction form.

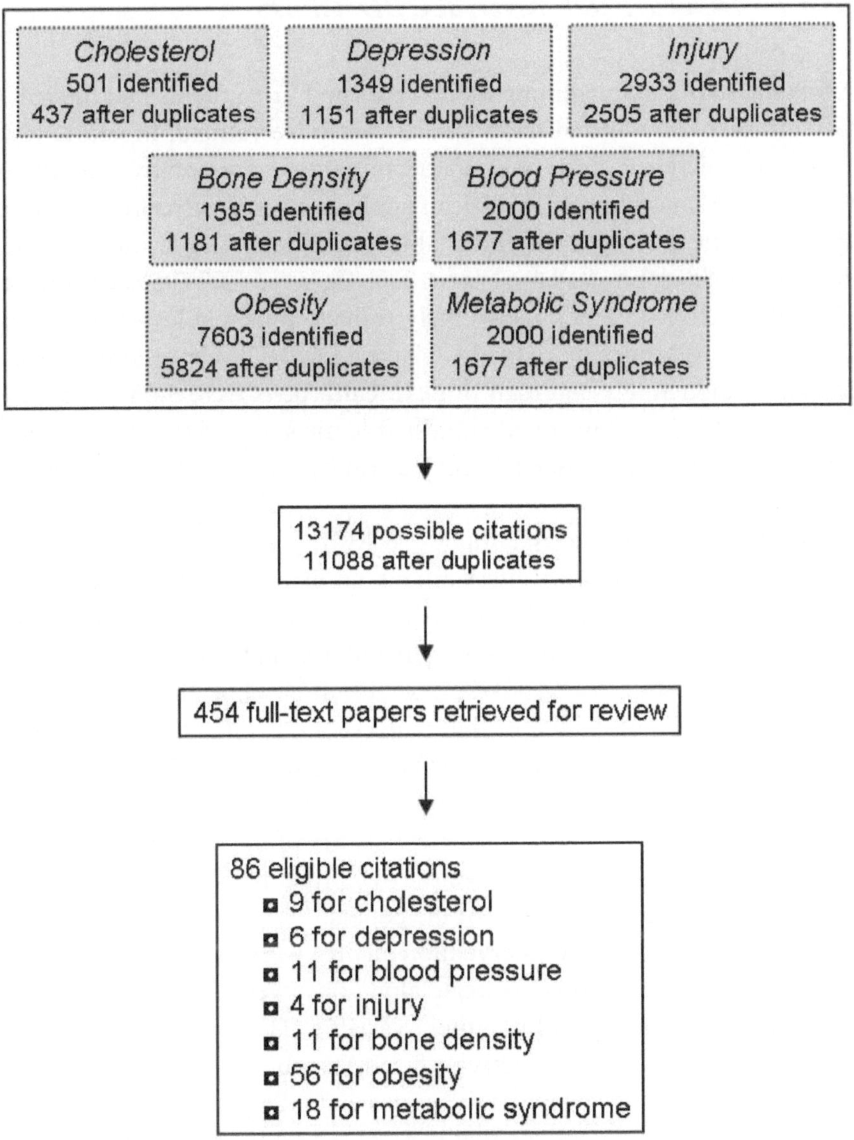

FIGURE 3: Flow of articles through the systematic review.

10.3.2 CHOLESTEROL AND BLOOD LIPIDS

A total of 9 articles examining blood lipids and lipoproteins met the inclusion criteria. Only one of these studies was observational in nature [28]. This cross-sectional study was conducted on a representative sample (n = 3110) of 12-19 year old American adolescents and measured cardiorespiratory fitness using a submaximal treadmill test. The results indicated that unfit girls, defined as the lowest 20% fit, were 1.89 (95% confidence interval: 1.12-3.17) times more likely to have hypercholesterolemia and 1.03 (0.74-1.43) times more likely to have a low HDL-cholesterol by comparison to moderately and high fit girls. Unfit boys were 3.68 (2.55-5.31) times more likely to have hypercholesterolemia and 1.25 (0.79-1.95) times more likely to have a low HDL-cholesterol by comparison to moderately and high fit boys.

A total of 8 experimental studies (6 RCT, 2 non-randomized) examined the effect of exercise interventions on changes in blood lipids and lipoproteins, as summarized in Table 4 [Additional file 4] [29-36]. For the most part, these studies were limited to children and youth with high cholesterol levels [30] or obesity [29,32,34,36] at baseline. The sample sizes were quite small and only 2 of these interventions included more than 37 participants [32,36]. The interventions ranged from 6 to 24 weeks in duration and included anywhere from 1 to 4 hours per week (9-34 minutes per day on average) of prescribed exercise. Six of the 8 exercise programs included various forms of moderate-to-vigorous physical activity as explained in the methods sections of the papers.

The results from these intervention studies were mixed. The 5 studies that were based on aerobic exercise alone observed significant improvements in at least one lipid/lipoprotein variable. The summary effects size measures (95% confidence interval) for the aerobic exercise interventions were -3.03 (-3.22, -2.84) for triglycerides and 0.26 (0.03, 0.49) for HDL-cholesterol. The interventions that were based on resistance training [33] and circuit training [34] reported small and/or insignificant changes for all of the lipid/lipoprotein variables examined, and the effect sizes within these studies tended to be quite small (eg, <0.5). Not surprisingly, the interventions that produced significant changes were also based on the studies that employed the largest sample sizes. This suggests that many of the studies were underpowered.

Due to the design of these interventions (eg, only one dose of exercise prescribed in a given study), the nature of the dose-response relation between exercise and blood lipids in children and youth remains unclear. Furthermore, the interventions that produced favorable effects on blood lipids did not tend to prescribe higher volumes or intensities of exercise by comparison to the interventions that did not produce significant changes. The favorable interventions were, however, based on 'high risk' participants, implying that low volumes of moderate-to-vigorous exercise may be beneficial for youngsters at the greatest risk.

The effects of age and sex have not been adequately addressed in the existing literature. Thus, conclusions cannot be made on the moderating effects of these demographic characteristics on the relation between physical activity and blood lipids in school-aged children and youth.

10.3.3 HIGH BLOOD PRESSURE

A total of 11 articles examining high blood pressure met the systematic review inclusion criteria. Three of these studies were observational in nature (2 cross-sectional, one prospective cohort) (Table 5) [Additional file 5] [28,37,38]. Of these 3 studies, one relied on self-reported measures of physical activity [37] and the remaining two measured cardiorespiratory fitness [28,38]. Within all 3 observational studies the relations between physical activity or fitness with hypertension were weak in magnitude (e.g., odds ratios <1.5), and in one case [28] was insignificant. Only one study examined more than 2 levels of physical activity or fitness (e.g., compared risk estimates across at least 3 groups), and thus was able to provide some insight into the dose-response relation. Within that study only participants within the least fit quartile were more likely to have hypertension relative to participants in the most fit quartile, a finding that was consistent in boys and girls [38].

Eight experimental studies, 4 of which were RCTs, examined the influence of exercise interventions on changes in blood pressure (Table 6)

[Additional file 6] [29,33,34,39-43]. Most of these studies were limited to children and youth with high blood pressure [39-42] or obesity [29,34]. The sample sizes were quite small; only one of these studies included more than 37 participants [42]. The interventions ranged from 4 to 25 weeks in duration. With one exception [43], the interventions included between 60 to 180 minutes/week of prescribed exercise. This equates to 9 to 30 minutes/day when averaged over a week.

Despite the small sample sizes, the results from these intervention studies were positive with reports of significant reductions in systolic blood pressure in response to aerobic exercise training, with effect sizes that all tended to be large (>0.80) [29,39,41-43]. Two of the aerobic based interventions also reported significant reductions (~6% to 11%) in diastolic blood pressure [34,39]. The summary effect size measures for the aerobic exercise interventions were -1.39 (-2.53, -0.24) for systolic blood pressure and -0.39 (-1.72, 0.93) for diastolic blood pressure. Unlike the aerobic-based exercise programs, only two of the four studies that employed other training modalities, such as resistance exercise, reported a significant effect on blood pressure [33,40], with small to modest effect sizes being observed. The summary effect size measures for the non-aerobic exercise interventions were -0.61 (-2.27, 1.05) for systolic blood pressure and -0.51 (-2.18, 1.06) for diastolic blood pressure.

Because the aerobic exercise intervention studies prescribed similar volumes and intensities of exercise, and because they found comparable reductions in blood pressure, the effects of the volume and intensity (moderate vs. vigorous) of exercise on blood pressure remain unclear. Due to limited variations in the age of the participants in these studies, the effects of age on the relation between exercise and blood pressure remains unclear. Most of the studies included both males and females, suggesting that aerobic exercise is effective at controlling blood pressure within box sexes.

10.3.4 METABOLIC SYNDROME

The metabolic syndrome has received considerable research attention in recent years in both adults and youngsters. Sixteen articles examining the metabolic syndrome met the inclusion criteria. The metabolic syndrome components (e.g., abdominal obesity, triglycerides, insulin, HDL-cholesterol, inflammatory markers, etc.) and criteria (e.g., cut-points used to define high-risk values) employed in these studies varied considerably. Eight of the 17 identified studies were observational in nature (7 cross-sectional, 1 prospective), as summarized in Table 7 [Additional file 7] [28,44-51]. Many of these observational studies examined large and heterogeneous samples of participants, suggesting that the findings are quite generalizable to the general population. Of the 3 cross-sectional studies that employed self-reported measures of physical activity, the reported relations with the metabolic syndrome were either weak or modest in strength, and all were non-significant [45,48,49]. The summary odds ratio for the least active group relative to the most active group in these 3 studies was 1.68 (95% confidence interval: 1.22, 2.31). By comparison, the study that used accelerometers to measure physical activity in an objective manner [51] and the 4 studies that used direct measures of cardiorespiratory fitness [28,46,47,50] all reported strong and significant relations with the metabolic syndrome. The summary odds ratio for the least fit group relative to the most fit group in the 4 studies that measured fitness was 6.79 (95% confidence interval: 5.11, 9.03). Further examination of these later studies revealed clear dose-response relations; however, the nature (e.g., linear or curvilinear) of the dose-response relation is unclear. In addition, comparison of the risk estimates in males and females suggests that the relation between physical activity and fitness with the metabolic syndrome is stronger in males. The influence of age on these relations remains uncertain.

Eight experimental studies, 5 of which were RCTs, examined the effect of exercise interventions on changes in markers of the metabolic syndrome, primarily in the form of fasting insulin and insulin resistance (Table 8) [Additional file 8] [32-34,36,52-55]. All but one of these studies was conducted in an overweight/obese sample [33]. The number of participants included in these studies was modest, with all but a single study being limited to 52 participants or less [36]. The exercise interventions ranged from 6 to 40 weeks in duration and included anywhere from 80 to 200 minutes per week (10-30 minutes per average day) of prescribed exercise. About half of the exercise programs were aerobic in nature.

The results from these 8 studies were mixed (Table 8). All of the 4 interventions that focused on aerobic exercise observed significant improvements in at least one of the insulin variables examined. Conversely, only one of the four interventions that employed resistance or circuit training observed any meaningful improvements [54]. The summary effect size measures (95% confidence interval) for fasting insulin in the aerobic and resistance exercise interventions were -0.60 (-1.71, 0.50) and -0.31 (-0.82, 0.19), respectively. No intervention studies systematically considered the influence of the dose or intensity of exercise, or sex and age effects, on markers of the metabolic syndrome. More research is needed to address these issues.

10.3.5 OVERWEIGHT AND OBESITY

The relation between physical activity and fitness with obesity in school-aged children and youth has been extensively studied. A total of 31 observational studies (24 cross-sectional, 3 prospective cohort, 2 case-control, 1 mixed) were retrieved that met the appropriate inclusion criteria, as summarized in Table 9 [Additional file 9] [56-86]. Overweight and obesity were classified using age- and gender-specific body mass index (BMI) criteria (e.g., BMI z-scores) in the majority of these observational studies. The majority of these studies assessed physical activity or sport participation using self- or parental-reported tools. These studies tended to report weak to modest relationships between physical activity and overweight/obesity, with many risk estimates being non-significant. Of the 25 available data points, the median odds ratio for overweight/obesity in the least active group relative to the most active group was 1.33. It is noteworthy that the studies that assessed moderate-to-vigorous intensity physical activities alone were more consistently and strongly related to obesity than the studies that included low intensity activities within the physical activity measure.

Four studies were identified that employed objective measures of physical activity, including one study that used pedometers [73] and 3 studies that used accelerometers [59,67,83]. These studies tended to report significant relations between physical activity with overweight/obesity that were strong in magnitude. Of the 8 available data points for cross-sectional findings, the median odds ratio was 3.79. An additional 4 studies measured the relation between cardiorespiratory fitness and obesity [75,76,82]. All of these studies reported significant relations between physical activity and fitness with overweight/obesity that were modest to strong in magnitude.

Several of the observational studies examining overweight and obesity presented analyses that were stratified by sex [56-58,60,64,67,71,73-75,77,79,81]. Although sex differences were rarely tested for using the appropriate statistical techniques, visual inspection of the risk estimates provided suggests that in 12 of the 14 studies the associations between physical activity and fitness with obesity were stronger in males than in females.

Many of the observational studies presented their results in a manner that permitted the dose-response relations with obesity to be examined [57,59,61,62,64,65,69,71,73,74,79,80,82,84]. From these studies it is apparent that a dose-response relation between physical activity and obesity exists. However, the pattern of this dose-response relation is unclear as some studies observed linear patterns and others observed curvilinear patterns.

In addition to the observational studies discussed above, 24 intervention studies, 17 of which were RCTs, examining changes in obesity measures were included in the systematic review (Table 10) [Additional file 10] [29,32,34-36,39,42,43,52-55,87-98]. It is important to note that in many of these studies the primary aim of the intervention was to improve other health measures (e.g., blood lipids, insulin resistance, and bone density) and not obesity measures per se. These studies examined several different measures of total (% fat, BMI, weight) and abdominal (waist circumference, trunk fat, visceral fat) adiposity. The studies ranged in length from 4 weeks to 2 years, with most being 4 to 6 months in duration. The amounts of exercise prescribed typically ranged from 2 to 3.5 hours per week, which averages out to 17 to 30 minutes per day. Half of the studies were limited to overweight and obese participants.

About 50% of the exercise interventions that were aerobic in nature observed significant changes in measures of BMI, total fat, and/or abdominal fat in response to training. Only 3 of the 17 studies that employed other training modalities (resistance training, circuit training, pilates, jumping exercises) observed significant improvements in measures of total fat, abdominal fat, or BMI in response to training. The effect sizes, even for the studies that found significant improvements, tended to be small (<0.50). For the interventions that were based on aerobic exercise, the summary effect size measures were -0.40 (-1.10, 0.31) for % body fat and -0.07 (-0.89, 0.75) for BMI. For the resistance exercise intervention, the summary effect size calculation for % body fat was -0.19 (-1.55, 1.18).

Variations in the effects of age, sex, and exercise dose on changes in obesity measures in response to exercise training have not been systematically addressed in the literature. Thus, no conclusions can be drawn on the potential moderating effects of these variables.

10.3.6 BONE MINERAL DENSITY

Many observational studies have examined the relation between physical activity and continuous measures of bone mineral density such as bone mineral content values in grams, bone density values in g/cm^2, and cortical bone area measures in cm^2 (see review [99]). However, no observational studies in the literature search met the systematic review criteria of predicting a low bone mineral density as a dichotomous outcome.

As summarized in Table 11 [Additional file 11], a total of 11 experimental studies examining changes in bone mineral density in response to exercise training were retrieved in the systematic review [55,88-94,100-103]. Two of these studies presented identical data on the same group of participants, and were therefore presented as a single study in the table [101,102]. The physical activity programs employed in these interventions typically consisted of moderate-to-high strain anaerobic activities such as impact resistance training, high impact weight bearing, and jumping. These programs were performed anywhere from 3 to 60 minutes in length on at least 2 or 3 days of the week, and lasted from a few months to 2 years in duration.

The results from these studies, although not undisputed, indicate that as little as 10 minutes of moderate-to-high impact activities performed on as little as 2 or 3 days of the week can have a modest effect on bone mineral density when combined with more general weight bearing aerobic activities that are also beneficial for cardiovascular risk factors and obesity prevention (e.g., jogging, play, etc.).

10.3.7 DEPRESSION

Only 6 studies on depression and related symptoms met the inclusion criteria. Table 12 [Additional file 12] outlines the 3 observational studies [104-106]. These were all cross-sectional in design, used self-reported measures of physical activity, and reported small and insignificant [104,106] or modest [105] relations between physical activity and depression. Interestingly, within the later study the relation between physical activity and depression were more evident at a moderate intensity of physical activity than at a vigorous intensity of physical activity [105].

The 3 experimental studies that examined changes in depression [107-109], all of which were RCTs based on aerobic exercise, are outlined in Table 13 [Additional file 13]. The volume of exercise prescribed in these studies was very modest (60 to 90 minutes per week). All three of these studies observed significant improvements in at least one depressive symptom measure in response to 8 to 12 week exercise programs. The effect sizes were small to modest in these studies, with very broad 95% confidence intervals. One of the studies included both high intensity and moderate intensity exercise programs, and only the high intensity program resulted in significant improvements in depression scores in comparison to the control group, which performed flexibility exercises [108].

10.3.8 INJURIES

Injuries are a leading cause of disability and mortality in young people. It has been reported that approximately 50% of medically treated injuries within 6th to 10th grade Canadian youth occur during physical activity [110]. Thus, it is not surprising that there is an extensive literature on physical activity and injuries in the pediatric population (see review [111]). However, most of the published information is limited to groups of participants that have all been injured or groups of participants comprised entirely of athletes (eg, football players, ballet dancers).

Only 3 articles examining injury met the inclusion criteria for this systematic review [112-114]. These studies were all cross-sectional in nature and relied on self- or parental-reported measures of physical activity and sports participation (Table 14) [Additional file 14]. These studies examined medically treated injuries; however, limited or no information on the severity of and long-term recovery from these injuries was presented. All 3 of the studies reported higher rates of injury in physically active children and youth compared with inactive children and youth. Furthermore, within all 3 of the papers there was clear evidence of a dose-response relation between physical activity participation and the likelihood of injury. That is, as the physical activity level increased, the likelihood of injury increased in a graded fashion. One study assessed vigorous sports, and within that study the risk estimates for injury within the most active group would be considered high [114]. Conversely the risk estimates for injury were modest within the 2 studies that measured moderate-to-vigorous intensity activities [112,113]. The quality of the evidence for the injury outcome, which is based on cross-sectional studies, is limited as cross-sectional research only provides a low level of evidence. Follow-up (incidence) studies that also take into consideration the volume of sports participation would provide a more powerful level of evidence.

10.3.9 QUALITY ASSESSMENT OF RCTS

The RCTs that are listed within the summary tables contained several significant limitations. The study samples were small, and non-representative. Although few of the studies addressed the issue of statistical power, the lack of power was clearly an issue. Specifically, for a number of the health outcomes, the RCTs in which significant findings were observed were also the RCTs with the largest sample sizes. Almost without exception, the RCTs included in the systematic review did not report adverse events for the physical activity interventions (e.g., injuries), provided little or no detail on the drop-outs, and did not perform intent-to-treat analyses. Given the consistency of these limitations across studies, Level 2 was the highest level that could be assigned to any of the recommendations.

10.4 DISCUSSION

10.4.1 RECOMMENDATIONS BASED ON SYSTEMATIC REVIEW

10.4.1.1 RECOMMENDATION #1: CHILDREN AND YOUTH 5-17 YEARS OF AGE SHOULD ACCUMULATE AN AVERAGE OF AT LEAST 60 MINUTES PER DAY AND UP TO SEVERAL HOURS OF AT LEAST MODERATE INTENSITY PHYSICAL ACTIVITY. SOME OF THE HEALTH BENEFITS CAN BE ACHIEVED THROUGH AN AVERAGE OF 30 MINUTES PER DAY. [LEVEL 2, GRADE A]

There is strong and consistent evidence based on experimental studies for several health outcomes that participating in as little as 2 or 3 hours of moderate-to-vigorously intense physical activity per week is associated with health benefits. Evidence from observational studies also demonstrates dose-response relations between physical activity and health, with differences in health risk between the least active (or fit) and the second least active (of fit) groups. Thus, it would seem appropriate to set minimal physical activity targets that reflect a low level of physical activity (see Recommendation #1). Furthermore, the current recommendation of 90 minutes more per day (Canadian) or 60 minutes per day (US, UK, Australian) may be quite intimidating, particularly for children and youth who are very inactive. From a behaviour modification perspective, having a target that seems out of reach may actually undermine physical activity participation [115].

That being said, with the exception of injuries, the dose-response evidence from observational studies for several health outcomes suggests that more physical activity will be better, and that additional health benefits can still be achieved at the higher end of the physical activity spectrum. Therefore, it would also seem appropriate to set higher physical activity targets (60 minutes and up to several hours) that would elicit more pronounced health benefits for those children and youth who are already somewhat active (see Recommendation #1). This approach is consistent with recommendations made by the U.S. National Association for Sports and Physical Education [116] and the Australia Department of Health and Ageing [117], both of whom have recommended that children and youth participate in at least 60 minutes, and up to several hours, of moderate to vigorous intensity physical activity every day.

This type of dual message provided in Recommendation #1 will hopefully encourage children and youth who are very inactive to engage in at least a modest amount of physical activity, while at the same time encourage moderately active children and youth to achieve even greater benefits by becoming more active. The minimal and optimal doses of physical activity required for good health in children and youth remain unclear, and more carefully conducted dose-responses studies are warranted in the pediatric age range.

Previous physical activity recommendations and guidelines for school-aged children and youth indicate that a high volume of physical activity needs to be performed everyday. The need for children and youth to engage in physical activity on a daily basis to maintain good health was not supported by the evidence reviewed here. In other words, it is unknown as to whether a child who accumulates 7 hours of activity over the week, with one hour being performed on each day, would have any greater health benefits than a child who accumulates 7 hours of activity over the week, with different amounts of activity being performed each day (including some days with no activity). Thus, the recommendation made in this systematic review calls for an "average" of at least 60 minutes per day instead of at least 60 minutes everyday. Future studies need to address whether a "days per week" recommendation is warranted. In addition, future studies within children and youth should consider whether the daily physical activity needs to be accumulated in bouts of at least a few minutes in duration (eg, 5 or 10 minutes). Most children accumulate the majority of their physical activity in a very sporadic manner (eg, a couple of minutes here and there), and new evidence suggests that this sporadic pattern of activity may not be as beneficial as bouts of activity that last at least 5 minutes in length [118].

Given the positive effect of physical activity on 6 of the 7 health outcomes examined, including observations from several large and diverse samples, this Recommendation was assigned a Grade A.

10.4.1.2 RECOMMENDATION #2: MORE VIGOROUS INTENSITY ACTIVITIES SHOULD BE INCORPORATED OR ADDED WHEN POSSIBLE, INCLUDING ACTIVITIES THAT STRENGTHEN MUSCLE AND BONE. [LEVEL 3, GRADE B].

Moderate intensity activity in children and youth has been defined in a variety of ways, depending on the method chosen to measure physical activity. The lower threshold of moderate intensity activity is usually defined as 4 METS (4 × resting metabolic rate), although it is not uncommon for investigators to use 3 METS. In general, the lower threshold of vigorous intensity activity is usually defined as 7 METS (7 × resting metabolic rate) in children.

The majority of observational studies have focused on measuring moderate-to-vigorous intensity physical activity. Furthermore, the relations between overall physical activity (including low intensity activities) and obesity do not appear to be as strong or consistent as the relations between moderate-to-vigorous intensity activity and obesity. In addition, the intervention studies included within this systematic review almost exclusively prescribed physical activity of at least a moderate intensity. Thus, while it is clear that moderate and vigorous intensity activities are associated with many health benefits, the same is not true for low intensity activity. Therefore, Recommendation #1 indicates that the physical activity should be of at least a moderate intensity. More consideration on the impact of low intensity activities on health should be given in future studies.

The next question to address is whether vigorous intensity activities provide benefits above and beyond that of moderate intensity activities. Regrettably, few studies have systematically addressed this question. The available information suggests that vigorous intensity activities provide additional health benefits beyond modest intensity activities. Furthermore, many of the experimental studies that observed significant changes in the health variables examined prescribed exercise that would fall within the vigorous intensity or upper-end of the moderate intensity range. Recommendation #2, therefore, suggests that vigorous intensity activities should be included when possible. This recommendation was assigned a lower level of evidence (Level 3) because of the limited amount of evidence and the inconsistency in the evidence that is available. This recommendation was given a lower grade (Grade C) because of the potential increase in injury risk associated with more vigorous intensity activities and sports. However, the injury data is weak and future studies, particularly intervention studies, should examine and report on injuries associated with physical activity in children.

10.4.1.3 RECOMMENDATION #3: AEROBIC ACTIVITIES SHOULD MAKE UP THE MAJORITY OF THE PHYSICAL ACTIVITY. MUSCLE AND BONE STRENGTHENING ACTIVITIES SHOULD BE INCORPORATED ON AT LEAST 3 DAYS OF THE WEEK. [LEVEL 2, GRADE A].

Many of the health outcomes examined, particularly obesity and the cardiometabolic health measures, responded almost exclusively to aerobic exercise interventions. It is also likely that most of the activity that was captured in the observational studies was aerobic in nature. Recommendation #3 therefore suggests that physical activity should focus on aerobic activities. However, bone health was more favorably affected by modest amounts of resistance training and other high-impact activities (jumping) that were performed on at least 2 or 3 days of the week. Thus, this recommendation indicates that a small amount of bone strengthening activities should be incorporated.

10.4.2 LIMITATIONS

This systematic review has several limitations, many of which related to practical issues around conducting the study (e.g., budgetary, human resource, and time constraints). First, because we did not include unpublished studies and studies that were published in a language other than English, and because we did not perform an extensive cross-referencing of the references lists from the papers that were retrieved in the electronic databases, several relevant papers may be been excluded. Second, the review was limited to 7 health outcomes and did not include several other outcomes that may be relevant for children and youth such as academic performance, emerging cardiometabolic risk factors (e.g., endothelial function, inflammatory markers), risky and aggressive behaviours (e.g., substance use and abuse, bullying and fighting), and measures of mental health and well-being outside of depression. Third, a large percentage of observational studies in the area were excluded because they did not report their findings in a dichotomous manner. Together, these limitations may have biased the Results and Recommendations that were made. Nonetheless, despite these limitations and the differences in methodology employed, the recommendations made here are remarkably comparable to the recommendations for children and youth that were part of the recently completed "Physical Activity Guidelines for Americans" project [21]. The reader is referred to the Expert Panel report for a more comprehensive discussion of the limitations of this systematic review [13].

10.5 CONCLUSION

In summary, the findings of this systematic review confirm that physical activity is associated with numerous health benefits in school-aged children and youth. The dose-response relations between physical activity and health that were observed in several observational studies suggest that the more physical activity, the greater the health benefit. However, the results from several experimental studies suggested that even modest amounts of physical activity can have tremendous health benefits in high-risk youngsters (e.g., obese, high blood pressure). To achieve substantive health benefits, the physical activity should be of at least a moderate intensity, and it should be recognized that vigorous intensity activities may provide an even greater benefit. Aerobic-based activities that stress the cardiovascular and respiratory systems have the greatest health benefit, other than for bone health, in which case high-impact weight bearing activities are required.

REFERENCES

1. Health Canada, Canadian Society for Exercise Physiology: Canada's Physical Activity Guide for Youth. Ottawa: Minister of Public Works and Government Services Canada; 2002.
2. Health Canada, Canadian Society for Exercise Physiology: Canada's Physical Activity Guideline for Children. Ottawa: Minister of Public Works and Government Services Canada; 2002.
3. Janssen I: Physical activity guidelines for children and youth. Can J Public Health 2007, 98(Suppl 2):S109-121.
4. Twisk JW: Physical activity guidelines for children and adolescents: a critical review. Sports Med 2001, 31(8):617-627.
5. Tolfrey K, Jones AM, Campbell IG: The effect of aerobic exercise training on the lipid-lipoprotein profile of children and adolescents. Sports Med 2000, 29(2):99-112.
6. Kelley GA, Kelley KS: Exercise and resting blood pressure in children and adolescents: a meta-analysis. Ped Exerc Sci 2003, 15:83-97.
7. Reilly JJ, McDowell ZC: Physical activity interventions in the prevention and treatment of paediatric obesity: systematic review and critical appraisal. Proc Nutr Soc 2003, 62(3):611-619.
8. Etnier JL, Nowell PM, Landers DM, Sibley BA: A meta-regression to examine the relationship between aerobic fitness and cognitive performance. Brain Res Brain Res Rev 2006, 52(1):119-130.
9. Cook DJ, Mulrow CD, Haynes RB: Systematic reviews: synthesis of best evidence for clinical decisions. Ann Intern Med 1997, 126(5):376-380.
10. Warburton DER, Charlesworth S, Ivey A, Nettlefold L, Bredin SSD: A systematic review of the evidence for Canada's Physical Activity Guidelines for Adults. Int J Behav Nutr Phys Act 2010, 7:39.
11. Paterson DH, Warburton DER: Physical activity and functional limitations in older adults: a systematic review related to Canada's Physical Activity Guidelines. Int J Behav Nutr Phys Act 2010, 7:38.
12. Tremblay MS, Kho ME, Tricco AC, Duggan M: Process description and evaluation of Canadian Physical Activity Guidelines development. Int J Behav Nutr Phys Act 2010, 7:42.
13. Kesaniemi A, Riddoch CJ, Reeder B, Blair SN, Sorensen TIA: Advancing the future of physical activity guidelines in Canada: an independent expert panel interpretation of the evidence. Int J Behav Nutr Phys Act 2010, 7:41.
14. Health Canada, Canadian Society for Exercise Physiology: Family Guide to Physical Activity for Youth 10-14 Years of Age. Minister of Public Works and Government Services Canada; 2002.
15. Health Canada, Canadian Society for Exercise Physiology: Family Guide to Physical Activity for Children 6-9 Years of Age. Minister of Public Works and Government Services Canada; 2002.

16. Health Canada, Canadian Society for Exercise Physiology: Teacher's Guide to Physical Activity for Youth 10-14 Years of Age. Minister of Public Works and Government Services Canada; 2002.
17. Health Canada, Canadian Society for Exercise Physiology: Teacher's Guide to Physical Activity for Children 6-9 Years of Age. Minister of Public Works and Government Services Canada; 2002.
18. Health Canada, Canadian Society for Exercise Physiology: Gotta Move! Magazine for Children 6-9 Years of Age. Minister of Public Works and Government Services Canada; 2002.
19. Health Canada, Canadian Society for Exercise Physiology: Let's Get Active! Magazine for Youth 10-14 Years of Age of Public Works and Government Services Canada. 2002.
20. Strong WB, Malina RM, Blimkie CJ, Daniels SR, Dishman RK, Gutin B, Hergenroeder AC, Must A, Nixon PA, Pivarnik JM, Rowland T, Trost S, Trudeau F: Evidence based physical activity for school-age youth. J Pediatr 2005, 146(6):732-737.
21. Physical Activity Guidelines Advisory Committee: Physical Activity Guidelines Advisory Committee Report, 2008. Washington, DC: U.S. Department of Health and Human Services; 2008.
22. Baquet G, van Praagh E, Berthoin S: Endurance training and aerobic fitness in young people. Sports Med 2003, 33(15):1127-1143.
23. Lau DC, Douketis JD, Morrison KM, Hramiak IM, Sharma AM, Ur E: 2006 Canadian clinical practice guidelines on the management and prevention of obesity in adults and children [summary]. CMAJ 2007, 176(8):S1-13.
24. Downs SH, Black N: The feasibility of creating a checklist for the assessment of the methodological quality both of randomised and non-randomised studies of health care interventions. J Epidemiol Community Health 1998, 52:377-384.
25. Oleckno WA: Essential Epidemiology: Principles and Applications. Long Grove, IL: Waveland Press; 2002.
26. Cohen J: Statistical power calculations for the behavioral sciences. 2nd edition. Hillsdale: Lawrence Erlbaum Associates; 1988.
27. Petitti DB: Meta-Analysis, Decision Analysis, and Cost-Effective Analysis. New York, NY: Oxford University Press; 1994.
28. Carnethon MR, Gulati M, Greenland P: Prevalence and cardiovascular disease correlates of low cardiorespiratory fitness in adolescents and adults. JAMA 2005, 294(23):2981-2988.
29. Kahle EB, Zipf WB, Lamb DR, Horswill CA, Ward KM: Association between mild, routine exercise and improved insulin dynamics and glucose control in obese adolescents. Int J Sports Med 1996, 17(1):1-6.
30. Hardin DS, Hebert JD, Bayden T, Dehart M, Mazur L: Treatment of childhood syndrome X. Pediatrics 1997, 100(2):E5.
31. Stergioulas A, Tripolitsioti A, Messinis D, Bouloukos A, Nounopoulos C: The effects of endurance training on selected coronary risk factors in children. Acta Paediatr 1998, 87(4):401-404.
32. Ferguson MA, Gutin B, Le NA, Karp W, Litaker M, Humphries M, Okuyama T, Riggs S, Owens S: Effects of exercise training and its cessation on components of

the insulin resistance syndrome in obese children. Int J Obes Relat Metab Disord 1999, 23(8):889-895.
33. Lau PWC, CW Y, Lee A, Sung RYT: The physiological and psychological effects of resistance training on Chinese obese adolescents. Journal of Exercise Science and Fitness 2004, 2(2):115-120.
34. Bell LM, Watts K, Siafarikas A, Thompson A, Ratnam N, Bulsara M, Finn J, O'Driscoll G, Green DJ, Jones TW, Davis EA: Exercise alone reduces insulin resistance in obese children independently of changes in body composition. J Clin Endocrinol Metab 2007, 92(11):4230-4235.
35. Heyman E, Toutain C, Delamarche P, Berthon P, Briard D, Youssef H, Dekerdanet M, Gratas-Delamarche A: Exercise training and cardiovascular risk factors in type 1 diabetic adolescent girls. Pediatr Exerc Sci 2007, 19(4):408-419.
36. Meyer AA, Kundt G, Lenschow U, Schuff-Werner P, Kienast W: Improvement of early vascular changes and cardiovascular risk factors in obese children after a six-month exercise program. J Am Coll Cardiol 2006, 48(9):1865-1870.
37. Dasgupta K, O'Loughlin J, Chen S, Karp I, Paradis G, Tremblay J, Hamet P, Pilote L: Emergence of sex differences in prevalence of high systolic blood pressure: analysis of a longitudinal adolescent cohort. Circulation 2006, 114(24):2663-2670.
38. Nielsen GA, Andersen LB: The association between high blood pressure, physical fitness, and body mass index in adolescents. Prev Med 2003, 36(2):229-234.
39. Hagberg JM, Goldring D, Ehsani AA, Heath GW, Hernandez A, Schechtman K, Holloszy JO: Effect of exercise training on the blood pressure and hemodynamic features of hypertensive adolescents. Am J Cardiol 1983, 52(7):763-768.
40. Hagberg JM, Ehsani AA, Goldring D, Hernandez A, Sinacore DR, Holloszy JO: Effect of weight training on blood pressure and hemodynamics in hypertensive adolescents. J Pediatr 1984, 104(1):147-151.
41. Danforth JS, Allen KD, Fitterling JM, Danforth JA, Farrar D, Brown M, Drabman RS: Exercise as a treatment for hypertension in low-socioeconomic-status black children. J Consult Clin Psychol 1990, 58(2):237-239.
42. Ewart CK, Young DR, Hagberg JM: Effects of school-based aerobic exercise on blood pressure in adolescent girls at risk for hypertension. Am J Public Health 1998, 88(6):949-951.
43. Jago R, Jonker ML, Missaghian M, Baranowski T: Effect of 4 weeks of Pilates on the body composition of young girls. Prev Med 2006, 42(3):177-180.
44. Yin Z, Davis CL, Moore JB, Treiber FA: Physical activity buffers the effects of chronic stress on adiposity in youth. Ann Behav Med 2005, 29(1):29-36.
45. Ramirez-Lopez G, Gonzalez-Villalpando C, Sanchez-Corona J, Salmeron-Castro J, Gonzalez-Ortiz M, Celis-de la Rosa A, Valles-Sanchez V: Weight, physical activity, and smoking as determinants of insulinemia in adolescents. Arch Med Res 2001, 32(3):208-213.
46. Andersen LB, Hasselstrom H, Gronfeldt V, Hansen SE, Karsten F: The relationship between physical fitness and clustered risk, and tracking of clustered risk from adolescence to young adulthood: eight years follow-up in the Danish Youth and Sport Study. Int J Behav Nutr Phys Act 2004, 1(1):6.
47. Eiberg A, Hasselstrom H, Gronfeldt V, Froberg K, Cooper A, Andersen LB: Physical fitness as a predictor of cardiovascular disease risk factors in 6- to 7-year-old Danish

children: The Copenhagen school-child intervention study. Pediatr Exerc Sci 2005, 17:161-170.

48. Hasselstrom H, Karlsson KM, Hansen SE, Gronfeldt V, Froberg K, Andersen LB: Peripheral bone mineral density and different intensities of physical activity in children 6-8 years old: the Copenhagen School Child Intervention study. Calcif Tissue Int 2007, 80(1):31-38.
49. Kelishadi R, Razaghi EM, Gouya MM, Ardalan G, Gheiratmand R, Delavari A, Motaghian M, Ziaee V, Siadat ZD, Majdzadeh R, Heshmat R, Barekati H, Arabi MS, Heidarzadeh A, Shariatinejad K: Association of physical activity and the metabolic syndrome in children and adolescents: CASPIAN Study. Horm Res 2007, 67(1):46-52.
50. Anderssen SA, Cooper AR, Riddoch C, Sardinha LB, Harro M, Brage S, Andersen LB: Low cardiorespiratory fitness is a strong predictor for clustering of cardiovascular disease risk factors in children independent of country, age and sex. Eur J Cardiovasc Prev Rehabil 2007, 14(4):526-531.
51. Andersen LB, Harro M, Sardinha LB, Froberg K, Ekelund U, Brage S, Anderssen SA: Physical activity and clustered cardiovascular risk in children: a cross-sectional study (The European Youth Heart Study). Lancet 2006, 368(9532):299-304.
52. Carrel AL, Clark RR, Peterson SE, Nemeth BA, Sullivan J, Allen DB: Improvement of fitness, body composition, and insulin sensitivity in overweight children in a school-based exercise program: a randomized, controlled study. Arch Pediatr Adolesc Med 2005, 159(10):963-968.
53. Nassis GP, Papantakou K, Skenderi K, Triandafillopoulou M, Kavouras SA, Yannakoulia M, Chrousos GP, Sidossis LS: Aerobic exercise training improves insulin sensitivity without changes in body weight, body fat, adiponectin, and inflammatory markers in overweight and obese girls. Metabolism 2005, 54(11):1472-1479.
54. Shaibi GQ, Cruz ML, Ball GD, Weigensberg MJ, Salem GJ, Crespo NC, Goran MI: Effects of resistance training on insulin sensitivity in overweight Latino adolescent males. Med Sci Sports Exerc 2006, 38(7):1208-1215.
55. Treuth MS, Hunter GR, Figueroa-Colon R, Goran MI: Effects of strength training on intra-abdominal adipose tissue in obese prepubertal girls. Med Sci Sports Exerc 1998, 30(12):1738-1743.
56. Gordon-Larsen P, Adair LS, Popkin BM: Ethnic differences in physical activity and inactivity patterns and overweight status. Obes Res 2002, 10(3):141-149.
57. Eisenmann JC, Bartee RT, Wang MQ: Physical activity, TV viewing, and weight in U.S. youth: 1999 Youth Risk Behavior Survey. Obes Res 2002, 10(5):379-385.
58. Kim J, Must A, Fitzmaurice GM, Gillman MW, Chomitz V, Kramer E, McGowan R, Peterson KE: Relationship of physical fitness to prevalence and incidence of overweight among schoolchildren. Obes Res 2005, 13(7):1246-1254.
59. Dencker M, Thorsson O, Karlsson MK, Linden C, Eiberg S, Wollmer P, Andersen LB: Daily physical activity related to body fat in children aged 8-11 years. J Pediatr 2006, 149(1):38-42.
60. Rosenberg DE, Sallis JF, Conway TL, Cain KL, McKenzie TL: Active transportation to school over 2 years in relation to weight status and physical activity. Obesity (Silver Spring) 2006, 14(10):1771-1776.

61. Laxmaiah A, Nagalla B, Vijayaraghavan K, Nair M: Factors affecting prevalence of overweight among 12- to 17-year-old urban adolescents in Hyderabad, India. Obesity (Silver Spring) 2007, 15(6):1384-1390.
62. Hernandez B, Gortmaker SL, Colditz GA, Peterson KE, Laird NM, Parra-Cabrera S: Association of obesity with physical activity, television programs and other forms of video viewing among children in Mexico city. Int J Obes Relat Metab Disord 1999, 23(8):845-854.
63. Tremblay MS, Willms JD: Is the Canadian childhood obesity epidemic related to physical inactivity? Int J Obes Relat Metab Disord 2003, 27(9):1100-1105.
64. Janssen I, Katzmarzyk PT, Boyce WF, King MA, Pickett W: Overweight and obesity in Canadian adolescents and their associations with dietary habits and physical activity patterns. J Adolesc Health 2004, 35(5):360-367.
65. Veugelers PJ, Fitzgerald AL: Prevalence of and risk factors for childhood overweight and obesity. CMAJ 2005, 173(6):607-613.
66. Ha A, Bae S, Urrutia-Rijas X, Singh KP: Eating and physical activity pracitces in risk of overweight and overweight children. Nutrition Research 2005, 25:905-915.
67. Ness AR, Leary SD, Mattocks C, Blair SN, Reilly JJ, Wells J, Ingle S, Tilling K, Smith GD, Riddoch C: Objectively measured physical activity and fat mass in a large cohort of children. PLoS Med 2007, 4(3):e97.
68. Li Y, Zhai F, Yang X, Schouten EG, Hu X, He Y, Luan D, Ma G: Determinants of childhood overweight and obesity in China. Br J Nutr 2007, 97(1):210-215.
69. Smith BJ, Phongsavan P, Havea D, Halavatau V, Chey T: Body mass index, physical activity and dietary behaviours among adolescents in the Kingdom of Tonga. Public Health Nutr 2007, 10(2):137-144.
70. Urrutia-Rojas X, Menchaca J: Prevalence of risk for type 2 diabetes in school children. J Sch Health 2006, 76(5):189-194.
71. Guerra S, Teixeira-Pinto A, Ribeiro JC, Ascensao A, Magalhaes J, Andersen LB, Duarte JA, Mota J: Relationship between physical activity and obesity in children and adolescents. J Sports Med Phys Fitness 2006, 46(1):79-83.
72. Ochoa MC, Moreno-Aliaga MJ, Martinez-Gonzalez MA, Martinez JA, Marti A: Predictor factors for childhood obesity in a Spanish case-control study. Nutrition 2007, 23(5):379-384.
73. Eisenmann JC, Laurson KR, Wickel EE, Gentile D, Walsh D: Utility of pedometer step recommendations for predicting overweight in children. Int J Obes (Lond) 2007, 31(7):1179-1182.
74. McMurray RG, Harrell JS, Deng S, Bradley CB, Cox LM, Bangdiwala SI: The influence of physical activity, socioeconomic status, and ethnicity on the weight status of adolescents. Obes Res 2000, 8(2):130-139.
75. Burke V, Beilin LJ, Durkin K, Stritzke WG, Houghton S, Cameron CA: Television, computer use, physical activity, diet and fatness in Australian adolescents. Int J Pediatr Obes 2006, 1(4):248-255.
76. Psarra G, Nassis GP, Sidossis LS: Short-term predictors of abdominal obesity in children. Eur J Public Health 2006, 16(5):520-525.
77. Yang X, Telama R, Viikari J, Raitakari OT: Risk of obesity in relation to physical activity tracking from youth to adulthood. Med Sci Sports Exerc 2006, 38(5):919-925.

78. Neutzling MB, Taddei JA, Gigante DP: Risk factors of obesity among Brazilian adolescents: a case-control study. Public Health Nutr 2003, 6(8):743-749.
79. O'Loughlin J, Paradis G, Renaud L, Meshefedjian G, Gray-Donald K: Prevalence and correlates of overweight among elementary schoolchildren in multiethnic, low income, inner-city neighbourhoods in Montreal, Canada. Ann Epidemiol 1998, 8(7):422-432.
80. Fiore H, Travis S, Whalen A, Auinger P, Ryan S: Potentially protective factors associated with healthful body mass index in adolescents with obese and nonobese parents: a secondary data analysis of the third national health and nutrition examination survey, 1988-1994. J Am Diet Assoc 2006, 106(1):55-64-64.
81. te Velde SJ, De Bourdeaudhuij I, Thorsdottir I, Rasmussen M, Hagstromer M, Klepp KI, Brug J: Patterns in sedentary and exercise behaviors and associations with overweight in 9-14-year-old boys and girls--a cross-sectional study. BMC Public Health 2007, 7:16.
82. Hanley AJ, Harris SB, Gittelsohn J, Wolever TM, Saksvig B, Zinman B: Overweight among children and adolescents in a Native Canadian community: prevalence and associated factors. Am J Clin Nutr 2000, 71(3):693-700.
83. Stevens J, Murray DM, Baggett CD, Elder JP, Lohman TG, Lytle LA, Pate RR, Pratt CA, Treuth MS, Webber LS, Young DR: Objectively assessed associations between physical activity and body composition in middle-school girls: the Trial of Activity for Adolescent Girls. Am J Epidemiol 2007, 166(11):1298-1305.
84. Kuriyan R, Bhat S, Thomas T, Vaz M, Kurpad AV: Television viewing and sleep are associated with overweight among urban and semi-urban South Indian children. Nutr J 2007, 6:25.
85. Muecke L, Simons-Morton B, Huang IW, Parcel G: Is childhood obesity associated with high-fat foods and low physical activity? J Sch Health 1992, 62(1):19-23.
86. Delva J, O'Malley PM, Johnston LD: Health-related behaviors and overweight: a study of Latino adolescents in the United States of America. Rev Panam Salud Publica 2007, 21(1):11-20.
87. Jette M, Barry W, Pearlman L: The effects of an extracurricular physical activity program on obese adolescents. Canadian Journal of Public Health 1977, 68(1):39-42.
88. Blimkie CJ, Rice S, Webber CE, Martin J, Levy D, Gordon CL: Effects of resistance training on bone mineral content and density in adolescent females. Can J Physiol Pharmacol 1996, 74(9):1025-1033.
89. Morris FL, Naughton GA, Gibbs JL, Carlson JS, Wark JD: Prospective ten-month exercise intervention in premenarcheal girls: positive effects on bone and lean mass. J Bone Miner Res 1997, 12(9):1453-1462.
90. McKay HA, Petit MA, Schutz RW, Prior JC, Barr SI, Khan KM: Augmented trochanteric bone mineral density after modified physical education classes: a randomized school-based exercise intervention study in prepubescent and early pubescent children. J Pediatr 2000, 136(2):156-162.
91. Nichols DL, Sanborn CF, Love AM: Resistance training and bone mineral density in adolescent females. J Pediatr 2001, 139(4):494-500.

92. MacKelvie KJ, Petit MA, Khan KM, Beck TJ, McKay HA: Bone mass and structure are enhanced following a 2-year randomized controlled trial of exercise in prepubertal boys. Bone 2004, 34(4):755-764.
93. Linden C, Ahlborg HG, Besjakov J, Gardsell P, Karlsson MK: A school curriculum-based exercise program increases bone mineral accrual and bone size in prepubertal girls: two-year data from the pediatric osteoporosis prevention (POP) study. J Bone Miner Res 2006, 21(6):829-835.
94. MacKelvie KJ, Khan KM, Petit MA, Janssen PA, McKay HA: A school-based exercise intervention elicits substantial bone health benefits: a 2-year randomized controlled trial in girls. Pediatrics 2003, 112(6 Pt 1):e447.
95. Kelly AS, Steinberger J, Olson TP, Dengel DR: In the absence of weight loss, exercise training does not improve adipokines or oxidative stress in overweight children. Metabolism 2007, 56(7):1005-1009.
96. Gutin B, Barbeau P, Owens S, Lemmon CR, Bauman M, Allison J, Kang HS, Litaker MS: Effects of exercise intensity on cardiovascular fitness, total body composition, and visceral adiposity of obese adolescents. Am J Clin Nutr 2002, 75(5):818-826.
97. Owens S, Gutin B, Allison J, Riggs S, Ferguson M, Litaker M, Thompson W: Effect of physical training on total and visceral fat in obese children. Med Sci Sports Exerc 1999, 31(1):143-148.
98. Lazaar N, Aucouturier J, Ratel S, Rance M, Meyer M, Duche P: Effect of physical activity intervention on body composition in young children: influence of body mass index status and gender. Acta Paediatr 2007, 96(9):1315-1320.
99. Ondrak KS, Morgan DW: Physical activity, calcium intake and bone health in children and adolescents. Sports Med 2007, 37(7):587-600.
100. Kontulainen SA, Kannus PA, Pasanen ME, Sievanen HT, Heinonen AO, Oja P, Vuori I: Does previous participation in high-impact training result in residual bone gain in growing girls? One year follow-up of a 9-month jumping intervention. Int J Sports Med 2002, 23(8):575-581.
101. Mackelvie KJ, McKay HA, Khan KM, Crocker PR: A school-based exercise intervention augments bone mineral accrual in early pubertal girls. J Pediatr 2001, 139(4):501-508.
102. Petit MA, McKay HA, MacKelvie KJ, Heinonen A, Khan KM, Beck TJ: A randomized school-based jumping intervention confers site and maturity-specific benefits on bone structural properties in girls: a hip structural analysis study. J Bone Miner Res 2002, 17(3):363-372.
103. McKay HA, MacLean L, Petit M, MacKelvie-O'Brien K, Janssen P, Beck T, Khan KM: "Bounce at the Bell": a novel program of short bouts of exercise improves proximal femur bone mass in early pubertal children. Br J Sports Med 2005, 39(8):521-526.
104. Brosnahan J, Steffen LM, Lytle L, Patterson J, Boostrom A: The relation between physical activity and mental health among Hispanic and non-Hispanic white adolescents. Arch Pediatr Adolesc Med 2004, 158(8):818-823.
105. Tao FB, Xu ML, Kim SD, Sun Y, Su PY, Huang K: Physical activity might not be the protective factor for health risk behaviours and psychopathological symptoms in adolescents. J Paediatr Child Health 2007, 43(11):762-767.

106. Haarasilta LM, Marttunen MJ, Kaprio JA, Aro HM: Correlates of depression in a representative nationwide sample of adolescents (15-19 years) and young adults (20-24 years). Eur J Public Health 2004, 14(3):280-285.
107. Annesi JJ: Correlations of depression and total mood disturbance with physical activity and self-concept in preadolescents enrolled in an after-school exercise program. Psychol Rep 2005, 96(3 Pt 2):891-898.
108. Norris R, Carroll D, Cochrane R: The effects of physical activity and exercise training on psychological stress and well-being in an adolescent population. J Psychosom Res 1992, 36(1):55-65.
109. Goldfield GS, Mallory R, Parker T, Cunningham T, Legg C, Lumb A, Parker K, Prud'homme D, Adamo KB: Effects of modifying physical activity and sedentary behavior on psychosocial adjustment in overweight/obese children. J Pediatr Psychol 2007, 32(7):783-793.
110. Pickett W: Injuries. In Young people in Canada: their health and wellbeing. Edited by Boyce WF. Ottawa: Health Canada; 2004:101-102.
111. Collard DC, Verhagen EA, Chin APMJ, van Mechelen W: Acute physical activity and sports injuries in children. Appl Physiol Nutr Metab 2008, 33(2):393-401.
112. Janssen I, Dostaler S, Boyce WF, Pickett W: Influence of multiple risk behaviors on physical activity-related injuries in adolescents. Pediatrics 2007, 119(3):e672-680.
113. Tsuang HCA, Guo YL, Lin YC, Su HJ: School type, stress and sport-related injuries in middle school students in central Taiwan. Safety Science 2001, 39:137-144.
114. Mattila V, Parkkari J, Kannus P, Rimpela A: Occurrence and risk factors of unintentional injuries among 12- to 18-year-old Finns--a survey of 8219 adolescents. Eur J Epidemiol 2004, 19(5):437-444.
115. Brawley LR, Latimer AE: Physical activity guides for Canadians: messaging strategies, realistic expectations for change, and evaluation. Can J Public Health 2007, 98(Suppl 2):S170-184.
116. Corbin CB, Pangrazi RP: Physical Activity for Children: A Statement of Guidelines for Children Aged 5-12. 2nd edition. Reston, VA: National Association for Sport and Physical Education; 2004.
117. Department of Health and Aging: National Physical Activity Guidelines for Australians. Canberra: Commonwealth of Australia; 1999.
118. Mark AE, Janssen I: Does physical activity accrued in bouts predict overweight and obesity beyond the total volume of physical activity in youth? Am J Prev Med 2009, 36:416-421.

There are several supplemental files that are not available in this version of the article. To view this additional information, please use the citation on the first page of this chapter.

CHAPTER 11

RETHINKING THE ROLE THAT SCHOOL MEALS PLAY FOR HEALTH AND NUTRITION EDUCATION: A EUROPEAN PERSPECTIVE

BENT EGBERG MIKKELSEN

The growth in obesity and other nutrition related disorders among young people demands a search for strategies that can counteract this development. According to the cross-national study on the Health Behaviour of School-aged Children (Meija et al 2013), a large number of young people do not meet the recommendations for good nutrition and physical activity. School based strategies are among the most promising, and the growing interest in school-based, public health nutrition strategies is reflected in the growing number of peer reviewed papers in the field (Campbell et al. 2001, Foster et al. 2008, Moore et al. 2014) as well as in the number of policy and strategy papers from both governments and intergovernmental organisations (WHO, 2006, EU commission, 2007, World Food Program, 2013, Wollgast et al 2014)

The rationale for taking action in schools is obvious. Lifestyle and behavioural patterns are founded early in life and studies have shown that

---

Original article, used with permission from Bent Egberg Mikkelsen.

health status has a tendency to track into adulthood (Whitaker et al. 1997; Wright et al. 2001). The same can be seen for behaviour (Birch et al 2007; Mikkilä et al 2005); studies have shown that children are more likely to accept new foods at a young age than later in life (Skinner et al 2002; Neumark-Sztainer et al 2011). Nearly all children attend school for up to 13 years, and studies have shown that close to 40% pupil's daily energy intake comes from food consumed during school hours (Bell & Swinburn 2004, Sanigorski et al 2005).

The new interest in School Meal Programs (SMPs) takes place at the same time European schools are undergoing other important reforms. The goal is to create schools with more competitive curricula. In many cases, this results in longer school days, which, in turn, create an increased need for food provision. Reforms are also affecting the pedagogy and approaches to learning. For instance, the new Danish school pedagogy introduces the idea of supportive teaching—a problem based approach to learning in which daily social practices such as food and cooking can become the object of the learning process.

This has resulted in a new interest in not only redesigning the way food is provided at school but also in considerations and experimentation on how food service and provision can be integrated more holistically into the life at school and in the learning and curricular activities. Food at school has traditionally been seen as a "mundane activity in prosaic settings" (Sonnino & Morgan, 2007) and there have been frequent reports of school meals being of poor quality (Nelson). However, the current interest in better school feeding has meant that School Meal Programs (SMPs) have found their way into high places. For example, both U.S. First Lady Michelle Obama and former British Prime Minister Tony Blair have been involved in attempts to improve the nutritional quality of school lunches in their own countries.

One of the results of the increasing interest school food and nutrition has been that there is an increased recognition of the complex food reality that young people at school are faced with. Traditional approaches have focused on school lunches provided in cafeterias, canteens etc., but increasingly people are focusing on the other aspects of the school food reality as well. These include fruit and vegetable and breakfast programs, as well as a range of curricular and learning approaches to the teaching of good nutrition. Such activities include a broad range of hands-on food activities. These are aimed at integrating, for instance, growing, harvesting, preparation, menu planning, and sensory activities to create a new way of learning and experience nutrition and food consumption. The literature about such activities is growing, and includes programs such as taste education, farm2School links, outdoor cooking, and school gardens, as well as cooking classes.

The increased understanding of the complex food environment in schools has also fuelled new research directions that can capture, and understand this diverse foodreality. FoodScapes Studies (FSS) is a growing area of research among scholars engaged in the study of foodways and offers well suited conceptual foundation for the holistic approach that is needed to understand the complex social system of the school and its opportunities for promoting good public health nutrition. The concept of foodscapes draws from different sources and has been further developed into the idea of 'foodscapes' and later to the idea of 'captive foodscapes' to illustrate the special importance of places where we eat regularly in "captive" daily life, such as schools (Mikkelsen, 2014) since they are of particular dietary relevance due to the high frequency of eating there.

The captive school foodscape can be understood as a web in which food, people, and space interact in particular ways. The goal of school nutrition programs is promote good food habits by teaching young people skills that focuse around the eating, serving and socializing of food. By adding meaning to food consumption, nutrition is given the power to become an important setting for change. The rethinking of European approaches to food, eating, and learning at school indicate that schools are increasingly recognized as meaningful settings for change by a broad range of stakeholders, including the people responsible for policy and decision making.

It is important to note that there is no single way to deal with food and eating at school. Studies have shown that there is considerable diversity to the national approaches to school feeding (Wollgast et al 2014, Mikkelsen 2014). One is the collective approach, in which the public provides free school lunches (Mikkelsen 2014). This is found in Sweden and Finland, whereas a semi-collective approach is found in countries such as France and the UK (Mikkelsen, 2014). In countries like Denmark, the Netherlands, and Norway a non-collective approach is found to school nutrition, and here there are no national regulations to provide school lunches. This means that school meal provision is decided by the individual schools and the buying of the food is determined by children and their parents.

When viewing food and nutrition at school as a foodscape, with different aspects connected as a web, it is possible to look at the issues more broadly and develop models of school nutrition that take into account more than the food student eat in the cafeteria. The foodscape approach acknowledges that students are influenced by multiple sources at school—not only the foods offered through school meal programs, but also foods offered through other services such as school fruit programs, milk programs, foods sold at vending machines and shops, and packed lunches and snacks brought from home. In addition, marketing is an important aspect of the food experience, as students encounter food in imagery form as wel as material form on their way to and from school, in the family sphere, and in media. A future approach to the rethinking of food at school should target the broad and complex social systems of the school and its environment. By taking a holistic approach instead of looking only at the school, we will broaden our understanding to look at the full range of food realities that young people meet.

REFERENCES

1. Birch L.L., Savaga, J.S. & Ventura. A (2007). Influences on the development of children's eating behaviors: From infancy to adolescence. Canadian Journal of Dietary Practice Research 68, pp. 1-56.
2. Bell AC & Swinburn BA (2004) What are the key food groups to target for preventing obesity and improving nutrition in schools? Eur J Clin Nutr., 58, 258-263.
3. Campbell K, Waters E, Meara SO et al. (2001) Interventions for preventing obesity in childhood. A systematic review, Obesity Reviews 2, 149–157
4. Foster GD, Sherman S, Borradaile KE et al. (2008). A policy-based school intervention to prevent overweight and obesity. Pediatrics. 121,794-802.
5. Commission of the EU. (2007). White Paper- a Strategy for Europe on Nutrition, Overweight and Obesity related health issues, Bruxelles
6. Council of Europe (2005). Resolution on healthy eating at school, Strasbourg
7. Kelder, S.H.; Perry, C.L.; Klepp, K.I. and Lytle, L.L. (1994): Longitudinal tracking of adolescent smoking, physical activity, and food choice behaviors. Am J Public Health. 84(7). 1121–1126.

8. Mikkelsen, B.E. (2014) School – a multitude of opportunities for promoting healthier eating. Public Health Nutrition, June issue
9. Mejia D, Berchtold A, Bélanger R et al (2013). Frequency and effects of meeting health-behavior guidelines among adolescents. European Journal of Public Health, 23, 8-13
10. Moore GF, Murphy S, Chaplin K et al (2014). Impacts of the Primary School Free breakfast Initiative on socio-economic inequalities in breakfast consumption among 9-11-year-old schoolchildren in Wales. Public Health Nutr. 17, 1280-9
11. Nelson, M. The School Food Trust: transforming school lunches in England, Nutrition Bulletin, Volume 36, Issue 3, p 381–389, September 2011
12. Neumark-Sztainer D, Wall M, Larson NI, Eisenberg ME, Loth, K. (2011) Dieting and disordered eating behaviors from adolescence to young adulthood: findings from a 10-year longitudinal study. J Am Diet Assoc. 111(7). Pp.1004-11.
13. Sanigorski AM, Bell AC, Kremer PJ et al (2005). Lunchbox contents of Australian school children: room for improvement. Eur J Clin Nutr. 59, 1310-1316.
14. Sonnino, R & Morgan, K (2007). The School Food Revolution: Public Food and the Challenge of Sustainable Development
15. Skinner, J., Carruth, B.R., Bounds, W. & Ziegler, P.J. (2002) Children's food preferences: A longitudinal analysis. Journal of the American Dietetic Association 102, 1638-1647.
16. World Food Program (2013) The State of School Feeding Worldwide, World Food Program. http://www.wfp.org/school-meals
17. Wollgast J, Nelson M, Kardakis T, Storcksdieck, S & Louro Caldeira S. (2014) Mapping of National School Food Policies across the EU28 plus Norway and Switzerland, EU Joinst Research Centre. https://ec.europa.eu/jrc/en/publication/eur-scientific-and-technical-research-reports/mapping-national-school-food-policies-across-eu28-plus-norway-and-switzerland
18. Whitaker, R.D., Wright, J.A., Pepe, M.S., Seidel. K.D. & Dietz, W.H. (1997) Predicting obesity in young adulthood from childhood and parental obesity. New England Journal of Medicine 337. pp. 869 – 73.
19. WHO (2006) European Charter on counteracting obesity adopted at the WHO European Ministerial Conference, Istanbul
20. Wright C.M., Parker L., Lamont, D. & Craft, A.W. (2001) Implications of childhood obesity for adult health: findings from a thousand families cohort study. British Medical Journal 323. pp. 1280 –

CHAPTER 12

FROM "BEST PRACTICE" TO "NEXT PRACTICE": THE EFFECTIVENESS OF SCHOOL-BASED HEALTH PROMOTION IN IMPROVING HEALTHY EATING AND PHYSICAL ACTIVITY AND PREVENTING CHILDHOOD OBESITY

CHRISTINA FUNG, STEFAN KUHLE, CONNIE LU, MEGAN PURCELL, MARG SCHWARTZ, KATE STOREY, AND PAUL J VEUGELERS

12.1 BACKGROUND

Childhood obesity is a growing epidemic and has become a public health priority in developed countries [1,2]. Over the past few decades, prevalence rates of childhood obesity have tripled, with recent estimates indicating that 16.9% and 8.6% of children are obese in United States and Canada respectively [3-6]. Obesity negatively impacts a child's self esteem and results in diminished quality of life [7]. Moreover, children with high body mass index (BMI) often become obese adults, who are at increased risk of developing obesity-related diseases, such as type 2 diabetes, cardiovascular disease, and certain types of cancer, and place significant financial burden on healthcare systems [8-10].

Poor diets and inadequate physical activity are widely acknowledged as the main drivers of the obesity epidemic [11-13]. As childhood obesity rates continue to rise, the effects of unhealthy eating, compounded by increasingly sedentary lifestyles, emphasize the need to identify comprehensive health promotion approaches to curb the worsening trends. Recent reviews suggest the use of school-based interventions to address the childhood obesity epidemic [14,15]. Schools are the ideal setting given their ability to reach nearly all children who spend a significant proportion of their time in schools [16]. Moreover, school-based programs influence children's learning environments at a young age where healthy habits can be taught and practiced, resulting in improved health and wellness later in life [17,18].

Based on the World Health Organization's Ottawa *Charter for Health Promotion* [19], Comprehensive School Health (CSH) is an integrated school-based health promotion framework that goes beyond classroom-based health education models to a more integrated approach involving education and the whole school environment. CSH is defined as "an internationally recognized framework for supporting improvements in students' educational outcomes while addressing health in a planned, integrated and holistic way" [20]. In the United States, CSH is more commonly referred to as "Coordinated School Health" [21] while the synonymous term "Health Promoting Schools" is often used to describe the same underlying concept of creating healthier environments for children in their schools in Australia and Europe [22,23]. In addition to improvements in academic outcomes, CSH has been shown to positively influence health behaviours and health outcomes of children [17,24-26]. In 2005, we reported on the Annapolis Valley Health Promoting Schools (AVHPS) project, a successful grassroots project that achieved healthy behaviours and a reduction in the prevalence of excess bodyweight among children in Nova Scotia, Canada [27]. The successful results from the AVHPS project is now recognized as a "best practice" in Canada [28] and have inspired the development of the Alberta Project Promoting active Living and healthy Eating (APPLE) Schools in Alberta, Canada.

Despite the promising potential of CSH, only few studies have evaluated its effectiveness, and this is essential to evidence-based decision-making [22,23]. As evidence-based decision-making in public health is currently not well established, there is a strong need for rigorous studies to provide evidence on the effectiveness and sustainability of promising programs [29]. APPLE Schools, therefore, provides the opportunity to not only further evaluate the effectiveness of a CSH program for the promotion of healthy body weights among children, but to also assess the transferability of "practice-based evidence" from a grassroots initiative to different settings within North America. The present study examines the changes in diet, physical activity, and weight status among grade 5 students in APPLE schools in comparison with students elsewhere in the province.

12.2 METHODS

12.2.1 APPLE SCHOOLS: THE INTERVENTION

Launched in 2008, the APPLE Schools project is a three-year intervention led by the School of Public Health at the University of Alberta. The project operates in 10 schools that were selected from five school jurisdictions in Alberta, all of which agreed to support healthy eating and active living initiatives among students. Inspired by the success of AVHPS, APPLE Schools incorporates many of the AVHPS elements and utilizes a similar CSH approach "to make the healthy choice the easy choice" [30]. However, APPLE Schools takes the AVHPS model one step further by tailoring the intervention to each of the APPLE Schools through the placement of a full-time School Health Facilitator in each school. These School Health Facilitators are responsible for implementing healthy eating and active living strategies while addressing the unique needs and barriers to health promotion in the school environment by engaging all stakeholders, including parents, staff and the community. School Health Facilitators contributed to the schools' health curriculum, both during instructional and non-instructional school time, engaged in developing cross curriculum links and taught across the curriculum. They facilitated professional development days for teachers and school staff, organized parent information nights, nutrition programs such as cooking clubs, after school physical activity programs, weekend events and celebrations, and circulated newsletters. Between 2008 and 2010, 8 of the 10 APPLE Schools implemented a nutrition policy and all 10 APPLE Schools adopted policies ensuring all their students receive a minimum of 30 minutes of physical activity per school day. Further, School Health Facilitators promoted community and parent involvement that led to community gardens, walk-to-school days, support for breakfast and lunch programs, and parent led extramural programs.

The commitment of APPLE Schools is to schools "in need". In the fall of 2007, school jurisdictions were asked to identify schools located in socioeconomically disadvantaged neighborhoods or that had otherwise challenges, included grade 5 in the grade configuration, had a principal supportive of the concept of CSH and the focus on healthy living, and schools with transient rates lower than 60%. The principals then agreed to: a) support the intervention by dedicating time directed to the project; b) commit to a three-and-a-half year involvement; c) participated in ongoing and new research; d) provide office space for the facilitator and access to infrastructure support; e) include the facilitator as part of the school staff; f) create supportive healthy living policies, and g) participate in meetings of other APPLE Schools administrators and facilitators. The recommendations by the school jurisdictions for 7 urban and 3 rural APPLE Schools with an average school size of 350 students were accommodated.

To examine the effectiveness of APPLE Schools, diet, physical activity, and health among students were measured through annual surveys using identical survey tools as the Raising healthy Eating and Active Living Kids in Alberta (REAL Kids Alberta) evaluation. In 2008, 345 home surveys and parental consent forms were distributed to parents. Of the 317 (92%) students who returned completed consent forms, 306 (97%) received parental consent to participate in the study. A total of 293 students completed the survey, resulting in a student participation rate of 85%. Similarly, data was collected among 344 and 394 consenting students and their parents from the 10 APPLE Schools in 2009 and 2010 respectively.

The student participation rate in 2009 and 2010 was 84%, which is considered high for school-based research.

12.2.2 REAL KIDS ALBERTA SURVEY

The Raising healthy Eating and Active Living Kids in Alberta (REAL Kids Alberta) is a large population-based survey that collects data on health, nutrition, physical activity, lifestyle factors, and measured height and weight among grade 5 students, and data on the school and home environment among their parents and school administrators. The aim of REAL Kids Alberta is to assess the impact of the provincial government's initiatives to promote healthy weights among children and youth in Alberta in 2008 and 2010 [31]. Details regarding the measures used as part of REAL Kids Alberta, including dietary intake, physical activity, and obesity, are provided below and are available through the project's website: http://www.REALKidsalberta.ca .

The REAL Kids Alberta evaluation used a one-stage stratified random sampling design. The sampling frame includes all elementary schools in Alberta with grade 5 students with the exception of private schools (4.7% of all Albertan students), francophone schools (0.6%), on-reserve federal schools (2.0%), charter schools (1.7%) and colony schools (0.8%) [32]. Schools were stratified according to the following geographical areas: 1) metropolitan: Calgary and Edmonton, each with populations of about 1 million people; 2) city: other municipalities with more than 40,000 residents; and 3) rural-town: municipalities with less than 40,000 residents. Schools were randomly selected within each of these geographical strata to achieve a balanced number of students in each stratum. Of the 184 invited schools, 148 (80.4%) participated in the study in 2008. Envelopes containing parental consent forms and a home survey were sent home to 5,321 students. Of the 3,704 (70%) students with completed consent forms, 3,645 (98%) received parental consent to participate in the study. Trained evaluation assistants visited each school to administer the student surveys and baseline data was collected among 3,421 students, resulting in a student participation rate of 64%. These surveys were repeated among grade 5 students of the same schools in 2010. However, within the random sample, 7 schools in 2010 refused to participate or were not available for other reasons (i.e. school closures); these schools were replaced by 10 additional schools. Therefore in 2010, 5,597 home surveys were distributed to parents from 151 randomly selected schools, of which 3,687 (66%) students returned consent forms to schools. Of these students, 3,656 (99%) received parental consent to participate and 3,469 were present to complete student surveys. A total of 3,398 participating students and their parents completed surveys, resulting in a participation rate of 61% in 2010.

12.2.3 SURVEY TOOLS

12.2.3.1 ASSESSMENT OF DIETARY INTAKE

Students completed the Harvard Youth/Adolescent Food Frequency Questionnaire (FFQ), which has been extensively validated for use in nutrition research among children and youth 3334. Student's caloric intake and intake of fruits and vegetables were calculated based on reported intake from the FFQ and from the Canadian Nutrient Files [35]. Overall diet quality was measured using the Diet Quality Index–International (DQI) score, a composite measure of diet quality ranging from 0 to 100 with higher scores indicating better diet quality and includes aspects of diet adequacy, variety, balance and moderation [36,37].

12.2.3.2 ASSESSMENT OF PHYSICAL ACTIVITY

Physical activity levels were measured using the Physical Activity Questionnaire for older Children (PAQ-C), which has been demonstrated to be a valid and reliable measure of general moderate to vigorous physical activity levels over a 7-day period [38,39]. The PAQ-C score ranges from 0 to 5 with higher scores indicating higher levels of physical activity.

12.2.3.3 ASSESSMENT OF OBESITY

Student standing height was measured to the nearest 0.1 centimeter after students had removed their shoes and body weight was measured to the nearest 0.1 kilogram on calibrated digital scales. Body mass index (BMI) was calculated as weight divided by height^2 (kg/m^2). Obesity was defined using the International Obesity Task Force (IOTF) BMI cut-off points that are adjusted to age and sex specific categories for children and youth [40].

12.2.4 SOCIOECONOMIC FACTORS

Information on household income (< $50,000; $50,001 - $100,000; and > $100,000) and parental education attainment levels (secondary or less, college, university or above) were determined from household questionnaires completed by parents.

12.2.5 STATISTICAL ANALYSIS

All statistical analyses pertaining to the Alberta population were weighted to account for the design effect and represent provincial estimates of the grade 5 student population in Alberta. Differences between baseline and two-year post-intervention characteristics were assessed using the Chi-square test, Rao-Scott Chi-square or t-test where appropriate. The Rao-Scott Chi-square test was applied to examine differences in weighted estimates by adjusting for the design effect [41,42].

As observations of students are nested within those of their schools, multilevel regression methods were used to examine the effect of CSH. Odds ratios (OR) and 95% confidence intervals (CI) were calculated from multilevel logistic regression models examining the independent association of obesity with the CSH intervention. Regression coefficients (β) and 95% CI were obtained from multilevel linear regression models with fruits and vegetables consumption, dietary quality, dietary energy intake, and physical activity level as outcomes. All analyses were adjusted for the confounding potential of gender, geographic residency, household income, and parental education. Analyses pertaining to dietary intake were further adjusted for energy intake; observations with reported dietary energy intakes less than 500 kcal or more than 5,000 kcal were excluded [43]. In subanalyses, we standardized the number of servings of fruit and vegetable consumption by assuming that each child consumes 2,000 kcal each day [43]. We used the interaction term (defined as the product of the year variable and the binary intervention variable Yes = APPLE Schools, No = Provincial sample) in the adjusted multilevel models to estimate the difference in regression coefficients as a measure of intervention effect: the change among students attending APPLE Schools relative to those attending other schools in Alberta. STATA version 11 (StataCorp, College Station, TX, USA) was used to perform the statistical analysis. This study, including data collection and parental informed consent forms, was approved by the Health Research Ethics Board at the University of Alberta.

12.3 RESULTS

Characteristics of the grade 5 students at baseline in 2008 and two-years post-intervention are shown in Table 1. With respect to gender, parental education, household income and place of residency, grade 5 students attending APPLE Schools in 2008 did not statistically differ from grade 5 students attending APPLE Schools in 2010. In 2010, relative to 2008, students attending APPLE Schools had higher intakes of fruits and vegetables, had lower caloric intakes, were more active, and were less likely to be obese (Table 1 and Figures 1 and 2). Temporal changes in provincial estimates of fruit and vegetable consumption, and caloric intake between 2008 and 2010 were less pronounced. Physical activity levels in the province increased between 2008 and 2010 but not with the same magnitude as APPLE Schools. Furthermore, in contrast to the 1.8% decline in the prevalence rates of obesity among APPLE Schools, the provincial obesity rates increased by 1.9% between 2008 and 2010 (Table 1).

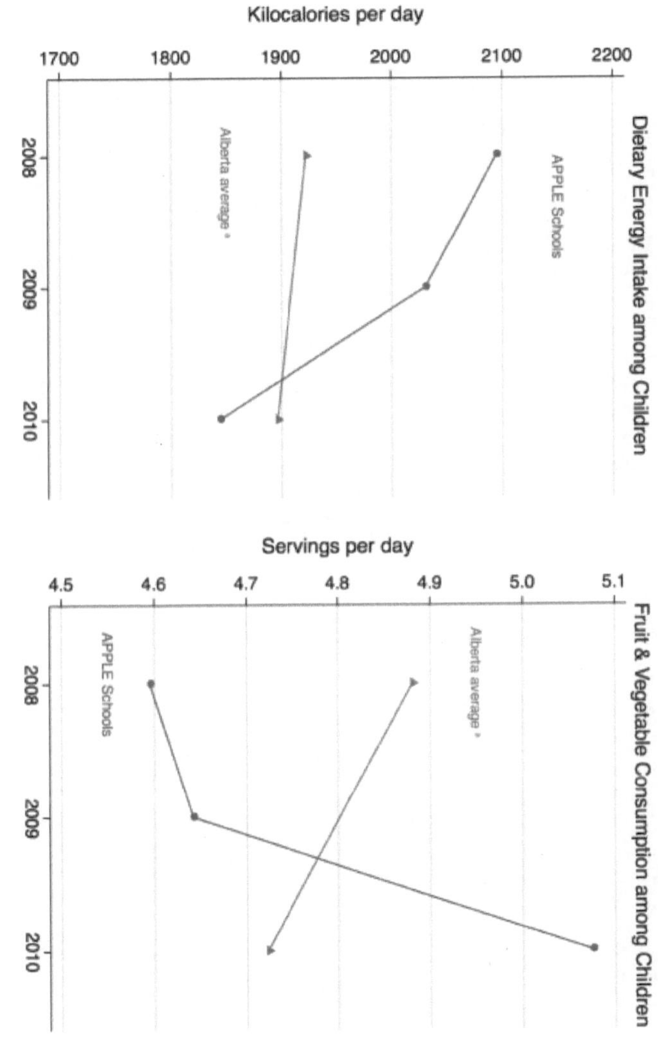

Note: APPLE Schools = Alberta Project Promoting Active Living and healthy Eating Schools.
* Data for Alberta, Canada from 2008-2010 REAL Kids Alberta (weighted to provide provincial estimates).

FIGURE 1: Dietary energy intake and fruits and vegetables consumption among children by intervention exposure.

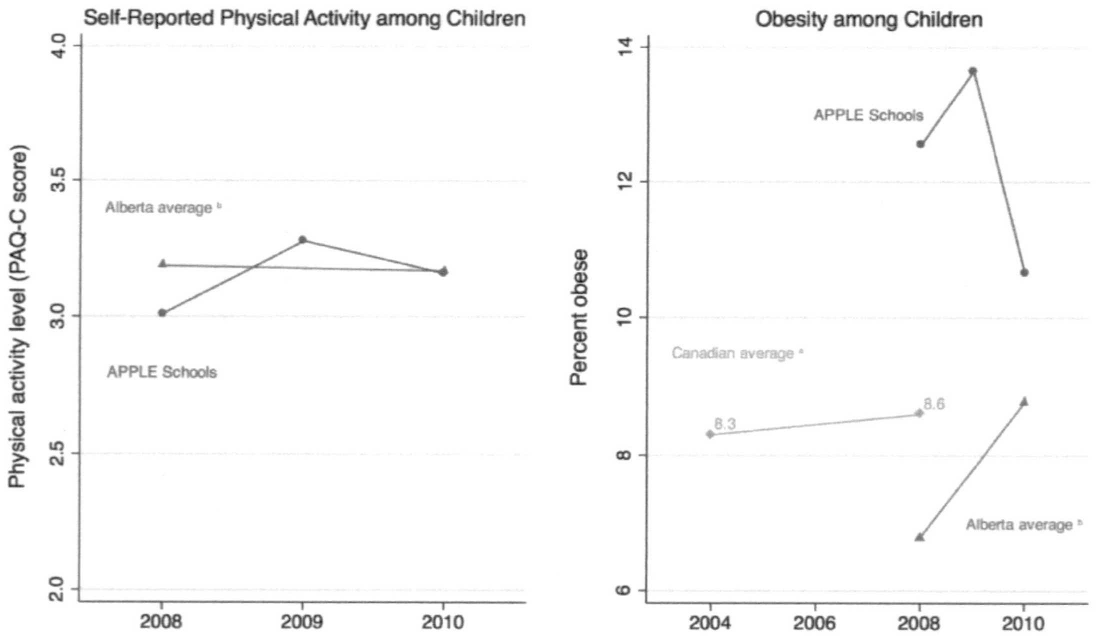

Note: APPLE Schools = Alberta Project Promoting Active Living and healthy Eating Schools; PAQ-C = Physical Activity Questionnaire for older Children.
[a] Data for Canada from the 2004 Canadian Community Health Survey: Nutrition (ages 2-17) and the 2007-2009 Canadian Health Measures Survey (ages 6-17); [b] Data for Alberta, Canada from 2008-2010 REAL Kids Alberta (weighted to provide provincial estimates).

FIGURE 2: Self-reported physical activity and prevalence of obesity among children by intervention exposure.

TABLE 1: Characteristics of grade 5 students attending APPLE Schools and other schools in Alberta in 2008 and 2010

	APPLE Schools			Provincial[a]		
Independent Variable	2008	2010	P[b]	2008	2010	P[b]
Gender			0.10			0.42
Girls	50.7	56.8		51.5	50.5	
Boys	49.3	43.2		48.5	49.5	
Parental Education			0.14			0.23
Secondary or less	30.5	24.1		27.2	25.3	
College	41.1	42.8		39.7	39.4	
University or above	28.5	33.2		33.1	35.3	
Household Income			0.62			0.41
Less than $50,000	34.5	31.0		24.3	24.4	
$50,001 - $100,000	37.4	41.6		39.8	37.9	
>$100,000	28.1	27.4		35.9	37.7	
Geographic Residency			0.53			0.91
Metropolitan	65.1	62.9		46.8	46.6	
City	0.0	0.0		15.2	14.9	
Rural-town	34.9	37.1		38.0	38.5	
Mean servings of fruits & vegetables per day	4.60	5.08	0.02	4.88	4.73	0.09
Mean dietary energy intake (kcal) per day	2094	1844	< 0.01	1924	1897	0.31
Mean DQI score	63.2	62.3	0.30	62.8	62.5	0.23
Mean PAQ-C score	3.01	3.16	< 0.01	3.19	3.17	0.41
Obese (%)	12.5	10.7	0.45	6.9	8.8	0.01

APPLE Schools = Alberta Project Promoting active Living and healthy Eating Schools; DQI = Diet Quality Index; PAQ-C = Physical Activity Questionnaire for older Children
[a] *Estimates weighted to be representative of the grade 5 student population*
[b] *p-values derived using the Chi-square test, Rao-Scott Chi-square or t-test where appropriate*

After controlling for the effect of a child's gender, household income, parental education, and location of residency, multilevel regression analysis showed that students attending APPLE Schools in 2010 had better diets compared to students attending APPLE Schools in 2008, as characterized by a statistically significant increase of 0.39 serving/day in fruits and vegetables consumption, a statistically significant decrease of 237 kcal/day in dietary energy intake, and an increase in overall diet quality. Students attending APPLE Schools in 2010 were also significantly more physically active than those in 2008. Moreover, we observed a 16% decline in the odds of being obese (adjusted OR, 0.84; 95% CI, 0.52, 1.36) among students attending the APPLE Schools two years into the intervention relative to baseline (2008). In contrast, students elsewhere in the province seemed to have exhibited opposite trends over the same two-year period. Adjusted regression analysis showed that students elsewhere in Alberta saw a decrease of 0.12 serving/day in the consumption of fruits and vegetables and a decrease in diet quality. At the provincial level, no substantial changes were observed in levels of physical activity and only a modest decline in energy intake was observed. Moreover, students attending schools elsewhere in Alberta saw a 37% increase in the odds of being obese (adjusted OR, 1.37; 95% CI, 1.11, 1.70).

The change in APPLE Schools relative to the change in Alberta represents the intervention effect. The change in fruits and vegetables consumption of students attending APPLE Schools relative to those attending other Albertan schools was 0.55 serving/day and borderline significant (Table 2: 95% CI, -0.02, 1.13). APPLE Schools students' changes in physical activity and calorie consumption were also statistically significant relative to changes elsewhere in the province (Table 2). The odds of being obese in 2010 relative to 2008 was 39% lower (Table 2 OR, 0.61; 95% CI, 0.35, 1.06) among students from APPLE Schools compared to students elsewhere in the province, although this was only borderline significant. This is equivalent to a multivariable-adjusted 2.2% reduction in the prevalence of obesity among APPLE Schools between 2008 to 2010 as compared to a multivariable-adjusted 2.8% increase in the prevalence of obesity elsewhere in Alberta over the same two-year period.

12.4 DISCUSSION

The present study demonstrates the effectiveness of a CSH intervention in fostering healthy behaviors in terms of improvements in healthy eating and active living. Over a two-year period, APPLE Schools changed their school environments and attending students reported increases in the consumption of fruits and vegetables along with decreases in energy intake, were more physically active, and exhibited less obesity compared to students elsewhere in the province.

TABLE 2: Effect of Comprehensive School Health on diet, physical activity and body weight among grade 5 students two years from baseline

	APPLE Schools[a]		Alberta Schools[b]		Intervention Effect: Change in APPLE Schools over time relative to the coinciding change in Alberta schools (95% CI)b	
Fruits and vegetables consumption per day (β and 95% CI)	0.39	(0.00, 0.78)	-0.12	(-0.29, 0.06)	0.55	(-0.02, 1.13)
Dietary energy intake (kcal) per day (β and 95% CI)	-236.51	(-366.22, -106.81)	-25.89	(-78.34, 26.56)	-212.11	(-315.07, -109.16)
DQI score (β and 95% CI)	0.96	(-0.28, 2.19)	-0.23	(-0.77, 0.31)	1.14	(-0.55, 2.83)
PAQ-C score (β and 95% CI)	0.13	(0.03,0.23)	0.02	(-0.01, 0.06)	0.10	(0.01, 0.20)
Obesity (Odds Ratio and 95% CI)	0.84	(0.52, 1.36)	1.37	(1.11, 1.70)	0.61	(0.35, 1.06)

APPLE Schools = Alberta Project Promoting active Living and healthy Eating Schools; DQI = Diet Quality Index; PAQ-C = Physical Activity Questionnaire for older Children [a] APPLE Schools were surveyed annually from 2008 to 2010; therefore analysis included additional measurements from 2009 [b] Estimates weighted to be representative of the grade 5 Alberta student population All estimates were adjusted for child's gender, household income, parental education, and rural residency. OR (Odds Ratio) were from multilevel logistic regression of obesity. β's were from multilevel linear regression representing the association of CSH programming with changes in consumption of fruits and vegetables, DQI score, dietary energy intake, and PAQ-C score. The reference category for all outcomes is 2008 baseline observations. All dietary outcomes were further adjusted for energy intake. The intervention effect was calculated using an interaction term between APPLE Schools (Yes/No) and year of observation (2008/2010). To facilitate interpretation of results, the odds of being obese was calculated from the adjusted multilevel models and converted into a probability by using the relation Prob = Odds/(Odds + 1). Data collected in 2009 in APPLE Schools was included in the multilevel regression analysis. However, 2009 observations were omitted from analyses comparing APPLE Schools with the provincial sample, as 2009 observations were not available for Alberta schools other than APPLE Schools

Public health research is increasingly aiming to identify “best practice” and “practice based evidence” rather than to demonstrate universal evidence because the success of public health programs is greatly affected by contextual factors [44]. The AVHPS project, a successful grassroots project, is recognized as a “best practice” of CSH in Canada [28]. However, to our knowledge, no earlier studies have addressed the transferability of “best practice,” or in other words, the extent to which the measured effectiveness of an applicable intervention could be achieved in another setting. To our knowledge, the present study is the first one where practice-based evidence of a CSH intervention was applied in a different setting while under rigorous evaluation. The demonstrated success of APPLE Schools in improving health behaviours and weight status indicates that the AVHPS model is replicable and transferable to other settings outside of the original schools in Nova Scotia, where it was developed as a grassroots initiative.

In light of the current obesity epidemic, there is a paucity of studies on the effectiveness of CSH programs [26]. Although few studies have thoroughly examined CSH interventions, our results are consistent with others that have reported on the benefits of CSH in terms of increased consumption of fruits and vegetables [45,46]. Similarly, our results are consistent with previous findings from the original AVHPS project on which the APPLE School program is based [27].

While we observed significant differences in diet and physical activity levels over a two-year period among students attending APPLE Schools, changes in obesity prevalence were only borderline significant. Longer follow-up and a larger number of schools are needed to establish improvements in longer term health outcomes such as body weights. Based on the encouraging results reported here, APPLE Schools is now expanding to include an additional 30 schools from Aboriginal and rural and remote communities throughout Alberta. This expansion will consider that schools vary in structure, organization, and objectives, and herewith that a standard implementation strategy for CSH is not plausible [23]. School Health Facilitators will be placed in new APPLE Schools as they were in the original 10 APPLE School to customize the CSH approach to suite the school’s needs. By tailoring the CSH approaches to each of the APPLE Schools, the intervention builds upon ongoing health promoting activities and policies. Ongoing evaluation will further establish the benefits of CSH and the APPLE Schools approach.

The 10 APPLE Schools were selected by school jurisdictions and were mostly located in socioeconomically disadvantaged neighborhoods. That these schools were "in need" of health promotion was reflected in the poor diets and low levels of physical activity among students attending these schools at baseline in 2008. However, two years into the intervention, students attending APPLE Schools had improved their eating behaviours and physical activity levels such that they approximated or exceeded the provincial average. Given the substantial morbidity and diminished quality of life associated with poor diet, physical inactivity and childhood obesity, studies are needed to demonstrate the cost-effectiveness of CSH prevention programs considering that obese children have higher health-care cost than normal weight children [47]. Such economic analyses will better guide public health decision makers in directing resources towards broader implementation of school-based interventions and may be instrumental in informing various policies across North America.

Strengths of the current study include its large representative sample, high response rate for school-based research, pre-intervention measurements, and the use of measured height and weight to assess body weight status. However, as with most population-based observational studies, the present study is subject to limitations. First of all, the 10 APPLE Schools were selected by school jurisdictions rather than randomly, which limits the generalizability of the results. Responses to questionnaires remain subjective and are prone to reporting error. Although individuals have a tendency to over-report levels of physical activity, it has been shown that self-reported measures of physical activity are correlated with objective measures among children [48]. Similarly, we acknowledge the imprecision associated with the assessment of dietary energy intake through the FFQ and therefore have standardized the number of servings of fruit and vegetable consumption based on energy intake. Despite the use of a validated FFQ for this age group, limitations of self-report apply to the assessment of dietary intake in which studies have shown that individuals are more likely to underreport energy intake [49]. Moreover, CSH aims to improve various aspects of the school environment such that they support improved dietary patterns and physical activity among students. The implementation was tailored and developed distinctively in each of the 10 APPLE Schools. Although randomized control trials provide the highest level of evidence for the evaluation of interventions, they may not be optimal for the evaluation of interventions that are tailored and develop distinctively. Furthermore, we opted for evaluation of prevalence rates that speak better to the needs of public health decision makers rather than incidence rates by following selected students over time.

12.5 CONCLUSIONS

In conclusion, the APPLE Schools program demonstrated positive results in the improvement of dietary habits and physical activity levels among grade 5 students in Alberta. This suggests that the AVHPS "best practice" approach to CSH is transferable outside of the original schools in Nova Scotia to another setting, a "next practice." This study adds to the limited evidence-base of the effectiveness of CSH and justifies investments for its broader implementation.

REFERENCES

1. Ebbeling CB, Pawlak DB, Ludwig DS: Childhood obesity: public-health crisis, common sense cure. Lancet 2002, 360:473-482.
2. Lobstein T, Baur L, Uauy R: Obesity in children and young people: a crisis in public health. Obes Rev 2004, 5:4-85.
3. Ogden CL, Carroll MD, Curtin LR, Lamb MM, Flegal KM: Prevalence of high body mass index in US children and adolescents, 2007-2008. JAMA 2010, 303:242-249.
4. Ogden CL, Carroll MD: Prevalence of Obesity Among Children and Adolescents: United States, Trends 1963-1965 Through 2007-2008. [http:/ / www.cdc.gov/ nchs/ data/ hestat/ obesity_child_07_08/ obesity_child_07_08.htm]
5. Statistics Canada: Canadian Health Measures Survey: Cycle 1 Data Tables. 2007 to 2009, no. 2. [http:/ / www.statcan.gc.ca/ bsolc/ olc-cel/ olc-cel?catno=82-623-XIE&lang=eng#f ormatdisp]
6. Shields M: Overweight and obesity among children and youth. Health Rep 2006, 17:27-42.
7. Wang F, Veugelers PJ: Self-esteem and cognitive development in the era of the childhood obesity epidemic. Obes Rev 2008, 9:615-623.

8. Dietz WH: Overweight in childhood and adolescence. N Engl J Med 2004, 350:855-857.
9. Manson JE, Bassuk SS: Obesity in the United States: a fresh look at its high toll. JAMA 2003, 289:229-230.
10. Must A, Strauss RS: Risks and consequences of childhood and adolescent obesity. Int J Obes Relat Metab Disord 1999, 23(Supp 2):s2-s11.
11. Andersen RE: The spread of the childhood obesity epidemic. CMAJ 2000, 163:1461-1462.
12. Hill JO, Wyatt HR, Reed GW, Peters JC: Obesity and the environment: Where do we go from here? Science 2003, 299:853-855.
13. Swinburn BA, Caterson I, Seidell JC, James WP: Diet, nutrition and the prevention of excess weight gain and obesity. Public Health Nutr 2004, 7:123-146.
14. Brown T, Summerbell C: Systematic review of school-based interventions that focus on changing dietary intake and physical activity levels to prevent childhood obesity: an update to the obesity guidance produced by the National Institute for Health and Clinical Excellence. Obes Rev 2009, 10:110-141.
15. Katz DL: School-based interventions for health promotion and weight control: not just waiting on the world to change. Annu Rev Public Health 2009, 30:253-272.
16. Booth M, O'Brodovich H, Finegood D: Addressing Childhood Obesity: The Evidence for Action. [http://publications.gc.ca/pub?id=329477&sl=0]
17. Stewart-Brown S: What is the evidence on school health promotion in improving health or preventing disease and, specifically, what is the effectiveness of the health promoting schools approach? [http://www.euro.who.int/__data/assets/pdf_file/0007/74653/E88185.pdf]
18. Story M, Kaphingst KM, French S: The role of schools in obesity prevention. The Future of Children 2006, 16:109-142.
19. Organization WH: Ottawa charter for health promotion. Can J Public Health 1986, 77:425-430.
20. Joint Consortium for School Health: What is Comprehensive School Health? [http://jcsh-cces.ca/index.php?option=com_content&view=article&id=40&Itemid=62]
21. CDC: Coordinated School Health. [http://www.cdc.gov/healthyyouth/cshp/]
22. Deschesnes M, Martin C, Hill AJ: Comprehensive approaches to school health promotion: how to achieve broader implementation? Health Promot Int 2003, 18:387-396.
23. Veugelers PJ, Schwartz ME: Comprehensive school health in Canada. Can J Public Health 2010, 101(Suppl 2):S5-S8.
24. Murray NG, Low BJ, Hollis C, Cross AW, Davis SM: Coordinated school health programs and academic achievement: a systematic review of the literature. J Sch Health 2007, 77:589-600.
25. Lister-Sharp D, Chapman S, Stewart-Brown S, Sowden A: Health promoting schools and health promotion in schools: two systematic reviews. Health Technol Assessment 1999, 3:1-207. OpenURL
26. Wanjirũ M, Flisher AJ: Evaluations of health promoting schools: a review of nine studies. Health Promot Int 2004, 19:357-368.
27. Veugelers PJ, Fitzgerald AL: Effectiveness of school programs in preventing childhood obesity: a multilevel comparison. Am J Public Health 2005, 95:432-435.

28. Public Health Agency of Canada: Canadian Best Practices Portal [http://cbpp-pcpe.phac-aspc.gc.ca/]
29. Swinburn B, Gill T, Kumanyika S: Obesity prevention: a proposed framework for translating evidence into action. Obes Rev 2005, 6:23-33.
30. APPLE Schools: Alberta Project Promoting active Living & healthy Eating (APPLE) Schools. [http://www.appleschools.ca/]
31. REAL Kids Alberta: Raising healthy Eating and Active Living Kids in Alberta. [http://www.realkidsalberta.ca/]
32. Alberta Education: Student population by grade, school and authority, Alberta 2006/07 school year. [http:/ / education.alberta.ca/ apps/ eireports/ pdf_files/ eis1004_2007/ eis1004_2007.pdf]
33. Rockett HRH, Breitenbach M, Frazier AL, Witschi J, Wolf AM, Field AE, Colditz GA: Validation of a youth/adolescent food frequency questionnaire. Prev Med 1997, 26:808-816.
34. Rockett HRH, Wolf AM, Colditz GA: Development and reproducibility of a food frequency questionnaire to assess diets of older children and adolescents. J Am Diet Assoc 1995, 95:336-340.
35. Government of Canada: The Canadian Nutrient File. [http:/ / www.hc-sc.gc.ca/ fn-an/ nutrition/ fiche-nutri-data/ cnf_aboutus-aproposdenous_fcen-eng. php]
36. Kant AK: Indexes of overall diet quality: a review. J Am Diet Assoc 1996, 96:785-791.
37. Kim S, Haines PS, Siega-Riz AM, Popkin BM: The Diet Quality Index-International (DQI-I) provides an effective tool for cross-national comparison of diet quality as illustrated by China and the United States. J Nutr 2003, 133:3476-3484.
38. Crocker PR, Bailey DA, Faulkner RA, Kowalski KC, McGrath R: Measuring general levels of physical activity: preliminary evidence for the Physical Activity Questionnaire for Older Children. Med Sci Sports Exerc 1997, 29:1344-1349.
39. Kowalski KC, Crocker PRE, Faulkner RA: Validation of the physical activity questionnaire for older children. Pediatr Exerc Sci 1997, 9:174-Äì186. OpenURL
40. Cole TJ, Bellizzi MC, Flegal KM, Dietz WH: Establishing a standard definition for child overweight and obesity worldwide: international survey. BMJ 2000, 320:1240.
41. Rao JNK, Scott AJ: The analysis of categorical data from complex sample surveys: Chi-squared tests for goodness of Fit and independence in Two-Way tables. J Am Statist Assoc 1981, 76:221-230.
42. Rao JNK, Scott AJ: On Chi-squared tests for multiway contingency tables with cell proportions estimated from survey data. Ann Statist 1984, 12:46-60.
43. Willett W: Nutritional Epidemiology. 2nd edition. New York: Oxford University Press; 1998.
44. Wang S, Moss JR, Hiller JE: Applicability and transferability of interventions in evidence-based public health. Health Promot Int 2006, 21:76-83.
45. Day ME, Strange KS, McKay HA, Naylor PJ: Action schools! BC-Healthy Eating: effects of a whole-school model to modifying eating behaviours of elementary school children. Can J Public Health 2008, 99:328-331.
46. Wang MC, Rauzon S, Studer N, Martin AC, Craig L, Merlo C, Fung K, Kursunoglu D, Shannguan M, Crawford P: Exposure to a Comprehensive School Intervention Increases Vegetable Consumption. J Adolesc Health 2010, 47:74-82.

47. Kuhle S, Kirk S, Ohinmaa A, Yasui Y, Allen AC, Veugelers PJ: Use and cost of health services among overweight and obese Canadian children. Int J Pediatr Obes 2011, 6(2):142-148.
48. Troiano RP, Berrigan D, Dodd KW, Masse LC, Tilert T, McDowell M: Physical activity in the United States measured by accelerometer. Med Sci Sports Exerc 2008, 40:181-188.
49. Livingstone MB, Black AE: Markers of the validity of reported energy intake. J Nutr 2003, 133(Suppl 3):895S-920S.

CHAPTER 13

SCHOOL HEALTH GUIDELINES TO PROMOTE HEALTHY EATING AND PHYSICAL ACTIVITY: RECOMMENDATIONS AND REPORTS

DIVISION OF ADOLESCENT AND SCHOOL HEALTH, NATIONAL CENTER FOR CHRONIC DISEASE PREVENTION AND HEALTH PROMOTION

13.1 BACKGROUND

Healthy eating and regular physical activity play a substantial role in preventing chronic diseases, including heart disease, cancer, and stroke, the three leading causes of death among adults aged >18 years (1–5). Poor diet and physical inactivity among younger persons can lead to an increased risk for certain chronic health conditions, including high blood pressure, type 2 diabetes, and obesity (1). During 2007–2008, 20% of U.S. children aged 6–11 years and 18% of persons aged 12–19 years were obese, percentages that have tripled since 1980 (6). Engaging children and adolescents in healthy eating and regular physical activity can lower their risk for obesity and related chronic diseases (7,8).

Reprinted with permission from the Centers for Disease Control and Prevention. School Health Guidelines to Promote Healthy Eating and Physical Activity: Recommendations and Reports. Division of Adolescent and School Health, National Center for Chronic Disease Prevention and Health Promotion. Morbidity and Mortality Weekly Report (MMWR), *(2011).*

The dietary and physical activity behaviors of children and adolescents are influenced by many sectors of society, including families, communities, schools, child care settings, health-care providers, faith-based institutions, government agencies, the media, and the food and beverage industries and entertainment industry. Each of these sectors has an important, independent role to play in improving the dietary and physical activity behaviors of young persons. Schools play a particularly critical role by establishing a safe and supportive environment with policies and practices that support healthy behaviors. Schools also provide opportunities for students to learn about and practice healthy eating and physical activity behaviors.

13.2 INTRODUCTION

In response to the childhood obesity epidemic, much research has been conducted on school-based obesity prevention and healthy eating and physical activity promotion and intervention since the last publication of the *Guidelines for School and Community Programs to Promote Lifelong Physical Activity Among Young People* (1997) and the *Guidelines for School Health Programs to Promote Lifelong Healthy Eating* (1996). The new guidelines in this report synthesize the scientific evidence and best practices during 1995–2009 and combine healthy eating and physical activity into one set of evidence-based guidelines for schools serving students in kindergarten through 12th grade (grades K–12); other educational programs within schools, such as prekindergarten, might also be able to apply these guidelines in their settings. These guidelines support the 2010 *Dietary Guidelines for Americans* (5), the *2008 Physical Activity Guidelines for Americans* (9), and the *Healthy People 2020* objectives related to healthy eating and physical activity among children and adolescents and schools (10). The guidelines establish a foundation for developing, implementing, and evaluating school-based healthy eating and physical activity policies and practices for students (Appendix A). Each of the nine guidelines is accompanied by a series of strategies for schools to implement.

The primary audience for this report includes state and local education and health agencies, federal agencies, and national nongovernmental organizations that focus on the health of students in school. Agencies can use these guidelines to establish professional development materials, programs, and resources for partners and constituents. Locally, physical education and health education teachers, school nutrition directors, school health councils, and other school staff members; health-care providers; community members; policy makers; parents; and students can use these guidelines to establish, implement, and assess healthy eating and physical activity policies and practices in schools. Finally, faculty members in institutions of higher education can use these guidelines to teach students of school health, public health, physical education, health education, exercise and wellness, physical activity, dietetics, nutrition education, nursing, elementary and secondary education, and other health- and education-related disciplines.

13.3 METHODS

This report updates and combines the previously published *Guidelines for School and Community Programs to Promote Lifelong Physical Activity Among Young People* (1997) and *Guidelines for School Health Programs to Promote Lifelong Healthy Eating* (1996) (11 ,12). The current guidelines and the corresponding strategies and actions were developed through a synthesis of scientific reports and expert opinion about effective and feasible practices in U.S. schools. Development of the guidelines involved an extensive literature search, development and use of a codebook by CDC staff members for rating the sufficiency of the scientific evidence and expert opinion, and an review by approximately 50 organizations and persons in the fields of school health, education, public health, nutrition, and physical activity. The use of practice-based expert opinion refines research-based guidelines to ensure that recommendations are accessible, given limited funding and resources; credible, allowing them to be implemented in various school settings and communities; and reasonable in terms of the expectations they set for professional practice and health outcomes (13).

13.3.1 LITERATURE SEARCH AND INCLUSION CRITERIA

CDC scientists conducted an extensive search for scientific reports, using five electronic citation databases: Medline, Cinahl, Sports Discus, PsychInfo, and ERIC. The coordinated school health approach was used to organize the literature search results for school-based nutrition and physical activity as they related to a healthy and safe school environment; nutrition services; physical education and school-based physical activity; health education; health services and counseling, psychological and social services; family and community involvement; and health promotion for staff members.

Scientific reports were included if they described practices to improve child and adolescent nutrition and physical activity that were based in schools or that addressed family or community involvement in schools. Two overall types of scientific reports were used to identify the new guidelines and corresponding strategies and actions: 1) reports that included cross-sectional, prospective, and randomized controlled trials that were designed to improve healthy eating and physical activity and prevent youth obesity and to promote wellness among school employees and 2) expert statements that included opinions, commentaries, or consensus statements from public health and education organizations or agencies about youth nutrition, physical activity, or obesity prevention. Scientific reports were included if they were published during 1995–2009 to update and expand on research described in the previous guidelines. Epidemiologic and surveillance data also were used to develop the introductory text.

Reports were excluded from consideration if they included only preschool children or college-age or older adults, were not in English, described clinical trials for weight-loss drugs or other nonbehavioral methods for weight loss, primarily addressed mental health issues such as eating disorders, or described interventions to improve performance in a specific sport or to improve functional ability after illness or injury. A total of 6,213 abstracts were screened to identify full scientific reports to be retrieved. A total of 1,325 full scientific reports and expert statements were retrieved and reviewed for consideration in the guidelines.

13.3.2 CHARACTERISTICS OF SCIENTIFIC REPORTS

A team of four CDC scientists used a database to record descriptions of each of the 1,325 scientific reports and expert statements, including health topics (e.g., nutrition, physical activity, and obesity prevention); component of the coordinated school health framework (e.g., physical education and health education); setting of the intervention (e.g., school, district, and community or county level); geographic location; age, sex, race/ethnicity, socioeconomic status, and health condition of participants; and topic of the report (e.g., policy and curricula). For reports describing evaluation studies, CDC scientists identified and documented the sample size, demographic makeup of study participants, duration of study, method of group assignment (e.g., random, quasiexperimental, or single group); length of follow-up after baseline measures; and outcomes of the study, such as impact on participant knowledge, attitude, behavior, or health status. Expert statements were described by type of statement (e.g., expert group statement, best practices document, or position statement), who convened the statement process, who funded the statement process, the nature of the convening group (e.g., established organization, ad hoc committee, federally sponsored committee, or CDC-funded grantee), and how evidence was presented in the expert statement.

13.3.3 RATING SUFFICIENCY OF EVIDENCE

After describing the characteristics of evaluation studies and expert statements, four CDC staff members rated the relevance of each for inclusion in the guidelines. Each study and expert statement was read, and its evidence was rated. For scientific reports, the rating process focused on rigor, confidence in the findings, efficacy, and feasibility. For expert statements, the rating process focused on the organization that published or wrote the report, conflicts of interest, and evidence to support the statement.

13.3.4 SCIENTIFIC REPORTS

Scientific reports were included if they had a rigorous study design with, at a minimum, a matched comparison group, strong study methods that contributed to confidence in the results, evaluation efficacy that included one or more positive results, and feasibility of implementing the intervention rated as medium or better. All four categories had to be rated as acceptable for a study to be included in the review for this guideline document.

In addition to the review of research and evaluation studies, CDC staff members identified, collected, and considered for inclusion all relevant reports from the Task Force on Community Preventive Services. Three task force reports on nutrition, physical activity, and obesity were relevant (i.e., applicable to school settings) and included recommendations from the task force.

13.3.5 EXPERT STATEMENTS

Best practice documents, position statements of individual persons or on behalf of organizations, and convened expert panels that covered topics related to youth physical activity and nutrition were included in the expert statements that were read and rated for sufficiency of evidence. Expert statements were included if 1) the experts had no conflicts of interest (i.e., financial support was reported and was provided by a federal agency or federal agency sponsor, a national nongovernmental organization such as the American Academy of Pediatrics, National Association for Sport and Physical Education, or American Dietetic Association, or a state-level health or education department); 2) the convening group was an established organization, federally sponsored committee, or a partner funded by the CDC Division of Adolescent and School Health; and 3) the expert statements could be associated with an evidence base (e.g., literature review and synthesis or meta-analysis).

13.3.6 CODING AND SYNTHESIS

To ensure standardized and reliable coding, four CDC staff worked in pairs to rate a subset of 40 reports. Discrepancies among coders were resolved through group discussion and consensus. The 1,325 scientific reports and expert statements were coded and categorized by each component for coordinated school health: healthy and safe school environment; nutrition services; physical education and school-based physical activity; health education; health services and counseling, psychological, and social services; family and community involvement; and school employee wellness. The CDC staff members concluded that there was enough scientific evidence on school-based nutrition and physical activity for each component of the coordinated school health framework to be an independent guideline. Furthermore, the CDC staff members identified enough scientific evidence to support the inclusion of two additional guidelines: 1) using a coordinated approach for nutrition and physical activity policies and practices and 2) professional development for school staff members. After identifying each guideline, the CDC staff members reviewed the scientific reports again to identify common strategies and actions within each guideline that resulted in positive associations with student knowledge, attitude, behavior, or health outcomes related to physical activity, diet, weight, or chronic disease risk factors. Expert statements also were reviewed for strategies and actions that are supported by opinions, commentaries, or consensus statements from public health and education organizations or agencies about youth nutrition, physical activity, or obesity prevention. Ultimately, 255 research and evaluation studies and 112 expert statements were rated as presenting evidence of sufficient relevance for a strategy or action to be included in the revision of the guidelines. An additional 343 descriptive articles were included in the document to support the background information (e.g., epidemiologic and surveillance data) included in the introduction and within each guideline.

13.3.7 EXPERT INPUT

In addition to the literature search and rating the sufficiency of the evidence, CDC convened a group of 10 experts in youth nutrition, physical activity, school health, school food service, education, and public health to review the scientific evidence and to provide individual input on proposed revisions of the guidelines. Input from the individual experts on the nine guidelines and corresponding strategies and actions were reviewed and integrated into the guidelines. CDC also garnered input from 53 federal and state education and public health agencies, as well as from nongovernmental organizations that represented policy makers, educators, parents, students, school nurses, physicians, and other health-care providers. Each of the 53 agencies provided a review of the guidelines and proposed revisions. The revised version was sent for review and revision to three experts in the field of school-based nutrition and physical activity who had not previously reviewed the document.

13.4 EPIDEMIOLOGIC ASPECTS OF HEALTHY EATING AND PHYSICAL ACTIVITY

13.4.1 LONG-TERM OUTCOMES OF HEALTHY EATING AND PHYSICAL ACTIVITY

This report was developed in response to the long-term and intermediate outcomes associated with inadequate physical activity and unhealthy eating. Healthy eating and physical activity have been associated with increased life expectancy, increased quality of life, and reduced risk for many chronic diseases (9,14–16). Healthy living through healthy eating and regular physical activity reduces the risk for the top three leading causes of death in the United States (heart disease, cancer, and stroke), as well as for certain chronic conditions, such as high blood pressure and type 2 diabetes (1,2,17).

13.4.2 CARDIOVASCULAR DISEASE

Cardiovascular disease (CVD) includes coronary heart disease, myocardial infarction, congestive heart failure, stroke, and other diseases and illnesses of the heart and blood vessels. Heart disease is the leading cause of death in the United States, and stroke is the third leading cause (18). Adult population subgroups disproportionately affected by CVD and its related risk factors include blacks, Hispanics, Mexican-Americans, and persons of low socioeconomic status (19). A healthy diet and regular physical activity can prevent and reduce metabolic risk factors that cause CVD, including hyperlipidemia (e.g., high cholesterol and triglyceride levels), high blood pressure, obesity, and insulin resistance and glucose intolerance (2,9,20). For example, dietary fiber can decrease the cholesterol concentration in the blood (21), and physical activity can help maintain normal blood glucose levels (9).

Studies indicate that CVD risk factors occur more frequently in obese children. Data from 2003–2006 National Health and Nutrition Examination Survey (NHANES) indicated that 3% of children and adolescents aged 8–17 years had increased blood pressure and that this risk was significantly greater among those who were obese (8%) (22). In a community-based sample of obese children aged 5–17 years, 70% had at least one CVD risk factor, such as a high cholesterol or triglyceride level, high blood pressure, or high insulin level, and 39% had two or more risk factors (23). However, among children of normal weight, 26% had at least one risk factor, and 13% had two or more risk factors (23).

13.4.3 CANCER

Cancer is the second leading cause of death in the United States, and black adults have a higher incidence rate of cancer than persons of any other racial/ethnic group (18,24). Some types of cancer can be prevented through regular physical activity and a diet consisting of various healthy foods with an emphasis on plant sources (e.g., fruits, vegetables, and whole grains) (17). A diet rich in plant foods is associated with a decreased risk for lung, esophageal, stomach, and colorectal cancer (17). Dietary factors that influence cancer risk include food type, variety, preparation, portion size, and fat content (17,25). Excess consumption of processed and red meats is associated with an increased risk for colorectal and prostate cancer (17).

Physical activity might contribute to cancer prevention through its role in regulating the production of hormones, boosting the immune system, and reducing insulin resistance (9). Regular physical activity can reduce the risk for developing cancers of the breast and colon, and some evidence indicates that physical activity can reduce the risk for developing endometrial and lung cancers (9). Healthy eating and physical activity also can contribute to cancer prevention by preventing obesity (9). Overweight and obesity are associated with increased risk for numerous types of cancer, including cancer of the breast, colon, endometrium, esophagus, kidney, pancreas, gall bladder, thyroid, ovary, cervix, and prostate, as well as multiple myeloma and Hodgkin's lymphoma (17).

13.4.4 DIABETES

Diabetes, a disease characterized by high blood glucose levels (26), was the seventh leading cause of death in the United States in 2007 (18). Diabetes is the leading cause of kidney failure, nontraumatic lower-extremity amputations, and new cases of blindness among adults and can affect the nervous system and oral health (26). Persons with diabetes have a two to four times higher risk for dying from CVD than those without diabetes (27,28). Diabetes is a result of defects in insulin production, insulin action, or both and is classified as either type 1 (insulin-dependent diabetes) or type 2 (usually non–insulin-dependent diabetes) (26). Although diet and physical activity can help control blood glucose levels and reduce complications from both types of diabetes, type 1 diabetes is an autoimmune disease of the pancreas, and little is known about prevention (29). In 2001, the prevalence of type 1 diabetes among a sample of U.S. persons aged 10–19 years was 2.28 cases per 1,000 persons (30).

Type 2 diabetes is the most common form of diabetes in adults (26). Healthy eating and regular physical activity can help prevent this type of diabetes (29,31,32). Type 2 diabetes was previously observed primarily among adults but has become more common among children and adolescents (26,29). In 2001, the prevalence of type 2 diabetes in a sample of U.S. persons aged 10–19 years was 0.42 cases per 1,000 persons (30) and was greatest among Asian/Pacific Islander, black, Hispanic, and American Indian persons (33). In the Pima Indian community, type 2 diabetes in children and adolescents aged 5–14 years increased significantly from 0.5 cases per 1,000 person-years in 1965–1977 to 3.3 cases per 1,000 person-years in 1991–2003 (32). According to the 2005–2006 NHANES, 16% (overall) of persons aged 12–19 years and 30% of obese persons aged

12–19 years had prediabetes, a condition in which blood glucose levels indicate a high risk for development of diabetes (26,34).

13.4.5 INTERMEDIATE OUTCOMES OF HEALTHY EATING AND PHYSICAL ACTIVITY

Poor diet and physical inactivity are risk factors for numerous conditions that affect overall health and quality of life, and many of these conditions can lead to chronic diseases. Intermediate outcomes such as obesity, metabolic syndrome, inadequate bone health, undernutrition, iron deficiency, eating disorders, and dental caries can begin in childhood, leading to earlier onset of disease and subsequent premature death.

13.4.6 OBESITY

Healthy eating and physical activity control body weight through a balance of energy expenditure and caloric consumption (35). Weight gain occurs when persons expend less energy through physical activity than they consume through their diet (35). As this imbalance continues over time, the risk for overweight and obesity increases (35). Overweight is defined as having excess body weight for a particular height from fat, muscle, bone, water, or a combination of these factors (36). Obesity is the condition of excess body fat (37). Body mass index (BMI) is a ratio of weight and height (kilograms/meters^2) and is the most widely used and recommended measure to estimate weight status. In adults, weight status is determined directly by BMI. Among adults aged ≥20 years, overweight is classified as BMI ≥25 to <30 kg/m^2; obesity is classified as BMI ≥30 kg/m^2. Weight status in persons aged 2–19 years is determined by comparing their BMI to other persons of the same sex and age in a reference population. BMI is calculated and plotted by age on a sex-specific growth chart to determine a BMI-for-age percentile. Among persons aged 2–20 years, overweight is classified as BMI ≥85th to <95 percentile for age and sex; obesity is classified as BMI ≥95th percentile for age and sex (38).

In 2008, the prevalence of obesity among children aged 6–11 years was 20%, nearly triple the prevalence in 1980 (7%) (6,39–41). The rate among persons aged 12–19 years more than tripled over the same period, increasing from 5% to 18% (6,39–41). A *Healthy People 2020* national health objective (nutrition and weight status [NWS]) is to reduce the proportion of children aged 6–11 years who are obese to 16% and reduce the proportion of persons aged 12–19 years who are obese to 16% by 2020 (objectives NWS 10.2 and NWS 10.3).

Since 1980, blacks aged <20 years have experienced greater BMI increases than both white and Mexican-American persons of the same age (42). During 2007–2008, non-Hispanic black females aged 2–19 years had significantly higher odds of being obese (23%) compared with non-Hispanic white females (15%); Hispanic males aged 2–19 years had significantly higher odds of being obese (24%) compared with non-Hispanic white males (16%) (6). Other evidence suggests that childhood obesity is significantly more common in American Indian/Alaska Native children than in white or Asian children (43). In addition, a greater percentage of adolescents from families in poverty are obese (23%) compared with those from families not in poverty (14%) (44). (Poverty is determined by the poverty-income ratio, which is the ratio of a family's income to the U.S. Census Bureau's poverty threshold. The threshold varies with the number and ages of family members and is revised yearly.)

Obesity in children and adolescents is associated with numerous immediate health risks, including high blood pressure, high blood cholesterol levels, type 2 diabetes, metabolic syndrome, sleep disturbances, orthopedic problems, and social and psychological problems, such as discrimination and poor self-esteem (7,35,45). These immediate health risks can have long-term consequences for children and adolescents, affecting them into adulthood. Insufficient public health and education efforts to decrease or minimize these health risks will affect both health-care and education systems.

Increasing rates of obesity among children and adolescents are of particular concern because those who are obese are more likely to become overweight or obese adults and have related chronic diseases (8). The probability of childhood obesity persisting into adulthood increases as children enter adolescence (46,47); even obesity during early childhood (ages 2–5 years) increases the risk for adult obesity (47–49). For example, a community-based study found that among boys aged 9–11 years, 4% of those with a childhood BMI <50th percentile (normal weight) and 22% of those with a childhood BMI of 50th–84th percentile (normal weight) became obese adults, whereas 76% of those who were obese (BMI ≥95th percentile) became obese adults. The findings were consistent for both sexes and all childhood age groups studied in the cohort (2–5 years, 6–8 years, 9–11 years, 12–14 years, 15–17 years) (47). Obesity in adults is associated with an increased risk for premature death, heart disease, type 2 diabetes, stroke, several types of cancer, osteoarthritis, and many other health problems (8,50). The risk factors and precursors to these diseases are being detected in obese children (23), and national concern exists that this trend might lower the age of onset of chronic conditions and diseases and possibly decrease the quality of life or shorten the lifespan of obese children (51).

13.4.7 METABOLIC SYNDROME

Metabolic syndrome is a clustering of metabolic risk factors that increases the risk for prematurely developing CVD and type 2 diabetes (52). Metabolic syndrome is defined as the presence of three or more of the following metabolic risk factors: abdominal obesity, high triglyceride levels, low high-density lipoprotein cholesterol (HDL-C) levels, high blood pressure, and high fasting glucose levels (52). Physical inactivity and obesity are established risk factors for metabolic syndrome, and a poor diet can accelerate the risk for developing CVD among persons with metabolic syndrome (52). A total of 27% of U.S. adults in 2004 (53) and 9% of adolescents in 2010 had metabolic syndrome (54), with Hispanic males having the highest prevalence among adolescents (54). In 2003, metabolic syndrome was significantly more prevalent among obese persons than among those of normal weight (55).

13.4.8 INADEQUATE BONE HEALTH

According to the 2004 Surgeon General's report on bone health and osteoporosis, diet and physical activity are responsible for 10%–50% of bone mass and structure (56). Adequate calcium and vitamin D intake, along with weight-bearing physical activity (e.g., walking, jogging, and weightlifting), provide bones with proper support for healthy growth. Physical activity places a mechanical load on the skeleton, and the body responds by strengthening bone mass to support the activity. In addition, both vitamin D and regular physical activity enhance the positive effects of calcium (56).

Bone growth during adolescence is particularly crucial for achieving optimal bone health because bone mass peaks in late adolescence (56,57). Adolescents who do not achieve optimal bone mass during this period will lack the adequate support to sustain normal losses of bone mass later in life. Low body weight, weight loss, physical inactivity, and dieting among children and adolescents can lead to low bone density. Low bone density leads to osteoporosis, which is the most common cause of fractures among adults. In older adults, fractures lead to physical disabilities, depression, reduced quality of life, and potentially death (56,57). In 2004, approximately 10 million U.S. adults aged >50 years had osteoporosis, and an additional 33 million U.S. adults had the precursor condition, osteopenia (low bone mass). These conditions disproportionately affect women (56). In addition, obesity in children and adolescents is associated with orthopedic complications such as fractures, musculoskeletal pain, impairment in mobility, and abnormal lower extremity alignment (58).

13.4.9 FOOD INSECURITY

Reduced food intake and disrupted eating patterns because a household lacks money and other resources for food is referred to as food insecurity. In 2008, approximately 49.1 million persons in the United States lived in food-insecure households, including 16.7 million children and adolescents, or 23% of all U.S. children and adolescents (59). Blacks and Hispanics have the highest prevalence of undernutrition (60), and food insecurity and hunger might be associated with lower dietary quality and undernutrition in children and adolescents, especially in adolescents (61). Undernutrition can have lasting effects on overall health, cognitive development, and school performance (62–65). Children and adolescents in food-insecure households have poorer health status and experience more frequent stomachaches and headaches than those from food-secure households (62). In addition to poor health outcomes, behavioral and psychosocial problems also have been associated with food insecurity and hunger in children and adolescents (62–64,66). Those who are food insecure have lower physical functioning and quality of life (67).

Children and adolescents experiencing hunger have lower math scores and are more likely to repeat a grade in school and receive special education services or mental health counseling than those not experiencing hunger (62,63). Children and adolescents experiencing hunger also are more likely to be absent and tardy from school than other children and adolescents (64). Schools have a long history of seeking out and developing strategies to address these concerns. The National School Lunch Program and School Breakfast Program were initiated, in part, as a way to reduce undernutrition among children and adolescents (68).

13.4.10 IRON DEFICIENCY

Iron deficiency is a condition resulting from too little iron in the body (69). Iron deficiency hampers the body's ability to produce hemoglobin, which is needed to carry oxygen in the blood. This deficiency can increase fatigue, shorten attention span, decrease work capacity, impair psychomotor development, affect physical activity, and reduce resistance to infection (70 ,71). Iron deficiency ranges from depleted iron stores without functional or health impairment to iron deficiency with anemia, which affects the functioning of several body systems (70). To prevent iron deficiency, children and adolescents need to consume adequate amounts of foods containing iron (e.g., meat, poultry, egg yolk, dried fruit, dried peas and beans, nuts, green leafy vegetables, whole grain breads, and fortified cereals), as well as foods high in vitamin C (e.g., citrus fruits, tomatoes, melons, peppers, greens, cabbage, broccoli, strawberries, kiwis, and potatoes), to help the body absorb iron efficiently (70). Among school-age children and adolescents with iron deficiency, anemia is associated with poor cognition and lower academic performance (72,73). Whether this association exists among iron-deficient children and adolescents without anemia is unclear (73).

A *Healthy People 2020* national health objective strives to reduce iron deficiency among young children (aged 1–4 years) and females of child-bearing age (aged 12–49 years) (objective NWS 21) (10). Among females aged 12–19 years, the prevalence of iron deficiency is 9% (74). In a national sample, children and adolescents who were overweight or obese were approximately twice as likely to be iron deficient than those of normal weight (75).

13.4.11 EATING DISORDERS

Eating disorders are psychological disorders characterized by severe disturbances in eating behavior. Anorexia nervosa is characterized by a refusal to maintain a normal body weight. Bulimia nervosa is characterized by repeated episodes of binge eating followed by compensatory behaviors such as self-induced vomiting (76). Disorders that do not meet all criteria for either anorexia nervosa or bulimia nervosa are referred to as eating disorders not otherwise specified.

Eating disorders are more common in females than males. Among females, the lifetime prevalence of anorexia nervosa is approximately 0.5%, and the lifetime prevalence of bulimia nervosa is 1%–3% (76). The prevalence of anorexia nervosa and bulimia nervosa in males is approximately one tenth that in females.

According to the American Psychiatric Association, the prevalence of anorexia nervosa and bulimia nervosa in U.S. children and younger adolescents is not well documented (77). However, children and adolescents report disordered eating behaviors that are clinically severe but do not meet full criteria for an eating disorder. For example, in 2009, in a nationally representative sample of high school students, 11% of students had gone without eating for >24 hours; 5% had taken diet pills, powders, or liquids without a physician's advice; and 4% had vomited or taken laxatives to lose weight or to keep from gaining weight during the 30 days before the survey (78). Eating disorders can cause severe complications, and mortality rates for these disorders are among the highest for any psychiatric disorder (79).

13.4.12 DENTAL CARIES

Dental caries is the most common chronic condition in children and adolescents, with the greatest prevalence in blacks and Mexican-Americans and in those who live in poverty (80). Pain from untreated caries can affect school attendance, eating, speaking, and subsequent growth and development (80). Dental caries is associated with sugar and full-calorie soda consumption (80,81). Children who are obese have been found to have higher rates of dental caries than their normal weight peers (82).

13.4.13 HEALTHY EATING RECOMMENDATIONS

The *Dietary Guidelines for Americans* have been published every 5 years since 1980 (5). These guidelines provide authoritative advice for persons aged ≥2 years on establishing dietary habits that promote health and reduce the risk for chronic disease. The guidelines recommend a diet rich in fruits and vegetables, whole grains, and fat-free and low-fat dairy products for persons aged ≥2 years. The guidelines also recommend that children, adolescents, and adults limit intake of solid fats (major sources of saturated and trans fatty acids), cholesterol, sodium, added sugars, and refined grains (5). National health objectives include increasing the consumption of fruits, vegetables, whole grains, and calcium among persons aged ≥2 years, reducing consumption of calories from solid fats and added sugars, reducing consumption of saturated fats, and reducing sodium consumption (objectives NWS-14 through NWS-21) (10).

13.4.14 EATING BEHAVIORS OF CHILDREN AND ADOLESCENTS

Available data indicate that most children and adolescents do not follow critical dietary guidelines. For example, the 2010 guidelines provide guidance on the amount of fruits and vegetables that children and adolescents should consume. The recommendation for persons aged 5–18 years is 21/2–61/2 cups of fruits and vegetables each day, depending on age and calorie requirements (5). However, most U.S. children and adolescents do not follow the recommendations for the numbers of daily servings or variety consumed (3). Furthermore, according to the 2009 national Youth Risk Behavior Survey (YRBS), only 22% of students in grades 9–12 reported consuming fruits and vegetables five or more times per day (78). The guidelines also recommend that children aged 4–8 years drink 2 cups of fat-free or low-fat milk or equivalent milk products per day and persons aged 9–18 years drink 3 cups per day (i.e., 1,300 mg/day), yet most children and adolescents do not drink the recommended amounts (3). A total of 15% of students in grades 9–12 drank three or more glasses of milk per day in 2009 (5,78). During 2007–2008, females aged 12–19 years had a particularly low intake of calcium, consuming an average of 878 mg of calcium daily, which is 67% of the recommended dietary allowance (5,83). In addition, from the 1970s through the mid-1990s, milk consumption among female adolescents decreased 36% (84).

The guidelines recommend that children and adolescents consume at least half of their daily grain intake as whole grains, which for many people is 2- to 3-oz equivalents, depending on age, sex, and calorie level (5). Whole grains are an important source of fiber and other nutrients. Persons aged 4–18 years do not eat the minimum recommended amounts of whole grains. During 2001–2004, the median intakes of whole grains in this age group ranged from 0.26–0.48 oz, far less than the recommended amounts (3).

During 2007–2008, the average percentage of calories from fat consumed by persons aged 6–19 years was 33%. Although these percentages are similar to those suggested by the dietary guidelines for total fat consumption (25%–35% of total calories), persons aged 6–19 years consumed more than the recommended amount of saturated fat (10% of total calories), ranging from 11%–12% (5,83).

Sodium intake, which is associated with increased blood pressure (85), has increased steadily during the last 35 years, in large part because of increased consumption of processed foods such as salty snacks and increased frequency of eating food away from home (84). The guidelines recommend a maximum daily intake of sodium of 2,300 mg or 1,500 mg, depending on age and other individual characteristics. African Americans; persons with hypertension, diabetes, or chronic kidney disease; and persons aged ≥51 years should have a sodium consumption of <1,500 mg/

day. These groups make up approximately half of the U.S. population aged ≥2 years. However, almost all persons in the United States consume more than the recommended amount of sodium. During 2007–2008, boys aged 6–11 years and 12–19 years had an average daily sodium intake of 3,169 mg and 3,990 mg, respectively. Girls aged 6–11 and 12–19 years had an average daily sodium intake of 2,717 mg and 3,013 mg, respectively (83).

Although the dietary guidelines do not have a recommendation for the maximum daily intake for added sugar, they do recommend that persons reduce their intake of added sugars (5). Children and adolescents tend to have diets high in added sugar (84), with added sugar contributing approximately 18% of their total daily calories (86). Sugar-sweetened beverages (such as soda and fruit drinks) are major contributors to added sugar consumption and contribute an average of 8% of energy intake among persons aged 2–18 years (86). Males aged 12–19 years consume an average of 22.0 oz of full-calorie soda per day, more than twice their intake of fluid milk (9.8 oz); females consume an average of 14.3 oz of full-calorie soda and 6.3 oz of fluid milk (87). Because many foods and beverages with added sugar tend to contain few or no essential nutrients or dietary fiber, the guidelines advise that one way to reduce intake of added sugar is to replace sweetened foods and beverages with those that are free of or low in added sugars (5). In addition, empty calories from added sugar and solid fats contribute 40% of daily calories for persons aged 2–18 years, affecting overall diet quality (86). Approximately half of these empty calories come from six sources, which include soda, fruit drinks, dairy desserts, grain desserts, pizza, and whole milk (86).

The guidelines recommend that persons in the United States, including children and adolescents, strive to achieve and maintain a healthy body weight. Specifically, children and adolescents are encouraged to maintain the calorie balance needed to support normal growth and development without promoting excess weight gain (5). During 1971–2000, a significant increase in caloric intake occurred in the United States (88). Changes in energy intake among children and adolescents varied by age. Studies indicate that the overall energy intake among children (aged 2–5 and 6–11 years) remained relatively stable from 1971 to the late 1990s and 2000 (84,89,90). However, the energy intake among persons aged 12–19 years increased significantly during the same period (84,90,91).

13.4.15 FACTORS THAT INFLUENCE THE EATING BEHAVIORS OF CHILDREN AND ADOLESCENTS

Multiple factors, including demographic, personal, and environmental factors, influence the eating behaviors of children and adolescents. Male adolescents report greater consumption of fruits and vegetables and higher daily intakes of calcium, dairy servings, and milk servings than females (78 ,92). Black adolescents are more likely than white or Hispanic adolescents to report eating fruits and vegetables five or more times per day (78). Children and adolescents from low-income households are less likely to eat whole grain foods (93).

Taste preferences of children and adolescents are a strong predictor of their food intake (94). Taste preference for milk, among both males and females, is associated with calcium intake (92). Taste preferences for fruits and vegetables are one of the strongest reported correlates of fruit and vegetable intake among males and females (94). Male and female adolescents who reported frequent fast-food restaurant visits (three or more visits in the past week) were more likely to report that healthy foods tasted bad, that they did not have time to eat healthy foods, and that they cared little about healthy eating (95).

Certain behaviors and attitudes among children and adolescents are related to healthy eating. For example, behavior-change strategies that are initiated by children and adolescents (e.g., setting goals for fruit and vegetable intake or rewarding themselves for eating fruits and vegetables) and positive feelings toward eating fruits and vegetables are predictors of fruit and vegetable intake (95). Among female adolescents, self-efficacy to make healthy food choices and positive attitudes toward nutrition and health are significantly related to calcium intake (92).

The home environment and parental influence are strongly correlated with youth eating behaviors. Home availability of healthy foods is one of the strongest correlates of fruit, vegetable, and calcium and dairy intakes (92,94). Family meal patterns, healthy household eating rules, and healthy lifestyles of parents influence fruit, vegetable, calcium and dairy, and dietary fat intake of adolescents (94–97).

The physical food environment in the community, including the presence of fast-food restaurants, grocery stores, schools, and convenience stores, influences access to and availability of foods and beverages (98). A lack of grocery stores in neighborhoods is associated with reduced access to fresh fruits and vegetables (99,100) and less healthy food intake (101). Low-income neighborhoods have fewer grocery stores than middle-income neighborhoods, predominantly black neighborhoods have half the number of grocery stores as predominantly white neighborhoods, and predominantly Hispanic neighborhoods have one third the amount of grocery stores as predominantly non-Hispanic neighborhoods (102). Furthermore, lower-income and minority neighborhoods tend to have more fast-food restaurants than high-income and predominately white neighborhoods (101)

During 1994–1998, approximately three in 10 children and adolescents consumed at least one fast-food meal per day; those who reported eating fast foods consumed more total calories than those who did not (103). Children and adolescents who report eating fast foods tend to consume more total energy, fat, and sugar-sweetened beverages and consume less milk, fruits, and nonstarchy vegetables (103). Children and adolescents are more likely than adults to report fast-food consumption (104).

The school environment also influences youth eating behaviors and provides them with opportunities to consume an array of foods and beverages throughout the school day. The widespread availability of foods and beverages served outside of the federal school lunch and breakfast programs is well-documented (105,106). These products, referred to as competitive foods and beverages because they are sold in competition with traditional school meals, often are sold in the school cafeteria and are available throughout school buildings, on school grounds, or at school-sponsored events. Results from a nationally representative survey found that in the 2004–2005 school year, one or more sources of competitive foods were available in 75% of elementary schools, 97% of middle schools, and 100% of high schools (106).

Food advertising and marketing influence food and beverage preferences and purchase requests of children and adolescents (i.e., when a child asks a parent to buy a specific item) and influence the dietary intake of children and adolescents (107). Children and adolescents are exposed to many forms of marketing, including television advertisements, advertising on the Internet and advergames (i.e., interactive, electronic games on a company-sponsored website that prominently feature one or more of the company's products or services), contests and prizes, television and movie product placement, marketing in schools (e.g., school score boards, vending machines, book covers, and homework incentives), and use of licensed characters to promote foods or restaurants. In a recent report to Congress, the Federal Trade Commission estimated that in 2006, approximately $1.6 billion was spent promoting foods, beverages, and fast-food restaurants to children (108). Because of the concern regarding the effect of food marketing on the diets of children and adolescents, Congress ordered the creation of an Interagency Working Group on Food Marketing to Children in 2009 to develop recommendations for foods marketed to persons aged <18 years.

13.4.16 PHYSICAL ACTIVITY RECOMMENDATIONS

Physical activity is defined as "any bodily movement produced by the contraction of skeletal muscle that increases energy expenditure above a basal level" (9). Examples of physical activity include walking, running, bicycling, swimming, jumping rope, active games, resistance exercises, and household chores. In the 2008 Physical Activity Guidelines for Americans, the U.S. Department of Health and Human Services (HHS) recommends that children and adolescents engage in ≥60 minutes of physical activity daily. Most of the ≥60 minutes/day should be either moderate- or vigorous-intensity aerobic physical activity. The guidelines indicate that children and adolescents should include vigorous intensity, muscle-strengthening, and bone-strengthening activities at least 3 days of the week. HHS also recommends encouraging children and adolescents to participate in activities that are age appropriate, are enjoyable, and offer variety (9). Healthy People 2020 national health objectives include an objective on increasing the proportion of adolescents who meet current federal physical activity (PA) guidelines for aerobic physical activity and for muscle-strengthening activity (objective PA 3) (10).

13.4.17 PHYSICAL ACTIVITY BEHAVIORS OF CHILDREN AND ADOLESCENTS

Despite national guidelines for physical activity, many young persons are not regularly physically active. In 2002, 62% of children and adolescents aged 9–13 years did not participate in any organized physical activity during nonschool hours, and 23% did not engage in any free-time physical activity (109). The 2009 national YRBS indicated that only 18% of high school students had been physically active for 60 minutes every day in the previous week (78). In 2009, although 56% of high school students reported being enrolled in physical education, only 33% of high school students nationwide attended physical education classes 5 days in an average school week, a decrease from 1991, when 43% of students attended physical education classes 5 days/week (78). Nationwide, 58% of high school students reported playing on at least one sports team run by their school or a community group in 2009 (78). As of 2005, <15% of children and adolescents walked or bicycled to and from school (110).

13.4.18 FACTORS THAT INFLUENCE THE PHYSICAL ACTIVITY OF CHILDREN AND ADOLESCENTS

Regular participation in physical activity among children and adolescents is related to demographic, personal, social, and environmental factors. Hispanic and non-Hispanic black students are less active than their non-Hispanic white counterparts (78). In 2009, 20% of non-Hispanic white high school students, compared with 16% of Hispanic students and 17% of non-Hispanic black students, had been physically active for 60 minutes every day in the previous week (78). This difference also is evident during childhood and continues through adulthood, with non-Hispanic white adults having the highest prevalence of activity compared with other ethnic groups (111).

Sex is correlated with physical activity levels, with males participating in more overall physical activity than females (112–118). The 2009 national YRBS indicated that 25% of males and 11% of females had been physically active doing any kind of physical activity for at least 60 minutes per day in the previous week (78). This trend continues through adulthood, with females remaining less physically active than males (119). Adolescent males also report a greater intention to be physically active in the future than females (120).

Children and adolescents who intend to be active in the future and who believe physical activity is important for a healthy lifestyle engage in more activity. Overall, personal fulfillment influences the motivation both of boys and girls to be physically active (121). Child and adolescent perceptions of their ability to perform a physical activity (i.e., self-efficacy) and perceived competence affects their participation in the activity (112,121–123). Girls are motivated by physical activities that they prefer and by their confidence in their ability to perform an activity (123). Boys are affected by their ability to perform a particular physical activity, as well as by social norms among both friends and parents (123).

Positive social norms and support from friends and family encourage youth involvement in physical activity among all children and adolescents (112,122,124–132). Parent and family support for physical activity can be defined as a child's perception of support (e.g., perceiving parents will do physical activity with them and sign them up for sports or other physical activities) to a parent's reported support (e.g., regular encouragement of physical activity or regularly placing value on being active). Youth perceptions and parent reports of support for physical activity are strongly associated with participation in both structured and nonstructured physical activity among children and adolescents (112,122,133–135).

The physical environment can be both a benefit and a barrier to being physically active. Environmental factors that might pose a barrier to physical activity include low availability of safe locations to be active, perceived lack of access to physical activity equipment, cost of physical activities, and time constraints (126,136–138). Youth perceptions of neighborhood safety (e.g., traffic, strangers, poorly maintained or unsafe facilities, poor lighting, or negative social influences) also are associated with physical activity participation (139–142). Parents' perceptions about environmental factors also influence physical activity among children and adolescents. For example, parents rate distance and safety as top barriers for their children walking to school (143).

The school environment can also influence the participation of children and adolescents in physical activity. In 2006, 4% of elementary schools, 8% of middle schools, and 2% of high schools provided daily physical education for the entire school year for students in all grades in the school (144). Although this is a critical opportunity for children and adolescents to participate in physical activity, schools do not provide it daily. In addition, many schools do not regularly provide other physical activity opportunities during the school day, such as recess. In 2006, 26% of elementary schools did not provide regularly scheduled recess for students in all grades in the school (144). When schools provide supportive environments by enhancing physical education (145,146) and health education (147), having staff members become role models for physical activity, increasing communication about the benefits of physical activity, and engaging families and communities in physical activity, children and adolescents are more likely to be physically active and maintain a physically active lifestyle (147–149).

13.4.19 TELEVISION VIEWING AND OTHER SCREEN-BASED MEDIA BEHAVIORS OF CHILDREN AND ADOLESCENTS

Television viewing, nonactive computer use, and nonactive video and DVD viewing are all considered sedentary behaviors. Television viewing among children and adolescents, in particular, has been shown to be associated with childhood and adult obesity (150–157). Potential mechanisms through which television viewing might lead to childhood obesity include 1) lower resting energy expenditure, 2) displacement of physical activity, 3) food advertising that influences greater energy intake, and 4) excess eating while viewing (158,159).

The American Academy of Pediatrics (AAP) recommends no more than 2 hours of quality television and video viewing (e.g., educational television programs) per day for children aged ≥2 years (160). Overall, persons aged 8–18 years spend an average of 7 hours and 11 minutes per day watching television, using a computer, and playing video games (161). In 2009, 33% of 9th- through 12th-grade students reported watching ≥3 hours of television on an average school day, and 25% reported using a computer ≥3 hours on an average school day (78). Black high school students most frequently reported excessive television viewing (≥3 hours/day) (56%), compared with their Hispanic (42%) and non-Hispanic white (25%) counterparts. Non-Hispanic black and Hispanic students also were more likely to report excessive computer use (≥3 hours/day) (30% and 26%, respectively) compared with non-Hispanic white students (22%) (78).

The home environment offers children and adolescents many opportunities for television viewing, including eating meals while watching television or having a television in their bedroom (162–165). The presence of a television in a child's bedroom is associated with more hours spent watching television (0.25 hours/day) (163), more time engaged in video games (0.31 hours/day), more time using computers (0.21 hours/day) (163), and obesity (162,164,166,167). The likelihood of having a television in the bedroom increases with a child's age (163,167).

Eating meals in front of the television is associated with more viewing hours (163). Children and adolescents are more likely to engage in unhealthy eating behaviors when watching television (155,168,169) and are exposed to television advertisements promoting primarily restaurants and unhealthy food products (151,170). Increased television viewing among children and adolescents is associated with consuming more products such as fast food, soft drinks, and high-fat snacks (151,156,165,171–173) and consuming fewer fruits and vegetables (151,155,174).

13.4.19.1 HEALTHY PEOPLE 2020 OBJECTIVES FOR HEALTHY EATING AND PHYSICAL ACTIVITY AMONG CHILDREN AND ADOLESCENTS

Healthy People 2020 national health objectives include a comprehensive plan for health promotion and disease prevention in the United States. *Healthy People 2020* includes objectives related to physical activity and healthy eating among children and adolescents and in schools (Appendix B) (10).

13.4.20 RATIONALE FOR SCHOOL HEALTH PROGRAMS TO PROMOTE HEALTHY EATING AND PHYSICAL ACTIVITY

13.4.20.1 HEALTHY EATING, PHYSICAL ACTIVITY, AND ACADEMIC PERFORMANCE

As of 2009, >95% of children and adolescents aged 5–17 years were enrolled in schools (175). Schools have direct contact with students for approximately 6 hours each day and for up to 13 critical years of their social, psychological, physical, and intellectual development (176). The health of students is strongly linked to their academic success, and the academic success of students is strongly linked with their health. Therefore, helping students stay healthy is a fundamental part of the mission of schools (177–180). School health programs and policies might be one of the most efficient means to prevent or reduce risk behaviors, prevent serious health problems among students, and help close the educational achievement gap (181,182). Schools offer an ideal setting for delivering health promotion strategies that provide opportunities for students to learn about and practice healthy behaviors. Schools, across all regional, demographic, and income categories, share the responsibility with families and communities to provide students with healthy environments that foster regular opportunities for healthy eating and physical activity. Healthy eating and physical activity also play a significant role in students' academic performance.

The importance of healthy eating, including eating breakfast, for the overall health and well-being of school-aged children cannot be understated. Most research on healthy eating and academic performance has focused on the negative effects of hunger and food insufficiency (62) and the importance of eating breakfast (65,183,184). Recent reviews of breakfast and cognition in students (73,185,186) report that eating a healthy breakfast might enhance cognitive function (especially memory), increase attendance rates, reduce absenteeism, and improve psychosocial function and mood. Certain improvements in academic performance such as improved math scores also were noted (65,183).

A growing body of research focuses on the association between school-based physical activity, including physical education, and academic performance among school-aged children and adolescents. A comprehensive

CDC literature review that included 50 studies synthesized the scientific literature on the association between school-based physical activity, including physical education, and academic performance, including indicators of cognitive skills and attitudes, academic behaviors (e.g., concentration, attentiveness, and time on task), and academic achievement (e.g., grade point average and test scores). The review identified a total of 251 associations between school-based physical activity and academic performance. Of all the associations examined, 51% were positive, 48% were not significant, and 2% were negative. Therefore, the evidence suggests that 1) substantial evidence indicates that physical activity can help improve academic achievement, including grades and standardized test scores; 2) physical activity can affect cognitive skills and attitudes and academic behavior (including enhanced concentration, attention, and improved classroom behavior); and 3) increasing or maintaining time dedicated to physical education might help and does not appear to adversely affect academic performance (187).

13.4.21 COORDINATED SCHOOL HEALTH APPROACH

Schools can promote the acquisition of lifelong healthy eating and physical activity behaviors through strategies that provide opportunities to practice and reinforce these behaviors. School efforts to promote healthy eating and physical activity should be part of a coordinated school health framework, which provides an integrated set of planned, sequential, and school-affiliated strategies, activities, and services designed to promote the optimal physical, emotional, social, and educational development of students. A coordinated school health framework involves families and is based on school and community needs, resources, and standards. The framework is coordinated by a multidisciplinary team such as a school health council and is accountable to the school and community for program quality and effectiveness (182).

School personnel, students, families, community organizations and agencies, and businesses can collaborate to successfully implement the coordinated school health approach and develop, implement, and evaluate healthy eating and physical activity efforts. Ideally, a coordinated school health framework integrates the efforts of eight components of the school environment that influence student health (i.e., comprehensive health education, physical education, and health services: mental health and social services, school nutrition services, healthy and safe school environment, school employee wellness, and family and community involvement) (188). The following guidelines reflect the coordinated school health approach and include additional areas deemed to be important contributors to school health: policy development and implementation and professional development for program staff.

13.5 SCHOOL HEALTH GUIDELINES TO PROMOTE HEALTHY EATING AND PHYSICAL ACTIVITY

This report includes nine general guidelines for school health programs to promote healthy eating and physical activity. Each guideline is followed by a series of strategies for implementing the general guidelines. Because each guideline is important to school health, there is no priority order. Guidelines presented first focus on the importance of a coordinated approach for nutrition and physical activity policies and practices within a health-promoting school environment. Then, guidelines pertaining to nutrition services and physical education are provided, followed by guidelines for health education, health, mental health and social services, family and community involvement, staff wellness, and professional development for staff.

Although the ultimate goal is to implement all guidelines recommended in this report, not every guideline and its corresponding strategies will be feasible for every school to implement. Because of resource limitations, some schools might need to implement the guidelines incrementally. Therefore, the recommendation is for schools to identify which guidelines are feasible to implement, based on the top health needs and priorities of the school and available resources. Families, school personnel, health-care providers, businesses, the media, religious organizations, community organizations that serve children and adolescents, and the students themselves also should be systematically involved in implementing the guidelines to optimize a coordinated approach to healthy eating and regular physical activity among school-aged children and adolescents.

The guidelines in this report are not clinical guidelines; compliance is neither mandatory nor tracked by CDC. However, CDC monitors the status of student health behaviors and school health policies and practices nationwide through three surveillance systems. These systems provide information about the degree to which students are participating in healthy behaviors and schools are developing and implementing the policies and practices recommended in the guidelines. The Youth Risk Behavior Surveillance System (YRBSS) monitors priority health-risk behaviors (e.g., unhealthy dietary behaviors and physical inactivity) and the prevalence of obesity and asthma among high school students. YRBSS includes a national, school-based survey conducted by CDC and state, territorial, tribal, and district surveys conducted by state, territorial, and local education and health agencies and tribal governments. YRBSS data are used to 1) measure progress toward achieving national health objectives for Healthy People 2020 and other program and policy indicators, 2) assess trends in priority health-risk behaviors among adolescents and young adults, and 3) evaluate the effect of broad school and community interventions at the national, state, and local levels. In addition, state, territorial, and local agencies and nongovernmental organizations use YRBSS data to set and track progress toward meeting school health and health promotion program goals, support modification of school health curricula or other programs, support new legislation and policies that promote health, and seek funding and other support for new initiatives. The CDC School Health Policies and Practices Study (SHPPS) is a national survey conducted periodically to assess school health policies and practices at the state, district, school, and classroom levels. SHPPS data are used to 1) identify the characteristics of each school health program component (e.g., physical education and activity and nutrition services) at the state, district, school, and classroom (where applicable) levels across elementary, middle, and high schools; 2) identify persons responsible for coordinating and delivering each school health program component and their qualifications and educational background; 3) identify collaborations that occur among staff members from each school health program component and with staff members from outside agencies and organizations; and 4) describe changes in key policies and practices over time. The School Health Profiles (i.e., Profiles) is a system of surveys assessing school health policies and practices in states, large urban school districts, territories, and tribal governments. State, local, and territorial education and health officials use Profiles data to 1) describe school health policies and practices and compare them across jurisdictions, 2) identify professional development needs, 3) plan and monitor programs, 4) support health-related policies and legislation, 5) seek funding, and 6) garner support for future surveys. Results from the surveys are described throughout this report.

13.5.1 GUIDELINE 1. USE A COORDINATED APPROACH TO DEVELOP, IMPLEMENT, AND EVALUATE HEALTHY EATING AND PHYSICAL ACTIVITY POLICIES AND PRACTICES

Physical education, health education, and other teachers; school nutrition service staff members; school counselors; school nurses and other health, mental health, and social services staff members; community health-care providers; school administrators; student and parent groups; and community organizations should work together to maximize healthy eating and physical activity opportunities for students (Box 1). Coordination of all these persons and groups facilitates greater communication, minimizes duplication of policy and program initiatives, and increases the pooling of resources for healthy eating and physical activity policies and practices (189–192).

13.5.1.1 COORDINATE HEALTHY EATING AND PHYSICAL ACTIVITY POLICIES AND PRACTICES THROUGH A SCHOOL HEALTH COUNCIL AND SCHOOL HEALTH COORDINATOR

Establish a school health council and designate a school health coordinator at the district level. Each district should have a school health council to help ensure that schools implement developmentally appropriate and evidence-based health policies and practices. Nationwide, in 2006, 73% of districts had one or more school health councils at the district level that offered guidance on the development of policies or coordinated activities on health topics (193). The school health council serves as a planning, advisory, and decision-making group for school health policies and programs. School health councils should include representatives from different segments of the school and community, including health and physical education teachers, nutrition service staff members, students, families, school administrators, school nurses and other health-care providers, social service professionals, and religious and civic leaders (193–195). The school health council provides input on decisions about how to promote health-enhancing behaviors, including healthy eating and physical activity among students. Some roles of school health councils include (194)

- needs assessment and resource mapping;
- program planning;
- advocacy;
- financial and resource planning;
- development of policies and practices, including those that address healthy eating and physical activity;
- assistance in reviewing and making recommendations about health-related curricula and instructional materials;
- communication of the importance of health and safety policies and activities to the superintendent, school board, schools, and community;
- coordination of school health programs and events within the school district and between schools and local community groups; and
- evaluation, accountability, and quality control of school health policies and programs.

Each district also should designate a school health coordinator who manages and coordinates health-related policies and practices across the district, including those related to healthy eating and physical activity. This person serves as an active member of the district-level school health council and communicates the district school health council's decisions and actions to school-level health coordinators and teams, staff, students, and parents (189,196–198). In 2006, 68% of districts had a person who oversaw or coordinated school health (e.g., a school health coordinator) (193). A district school health coordinator also should

- work closely with school-level health coordinators to ensure consistent implementation of health policies and practices across schools;
- coordinate professional development for school health staff members;
- secure funding and other resources to support school health and safety policies and activities;

- facilitate linkages between the district's health-related programs and services and health-related resources in the community; and
- coordinate evaluation of policies and practices.

Establish a school health team and designate a school health coordinator at the school level. Each school should establish a school health team, representative of school and community groups, to work with the greater school community to identify and address the health needs of students, school administrators, parents, and school staff. Nationwide, in 2006, 40% of schools had a school health council that offered guidance on the development of policies or coordinated activities on health topics (193). A school health team

- ensures that district-level policies and practices are implemented efficiently;
- communicates and coordinates with the district-level school health coordinator;
- assists with evaluating school health policies and practices;
- recommends new or revised health and safety policies and activities;
- assists in reviewing and making recommendations about health-related curricula and instructional materials;
- seeks funding or leverages resources to support school health and safety priorities; and
- communicates the importance of school health and safety policies and activities within the school, as well as to parents and the community.

Every school also should designate a school health coordinator to manage the school health policies, practices, activities, and resources, including those that address healthy eating and physical activity. In 2006, 61% of schools had someone at the school to oversee or coordinate school health (e.g., a school health coordinator) (193). School health coordinators might:

- facilitate collaboration among school staff responsible for the health and safety of students;
- facilitate linkages between the school's health-related programs and services and health-related resources in the community (189,196,197);
- serve as a liaison between the school and those who oversee school health and safety programs at the district level and in other schools;
- communicate school health and safety priorities to the principal, staff, parents, community organizations, and students;
- help secure funding or other resources to support school building health and safety activities;

- manage school health funds;
- assist in the development of school health and safety policy materials and in the selection of educational materials;
- organize and conduct school health team meetings;
- facilitate the provision of professional development activities for school health staff; and
- assist with the assessment of student health needs and evaluation of school health policies and activities.

13.5.1.2 ASSESS HEALTHY EATING AND PHYSICAL ACTIVITY POLICIES AND PRACTICES

An assessment of current school-based healthy eating and physical activity policies and practices is necessary to provide baseline information about strengths and weaknesses. An assessment can also identify how district-level policies are being implemented at the school level and in the development of community-specific strategies. An assessment enables the school health council, school health coordinator, parents, school administrators, and school board members to develop a data-based plan for improving student health. The CDC School Health Index: A Self-Assessment and Planning Guide (available at http://www.cdc.gov/healthyyouth/shi), a tool based on scientific evidence and best practices in school health, helps schools identify strengths and weaknesses of school policies and practices related to nutrition, physical activity, and other important health topics. Schools and school districts can refer to the School Health Index for a comprehensive list of policies and practices that promote healthy eating and physical activity in schools. The School Health Index guides schools through the development of an action plan to improve their school health policies and practices (199,200). Results from the School Health Index assessment and action plan can help schools determine where, what, and how to incorporate health promotion programs and policies into their overall school improvement plan. Inclusion in the school improvement plan helps ensure that health is a regular item on agendas of district school board meetings and school-based management committees.

Completing the School Health Index can lead to positive changes in the school health environment. For example, after completing the School

Health Index, some schools have hired a physical education teacher for the first time, added healthier food choices to school meal programs, and incorporated structured fitness breaks into the school day (201–203). An assessment might also involve collection of data on current eating and physical activity behaviors of students, community-based nutrition and physical activity programs, and student, staff, and parent needs (189).

13.5.1.3 USE A SYSTEMATIC APPROACH TO DEVELOP, IMPLEMENT, AND MONITOR HEALTHY EATING AND PHYSICAL ACTIVITY POLICIES

School health policies are official statements from education agencies and other governing bodies (e.g., state legislatures) at the state, district, or school level. They identify what should be done, why it should be done, and who is responsible for doing it. School health policies can (204)

- provide evidence of leadership, commitment, and support for school health, including healthy eating and physical activity, from school boards, school administrators, and other decision makers;
- drive positive changes in healthy eating and physical activity programs;
- sustain and expand healthy eating and physical activity programs or activities;
- establish accountability by identifying who is responsible for healthy eating and physical activity programs and policies; and
- establish performance measures.

School health policies should comply with federal, state, and local laws and mandates. School health councils, teams, and coordinators can lead the development, implementation, and monitoring of policies (194,196).

The Child Nutrition and WIC Reauthorization Act of 2004 required that each school district participating in the federally supported meal program establish a local school wellness policy for the first time by school year 2006 (205). By 2007–2008, most school districts had a local wellness policy; however, the quality of policies varied across school districts. In addition, many of the policies lacked plans for implementing and monitoring the status of the wellness policy (206).

The Healthy, Hunger-Free Kids Act of 2010 (207) updated requirements for local school wellness policy to include, at a minimum,

- goals for nutrition promotion and education, physical activity, and other school-based activities that promote student wellness;
- nutrition guidelines for all foods available on each school campus under the jurisdiction of the local educational agency during the school day that are consistent with requirements in the act and that promote student health and reduce childhood obesity;
- a requirement that the local education agency permit parents, students, representatives of the school food authority, teachers of physical education, school health professionals, the school board, school administrators, and the general public to participate in the development, implementation, and periodic review and update of the local school wellness policy;
- a requirement that the local education agency inform and update the public on local school wellness policy content and implementation;
- a requirement that the local education agency periodically measure and make available to the public an assessment on the implementation of the local school wellness policy, including the level of school implementation, how the local school wellness policy compares with model policy, and a description of progress made toward goals; and
- a requirement that the local education agency designate one or more local education agency officials or school officials to ensure that each school complies with the local school wellness policy.

The act also requires that the U.S. Department of Agriculture (USDA), in conjunction with the CDC director, "prepare a report on the implementation, strength, and effectiveness of the local school wellness policies" (207).

States, districts, and schools should use a systematic approach when developing, implementing, and monitoring healthy eating and physical activity policies. They can use the following strategies throughout the policy process.

Identify and involve key stakeholders from the beginning of the policy process. One person, such as the school health coordinator (at the district or school level, depending on the level at which the policy is to be implemented), should assume or be designated with overall responsibility for coordinating and implementing healthy eating and physical activity policies. This person also can help identify and involve key stakeholders, including the school health council or team. Key stakeholders in district- and school-level policy processes include students, families, school nutrition service staff, physical education teachers, health education teachers, school nurses, school principals and other administrators, staff from local health departments, health-care providers, and staff from local community organizations and businesses. This group of stakeholders will contribute to the development, implementation, and monitoring of healthy eating and physical activity policies.

Draft the policy language. Policy language should be specific, simple, clear, and accurate; avoid education, health, and legal jargon; and be easy for readers with diverse backgrounds to understand and apply. Policy language should be consistent with state, district, and school visions for student learning and health and other policies in the same jurisdiction. A written policy should describe (204)

- who establishes the policy and the underlying legal authority;
- the rationale for the policy, including emphasis on the effects of health on academic achievement;
- the priority population (e.g., students and school staff members) to which the policy applies;
- definitions of key terms;
- a list and descriptions of the major activities to be conducted;
- who will be responsible for implementing the policy;
- who will enforce the policy and how they will do so;
- positive incentives for compliance and consequences for noncompliance;
- an evaluation plan, including how the effect of the policy will be measured and how the evaluation information will be used; and
- a timeline indicating when the policy will be adopted, take effect, and expire.

Resources to guide policy development include the National Association of State Boards of Education's (NASBE's) Fit, Healthy, and Ready to Learn (204), USDA's local wellness policy website (208), and the Action for Healthy Kids policy development tool (209). NASBE's state school health policy database includes a comprehensive set of laws and policies from 50 states on approximately 40 school health topics (available at http://www.nasbe.org/healthy_schools/hs).

Adopt, implement, and monitor healthy eating and physical activity policies. After the draft policy is completed, the process of adopting the policy begins (204,210). To ensure greater support for policy adoption, school health council members or other policy makers should be given time to share the draft policy with their partners and gather reactions. Public hearings or other meetings that gather wider input from the school and community might be beneficial or required. Such hearings allow every interested person or organization to provide input on the policy.

Policy adoption typically requires that the drafted policy be presented to the policy-making body (e.g., the school board or school administrators). The presentation should include background information about why the policy is needed (e.g., data about the eating and physical activity habits of students) and concise information about the policy. Policies likely will require final approval by the school board, the district superintendent, or both.

Implementation of policies should be a cooperative effort that includes the school health coordinator, school health council, and school staff members. All school staff members and teachers, in particular, need sufficient time to implement the policy and make agreed-on changes in the school environment to support the policy (211). Those responsible for implementation should be prepared to address challenges, such as perceptions that the policy is low priority, limited resources for full implementation, changes in school administrators and school staff members, and concerns such as lost revenue from certain food and beverage sales and resolving scheduling conflicts for use of physical activity facilities because of increasing numbers of physical activity programs (210). Parental and community concerns might be mitigated by making incremental changes and ensuring that the media receive positive stories about the response to the policy. Monitoring policy implementation allows school staff members to determine whether the policy yielded the expected results and which changes could be made to improve the results.

Establishing policy is an important component of many of the nine guidelines. Following is a list of key healthy eating and physical activity policies that are described in the remaining guidelines:

- Provide nutritious and appealing school meals that comply with the U.S. Dietary Guidelines for Americans.
- Ensure that foods and beverages sold or served outside of school meal programs follow the *Dietary Guidelines for Americans* and are consistent with the most recent scientific guidelines for nutrition standards.
- Require daily planned and sequential physical education from grades K–12.
- Require daily recess for elementary schools.
- Require planned and sequential health education from prekindergarten through grade 12.
- Require physical education specialists, health education specialists, and certified food service staff members to be hired for grades K–12.

- Provide school staff members with comprehensive professional development to deliver quality health education, physical education, food services, and health services.

13.5.1.4 EVALUATE HEALTHY EATING AND PHYSICAL ACTIVITY POLICIES AND PRACTICES

Evaluation can be used to assess and improve policies and practices that promote increased physical activity and healthier eating among students and faculty members. All groups involved in and affected by school efforts to promote lifelong physical activity and healthy eating should have the opportunity to contribute to evaluation. Education agencies and schools should designate a person to take the lead on evaluation activities. Schools may choose to enlist local universities, the health department, or the education department to assist with the evaluation of school policies and practices.

Evaluation can serve various purposes, including 1) improving the content, support for, and implementation of physical activity and healthy eating policies and practices; 2) documenting changes in the school environment, physical education and health education curricula, physical activity and healthy eating services for students and school staff members, physical activity and dietary habits, and health outcomes such as blood pressure and blood glucose levels; 3) identifying strengths and weakness of policies and practices and making a plan for improvement; and 4) responding to new and changing needs of students and school staff members. Although evaluations should not be used to audit or rank schools or penalize school staff members (199,200), evaluations can be used to motivate schools to make changes and monitor school-level implementation of school district, state, and federal policies.

Two fundamental types of evaluation are process and outcome. In process evaluation, educators collect and analyze data to determine who, what, when, where, and how much of program activities have been conducted. Process evaluation is the foundation of evaluation because it specifies the activities involved in policies, programs, and practices, and whether they were implemented as intended. In addition, process evaluation allows education agency staff members to assess how well a policy, program, or practice has been implemented and what strengths and improvements are necessary.

Outcome evaluation explores whether intended outcomes or specific changes occur as a direct result of policies, programs, or practices. Outcomes might include changes at the school level (e.g., changes in school environment, norms, or curricula) and at the individual level (e.g., student knowledge, attitudes, skills, and behaviors). Outcome evaluation can require a great deal of time, money, and expertise, and individual schools are unlikely to be able to conduct outcome evaluations on their own. A full-fledged outcome evaluation might be beyond the reach of most schools and is more likely the purview of state and local education agencies. However, some outcome-related questions can be answered using simple methods available to most schools. Outcome evaluation can focus on short- or long-term outcomes of policies, programs, or practices, including changes in practices at the school level or changes in student knowledge, attitudes, skills, behaviors, or health outcomes.

Conduct process evaluation of nutrition and physical activity policies and practices. Schools should conduct a process evaluation of their healthy eating and physical activity policies and practices. Process evaluation topics for schools might include the following:

- Did schools establish a school health council and conduct an assessment of their existing healthy eating and physical activity policies and practices?
- Did schools communicate about the development, implementation, and monitoring of healthy eating and physical activity policies to school administrators, school staff members, and others affected by the policies?
- Did schools develop a communications and marketing plan to promote participation in school breakfast, lunch, and other feeding programs that provide foods consistent with the Dietary Guidelines for Americans?
- Did schools provide training to physical education teachers on instructional strategies that would keep all students active for most of physical education class time?

Conduct outcome evaluation of healthy eating and physical activity policies, programs, and practices. In addition to the process evaluation topics, schools might evaluate changes that occurred after a policy, program, or practice was implemented. Outcome evaluation topics include the following:

- Did all foods and beverages sold in school stores, vending machines, and a la carte lines adhere to strong nutrition standards for all foods in schools?
- Did students' consumption of fruits and vegetables increase after their school increased the availability of fruits and vegetables?
- Did all students in all grades participate in daily recess throughout the school year?
- Did students' levels of physical activity increase after they participated in physical education?

CDC's *Framework for Program Evaluation in Public Health* summarizes and organizes essential elements of program evaluation (212). The *Physical Activity Evaluation Handbook* illustrates the six steps of program evaluation in the framework with physical activity program examples (213). *Understanding Evaluation: The Way to Better Prevention Programs* describes evaluation activities that school districts and community agencies can use to assess various programs (214). State and local education agencies and schools can consult with evaluators at universities, school districts, or state departments of education and health to identify methods and materials for evaluating their efforts.

13.5.2 GUIDELINE 2. ESTABLISH SCHOOL ENVIRONMENTS THAT SUPPORT HEALTHY EATING AND PHYSICAL ACTIVITY

The physical surroundings and psychosocial climate of a school should encourage all students to make healthy eating choices and be physically active. The physical environment includes the entire school building and the area surrounding it; facilities for physical activity, physical education, and food preparation and consumption; availability of food and physical activity options; and conditions such as temperature, air quality, noise, lighting, and safety (215). The psychosocial environment includes the social norms established by policies and practices that influence the physical activity and eating behaviors of students and staff members (216). Developing and maintaining a supportive school environment can improve the sustainability of healthy eating and physical activity policies and practices that support healthy lifestyles (147,217,218) (Box 2).

13.5.2.1 PROVIDE ACCESS TO HEALTHY FOODS AND PHYSICAL ACTIVITY OPPORTUNITIES AND TO SAFE SPACES, FACILITIES, AND EQUIPMENT FOR HEALTHY EATING AND PHYSICAL ACTIVITY

Provide adequate and safe spaces and facilities for healthy eating. Students should have access to a well-maintained cafeteria that is clean, is pleasant, has appropriate seating arrangements, and does not exceed 100% capacity (215,219–221). School nutrition services should serve healthy food in an environment that allows students to pay attention to what they are eating and enjoy social aspects of dining (215,220–223). Students can enjoy meal time more when they feel relaxed and are able to socialize without feeling rushed. Actions to support safe and healthy eating include

- ensuring sufficient time to receive and consume a meal, with at least 10 minutes for eating breakfast and 20 minutes for eating lunch after being seated (215,224);
- providing recess before lunch, which can reduce plate waste, increase student consumption of food (225), decrease student wait time in line, and reduce student discipline referrals (226);
- providing opportunities for students to wash or sanitize their hands in a convenient place before eating;
- providing tables and chairs of appropriate size, with space to accommodate all students with special needs (e.g., students who use wheel chairs and students with food allergies);
- maintaining an appropriate ambient noise level using acceptable and positive enforcement practices (e.g., no whistles and no orders to eat in silence [silent lunch]); and
- implementing rules for safe behavior.

Other food environment activities, such as school gardens, school salad bars, and farm-to-school programs, can enrich the eating and educational experience by providing quality produce and opportunities for hands-on multidisciplinary learning (227–231). In 2002, the National School Lunch

Act (232) was amended with a provision encouraging institutions participating in the school lunch and breakfast programs "to purchase unprocessed agricultural products, both locally grown and locally raised, to the maximum extent practicable and appropriate" (233). In addition to integrating local agriculture products, such as fruits, vegetables, and eggs, into the school cafeteria, farm-to-school activities include hands-on education through school garden programs and field trips to local farms, classroom nutrition education, and alternative fundraising using local produce (234). School garden programs have the potential to strengthen the healthy development of students through improved knowledge about fruits and vegetables (228,231,235), increased preference for fruits and vegetables (228,231,235), and increased consumption of fruits and vegetables (230,231,235,236).

Schools also should ensure that students have access to safe, free, and well-maintained drinking water fountains or dispensers during school meals, as required by the Healthy, Hunger-Free Kids Act (237), as well as throughout the school day (238). This provides a healthy alternative to sugar-sweetened beverages and can help increase students' overall water consumption (239,240). The National Policy and Legal Analysis Network (NPLAN) to Prevent Childhood Obesity has resources for developing policies and best practices to increase access to free drinking water in schools (available at http://www.nplanonline.org/childhood-obesity/products/water-access).

Ensure that spaces and facilities for physical activity meet or exceed recommended safety standards. The following should be in place to support safe and enjoyable student physical activity: 1) safe and age-appropriate playgrounds and equipment for physical education, physical activity, and recess during the school day (187,241–244); 2) safe routes to school, particularly for students living ≤1 mile from school (110); and 3) access to extracurricular programs such as intramurals and interscholastic sports that are age appropriate, are safe, provide proper equipment when needed, and are available for all students (241,242,245,246).

All spaces and facilities for physical activity, including playing fields, playgrounds, gymnasiums, swimming pools, multipurpose rooms, cafeterias, and fitness centers, should be regularly inspected and maintained, hazardous conditions should be corrected immediately, and a comprehensive safety assessment should be done at least annually (247,248). Regular inspection and maintenance of indoor and outdoor play surfaces should ensure that environmental safety devices are provided and maintained, including (244,248)

- padded goal posts (249) and gym walls;
- breakaway bases for baseball and softball (250,251);
- slip-resistant surfaces near swimming pools;
- sidewalks that are clear of debris and other hazards;
- securely anchored portable soccer goals that are stored in a locked facility when not in use;
- shade structures that are used for sun safety;
- bleachers that minimize the risk for falls; and
- pools and spas designed, constructed, and retrofitted to eliminate entrapment hazards (including evisceration or disembowelment, body entrapment, and hair entrapment or entanglement).

Develop, teach, implement, and enforce safety rules. Safe physical activity requires proper conditioning and use of appropriate equipment where needed. Dangerous behaviors (e.g., spearing in football, high-sticking in hockey, throwing a bat in baseball, and use of alcohol and other drugs by athletes) can be prohibited by establishing and enforcing rules (252,253). Explicit safety rules should be taught to and followed by students in physical education, extracurricular physical activity programs, and community sports and recreation programs (244,246,254). Adult supervisors should consistently reinforce safety rules, which should be posted in key locations. One person, such as the school health coordinator or lead physical education teacher, should be responsible for ensuring that safety measures are in place and updated as needed (198,255); however, minimizing physical activity–related injuries and illnesses among children and adolescents is the joint responsibility of teachers, administrators, coaches, athletic trainers, school nurses, other school and community personnel, parents, and students (254,256).

Maintain high levels of supervision during structured and unstructured physical activity programs. Trained staff members or volunteers, including coaches, teachers, parents, paraprofessionals, and community members, should supervise all physical activity programs. Staff members should be aware of the potential for physical activity–related injuries and illnesses among students so that the risks for and consequences of these injuries and illnesses can be minimized. To prevent injuries during structured physical activity schools can

- require physical assessment before participation (257);
- provide developmentally appropriate activities (246);
- ensure proper conditioning and avoid excesses in training (258–260);
- provide student instruction regarding the biomechanics of specific motor skills (260);
- appropriately match participants according to size and ability;
- adapt rules to the skill level of students and the protective equipment available (259);
- modify rules to eliminate unsafe practices;
- ensure that injuries, including concussions, are healed before allowing further participation; and
- establish criteria, including clearance by a health-care provider, for reentering play after an injury to ensure that injuries are fully healed.

Children and adolescents also could be provided with, and required to use, protective clothing and equipment appropriate for the type of physical activity and the environment (259). Protective clothing and equipment includes footwear appropriate for the specific activity; helmets for bicycling; helmets, face masks, mouth guards, and protective pads for football and ice hockey; shin guards for soccer; knee pads for in-line skating; and reflective clothing for walking and running. As a general recommendation, all protective equipment should 1) be in good condition; 2) be inspected and maintained frequently; 3) be replaced if worn, damaged, or outdated; 4) provide a good fit for the athlete; and 5) be appropriate for the sport and position. In addition, children and adolescents need to be trained to use equipment correctly; this is particularly true of helmets (261).

To prevent injuries during unstructured play time, schools should consider implementing training sessions for staff members focusing on observation techniques, behavior management, appropriate supervision, and emergency response procedures (244). Additional information that schools might want to integrate into training sessions can be found in the *Consumer Product Safety Commission Handbook for Public Playground Safety* (243). In general, playground supervisors should 1) repetitively teach children playground rules; 2) prevent, recognize, and stop children's dangerous and risky behavior; 3) help children to identify, acknowledge, and prevent their risky behavior; and 4) model appropriate safety behavior (243,262). When possible, schools can support those supervising unstructured physical activity by following the National Program for Playground Safety (NPPS) recommendations that the playground supervision ratio of teachers to students be equal to the indoor classroom ratio (263).

Increase community access to school physical activity facilities. Schools should provide community access to physical activity facilities, such as gymnasiums, tracks, baseball and softball fields, basketball courts, outdoor play areas, and indoor fitness centers during the school day and out-of-school time (242,264,265). In 2006, adults used school physical activity or athletic facilities during out-of-school–time hours for community-sponsored sports teams in 47% of all schools, for open gym in 31% of schools, and for physical activity classes or lessons in 23% of schools (144).

Establishing a formal policy or agreement, such as a joint use agreement, between schools and community organizations can help increase student, family, and community access to physical activity facilities and programs. A joint use agreement is a policy that allows two or more entities (e.g., schools, community organizations) to share use of their facilities. Joint use agreements provide details about the facilities to be shared, as well as scheduling, management, maintenance, and costs of the shared facilities. Roles, responsibilities, and liability terms also are typically outlined within joint use agreements (266). Access to these facilities can help to increase visibility of schools, provide community members a safe place for physical activity, and might increase partnerships with community-based physical activity programs (266,267). The National Policy and Legal Analysis Network to Prevent Childhood Obesity (available at http://www.nplanonline.org/nplan/joint-use) and the Prevention Institute (available at http://www.jointuse.org) offer free resources to assess school facilities for community use and establish joint use agreements.

Frequently, schools have the facilities but lack the personnel to deliver extracurricular physical activity programs. Community resources can expand existing school programs by providing program staff members as well as intramural and club activities on school grounds. For example, community agencies and organizations can use school facilities for after-school physical fitness programs for students, weight management programs for overweight or obese students, and sports and recreation programs for students with disabilities or chronic health conditions.

13.5.2.2 ESTABLISH A CLIMATE THAT ENCOURAGES AND DOES NOT STIGMATIZE HEALTHY EATING AND PHYSICAL ACTIVITY

Adopt marketing techniques to promote healthy dietary choices. Marketing techniques can be used to promote healthy foods and beverages among students. The following techniques have been used in schools to increase the likelihood of students choosing healthier foods and beverages:

- placing nutritious products so that they are easy for students to choose, such as featuring fruits and vegetables, low-fat and fat-free milk and other dairy products, and whole grains in prominent places in cafeteria lines (268)
- promoting healthy eating through environmental strategies such as prompts, parental outreach, and point-of-purchase promotions (269,270) because point-of-purchase signage and parental newsletters highlighting parents' healthy eating behaviors influence children's food selections (269,271)
- applying pricing strategies, such as lowering the price of nutritious items and, if offered, raising the price of less nutritious items, because this practice encourages students to purchase more healthy items (269,272–274)

Use student rewards that support health. Student achievement or positive classroom behavior should only be rewarded with nonfood items or activities. In 2006, only 17% of all schools prohibited faculty and staff members from using food or food coupons as a reward for good behavior or good academic performance (105). The use of food as rewards, especially foods with little nutritional value, might increase the risk that children associate such foods with emotions, such as feelings of accomplishment (268,275). Providing food based on performance or behavior connects the experience of eating food to the student's perceptions and mood. Rewarding students with food during class also reinforces eating outside of meal or snack times. This practice can encourage students to eat treats even when they are not hungry and instill lifetime habits of rewarding or comforting themselves with unhealthy eating, resulting in overconsumption of foods high in added sugar and fat (276–278). Although few studies have examined the effect of using food rewards on students' long-term eating habits, the IOM Nutrition Standards for Foods in Schools report determined that such use of foods in schools is inappropriate (238) because this practice establishes an emotional connection between foods and accomplishments.

When an extrinsic reward system is used, rewards should be nonfood items or activities (e.g., stickers, books, or extra time for recess) to recognize students for their achievements or good behavior. The Center for Science in the Public Interest lists examples of constructive student rewards (available at http://cspinet.org/new/pdf/constructive_classroom_rewards.pdf).

Do not use physical activity as punishment. Teachers, coaches, and other school and community personnel should not use physical activity as punishment or withhold opportunities for physical activity as a form of punishment. Nationwide in 2006, in 32% of schools, school staff members were allowed to use physical activity (e.g., running laps or doing push-ups) to punish students for bad behavior in physical education. In 23% of schools, staff members were allowed to exclude students from all or part of physical education as punishment for bad behavior in another class (144). Using physical activity as a punishment (e.g., forcing students to perform push-ups or sit-ups for bad behavior in physical education) might create negative associations with physical activity in the minds of students (279). Exclusion from physical education or recess for bad behavior in a classroom deprives students of physical activity experiences that benefit health and can contribute toward improved behavior in the classroom (280,281). Disciplining students for unacceptable behavior or academic performance by not allowing them to participate in recess or physical education prevents students from 1) accumulating valuable free-time physical activity and 2) learning essential physical activity knowledge and skills.

13.5.2.3 CREATE A SCHOOL ENVIRONMENT THAT ENCOURAGES A HEALTHY BODY IMAGE, SHAPE, AND SIZE AMONG ALL STUDENTS AND STAFF MEMBERS, IS ACCEPTING OF DIVERSE ABILITIES, AND DOES NOT TOLERATE WEIGHT-BASED TEASING

The psychological environment at a school should support all students in making healthy eating choices and being physically active, regardless of race/ethnicity, income, sex, and physical ability (215). Schools can take numerous steps to help shape a health-promoting psychological environment. For example, they can adopt and enforce a universal bullying prevention program that addresses weight discrimination and teasing (215,282,283), ensure that students of all sizes are encouraged to participate in a wide variety of physical activities (279), display posters or other visual materials that feature a diverse combination of students being active and eating healthy, and avoid practices that single out students on the basis of body size or shape (283). Schools should avoid elimination games such as dodge ball, bombardment, and elimination tag that limit opportunities for all students to be active (284). School health, mental health, and social services staff members can play a key role in helping to communicate and promote these practices.

The school nutrition policy should ensure a safe environment for students with chronic health conditions. The policy should cover all venues where foods and beverages are available, during the regular and extended school day, and all families and staff members should be informed of the policy (215). Nutrition service staff members should be provided with information and support to assist students who are on nutrition programs or diets prescribed by their health-care provider. USDA provides guidance on accommodating children with special dietary needs, supported by the USDA nondiscrimination regulation (285), allowing for substitutions or modifications in the National School Meals Program for children whose disabilities restrict their diet as certified by a licensed physician (286). The school nutrition service staff members also should consider making food substitutions for students with food allergies, for students with food intolerances, or on a case-by-case basis for students who are medically certified as having a special medical dietary need (286).

The school environment should support students with disabilities and chronic health conditions in being physically active and making healthy eating choices. A chronic health condition is defined as any illness, disease, disorder, or disability of long duration or frequent recurrence, including asthma, diabetes, serious allergies, epilepsy, and obesity (287). Schools should establish policies that allow full participation by all students in physical activity, including extracurricular activities, and ensure access to preventive and quick-relief medications as indicated by a student's Individualized Health Care Plan, 504 plan, Individualized Education Plan (IEP), or all of these as appropriate (204,288–297). Coordination between health services staff members, special education, nutrition services staff members, and health and physical education staff members can help ensure that these policies are established.

13.5.3 GUIDELINE 3. PROVIDE A QUALITY SCHOOL MEAL PROGRAM AND ENSURE THAT STUDENTS HAVE ONLY APPEALING, HEALTHY FOOD AND BEVERAGE CHOICES OFFERED OUTSIDE OF THE SCHOOL MEAL PROGRAM

Schools are in a unique position to promote healthy dietary behaviors and help ensure appropriate food and nutrient intake among their students. Many schools provide students with access to foods and beverages in various venues across the school campus, including meals served in the cafeteria as part of the federally reimbursable school meal program and competitive foods (i.e., foods and beverages that are sold, served, or given to students but are not part of the school meal program). Schools should model and reinforce healthy dietary behaviors by ensuring that only nutritious and appealing foods and beverages are provided in all venues accessible to students (Box 3).

13.5.3.1 PROMOTE ACCESS TO AND PARTICIPATION IN SCHOOL MEALS

Schools should provide students with access to breakfast, lunch, and other important programs (e.g., after-school snack programs and summer feeding programs) and promote participation in these programs by all students (298,299). A school meal program offers students the opportunity to apply knowledge and skills learned through nutrition education, can affect students' food choices by providing nutrient information of the foods available, and can encourage students to make healthy choices (98,300,301).

The USDA's Food and Nutrition Service administers the federally sponsored school meal programs including the National School Lunch Program and the School Breakfast Program. Although schools are not required to participate in these programs, 94% of schools, both public and private, participate in the National School Lunch Program (68). Among public schools offering the National School Lunch Program, approximately 81% also offer the School Breakfast Program (302). School districts and independent schools that choose to take part in the federal school meal programs receive cash reimbursements and entitlement funds for USDA Foods (commodities), provided that the meals they serve meet federal requirements and that they offer free or reduced price lunches to eligible students.

The School Breakfast Program and National School Lunch Program play major roles in the diets of children and adolescents in the United States. Approximately 30 million students participate in the National School Lunch Program every school day, with approximately 63% of school lunches served free or at a reduced price for students from low-income families (303). An average of 10 million children participate in the School Breakfast Program each school day, and 82% of these breakfasts are provided free or at a reduced price to students from low-income families (304). On a typical school day during the 2004–2005 school year, among students who participated in both the School Breakfast Program and the National School Lunch Program, an average of 47% of their calories came from meals and snacks consumed at school (305). Students who participate in school meal programs have been found to consume more milk, fruits, and vegetables and have better nutrient intake than those who do not participate (306,307). However, participants in the School Breakfast Program and National School Lunch Program also have higher sodium intake from school meals than those who do not participate (308). In addition, regular participation in the School Breakfast Program is associated with lower BMI among students (309).

Student participation in school meal programs, particularly breakfast, has been shown to be associated in the short term with improved student functioning on a broad range of psychosocial and academic measures (65,310–312). Studies of students who participated more often in school breakfast programs showed increases in test scores and significant decreases in the rates of school absence and tardiness compared with students whose participation remained the same or decreased (65,313).

Encourage participation in school meal programs among all students. Participation rates in school meal programs vary by sex, income, age, and race/ethnicity. In the 2004–2005 school year, boys participated in the National School Lunch Program at a higher rate than girls, elementary school students participated at a higher rate than middle and high school students, students who were eligible for free and reduced-price meals participated at a higher rate than students who were not income eligible, rural students participated at a higher rate than urban students, and students whose parents did not attend college participated at a higher rate than those parents who did. In the 2004–2005 school year, boys participated in the School Breakfast Program at a higher rate than girls, non-Hispanic black students participated at a higher rate than Hispanic students and non-Hispanic white students, elementary school students participated at a higher rate than middle and high school students, students who were eligible for free and reduced-price meals participated at a higher rate than students who were not income eligible, students who spoke Spanish in the home participated at a higher rate than students who spoke English, and rural students participated at a higher rate than urban students (314). Participation decreased as grade level increased, decreasing from 73% among elementary students to 60% among middle school students and 44% among high school (314).

All students are eligible to participate in the school meal program; however, schools receive a smaller reimbursement for students who exceed income limits than for students from low-income families. Increased effort is needed to ensure that participation in a school meal program that complies with the *Dietary Guidelines for Americans* is promoted and supported.

To encourage increased participation in school meal programs by all students, schools can use the following strategies:

- Offer breakfast to all students at no cost to increase overall participation in the school breakfast program (315).
- Offer breakfast through alternative service methods (e.g., breakfast carts, breakfast in the classroom, breakfast after first period, and "grab and go").
- Use Provision 2 and Provision 3 (316) of the National School Lunch Act to reduce paperwork and applications and to simplify meal counting and claiming procedures. Schools using Provision 2 and Provision 3 establish claiming percentages for reimbursement and serve meals free to all participating students for 4 years.
- Use direct certification to automatically qualify students who participate in Temporary Assistance to Needy Families, the Supplemental Nutrition Assistance Program (formerly the Food Stamp Program), and the Food Distribution Program on Indian Reservations for free meals without requiring additional applications.

- Eliminate the reduced-price category for breakfast. This option, as well as direct certification, Provision 2 and Provision 3, and alternate service methods are described in USDA Food and Nutrition Service School Breakfast Toolkit (available at http://www.fns.usda.gov/cnd/breakfast/expansion).
- Eliminate any social stigma attached to, and prevent the overt identification of, students who are eligible for free and reduced-price school meals (317).
- Ensure that meals meet students' cultural preferences; for example, encourage students and parents to participate in planning meals and incorporating cultural and regional preferences.
- Obtain input from students about menu choices through taste-testing and the school health council.
- Serve meals at an appropriate time, such as 11:00 a.m.–1:00 p.m., in a supportive, comfortable, and attractive environment with a minimal wait time (222).
- Have school nutrition staff members and teachers collaborate to design and implement nutrition education programs that promote healthy eating messages to the entire school community (299).

13.5.3.2 PROVIDE NUTRITIOUS AND APPEALING SCHOOL MEALS THAT COMPLY WITH THE DIETARY GUIDELINES FOR AMERICANS

The school meal program should provide various healthy, appetizing, and culturally appropriate choices to help students meet their nutritional needs. Meals served in the National School Lunch Program and School Breakfast Program must meet federally defined nutrition standards based on the *Dietary Guidelines for Americans* for schools to be eligible for federal subsidies. On average per week, current school lunches must have no more than 30% of calories from fat, with <10% from saturated fat, and must provide one third of the Recommended Dietary Allowances of protein, vitamin A, vitamin C, iron, calcium, and calories. Decisions about the specific foods to offer and how to prepare them are made by local school food authorities. The Healthy, Hunger-Free Kids Act of 2010 requires USDA to update the meal patterns and nutrition standards for the National School Lunch Program and School Breakfast Program based on recommendations made by the Food and Nutrition Board of the National Research Council of the National Academies of Sciences (318). The 2009 IOM report *School Meals: Building Blocks for Healthy Children* (319) recommendations reflect current dietary guidance including increasing the requirements for fruits, vegetables and whole grains, requiring only fat-free and low-fat milk, and decreasing the amount of sodium and trans fat in school meals. Schools that provide meals that meet these recommendations will receive an additional $0.06 (6 cents) for each qualifying meal served (318).

Schools also should take necessary action to prevent or minimize the risk for foodborne illness among participants in the National School Lunch Program and School Breakfast Program. School food authorities are required to develop and implement a food safety program based on a hazard analysis critical control point system (320). This law allows school food authorities to identify potential food hazards, identify critical points where hazards can be eliminated or minimized through control measures, and establish monitoring procedures and corrective action. The National Food Service Management Institute and USDA's Food and Nutrition Service offer various trainings and resources to assist school food authorities in implementing food safety programs.

Ensure that meals meet federally defined nutrition standards. Schools have made considerable progress in meeting federal nutrition requirements for school meals. A national study conducted during the 2004–2005 school year found that approximately 85% of public schools offering the National School Lunch Program served meals that met the standards for protein, vitamins, and minerals; 88% offered a vegetable (not including French fries) every day; 50% offered fresh fruit every day; and 62% offered canned fruit every day (306,321). However, although three fourths of schools met the fat standards in school breakfasts, less than one third of schools met the standards for calories from fat or saturated fat in the average lunch (321). For both breakfast and lunch, average levels of sodium were higher and fiber was lower than the *Dietary Guidelines for Americans* recommendations (321). Schools can choose to take USDA's Healthier U.S. School Challenge to create healthier food and beverage choices. Schools that engage in the Healthier U.S. School Challenge commit to meeting specified criteria including stricter nutrition standards such as increasing the number of servings of whole-grain foods, dark green and orange vegetables, and dry beans and peas.

The USDA A *Menu Planner for Healthy School Meals* provides information on how to plan, prepare, serve, and market healthy school meals

(322). School nutrition services staff members may modify menus to include healthier foods, such as serving more fruits, vegetables, and whole grains, and offering a greater variety of low-fat foods, including fat-free and low-fat milk. Other ideas include serving foods such as salsas for fresh flavor and less fat; making reductions and substitutions, such as reducing salt and using low-fat mayonnaise and salad dressings; and preparing foods in different ways, such as baking rather than frying French fries or serving baked potatoes instead (322,323).

Ensure that schools have kitchen facilities and equipment needed to cook quality, appealing meals. Support should be provided to schools to upgrade kitchen facilities with state-of-the-art equipment, which can help ensure that school meals are appealing to children and that they are prepared using the most healthy cooking techniques and food products available. Serving baked instead of fried foods can make a substantial difference in the amount of calories, fat, and saturated fat that children consume. For example, baked French fries have 55% less total fat and 34% less saturated fat than deep-fried French fries (324). Ovens, instead of deep-fat fryers, are needed to bake fries, but not all schools have such equipment and need financial support to purchase these types of items (190,325,326).

Outdated kitchen equipment, limited and inadequate kitchen facilities, and food budgets are substantial barriers for school nutrition staff members to provide healthy and appealing school meals (323,327–330). Recent trends associated with the need to update kitchen equipment in school nutrition programs include an increased emphasis on health and wellness, food security and emergency preparedness, smaller and more mobile equipment (e.g., for salad bars), blended technologies (e.g., combination oven-steamers), and machines that vend complete reimbursable school meals (331). The National Food Service Management Institute (available at http://www.nfsmi.org) offers training and resources on effective equipment purchasing guidance and financial management practices of operating a school nutrition program.

Use healthy food preparation methods and purchasing techniques. Healthy food preparation methods play an important role in providing nutritious and appealing meals and include practices such as substitution techniques (i.e., substituting one type of ingredient for another), reduction techniques (i.e., reducing the amount of an ingredient), fat-reduction techniques when preparing meat and poultry, and vegetable preparation techniques. When making substitutions or reductions in ingredients, schools should standardize the recipe to account for the changes in yield and meal pattern requirements. Standardized recipes help to ensure that the products are prepared consistently, provide a defined yield, and list the meal pattern contribution. Schools should seek out and taste test standardized recipes that are low in fat, oil, salt, and sugar to ensure that they are acceptable to students. Schools may consider USDA Foods (commodities), which have been modified to reduce sodium and fat, including saturated fat, as substitutions for less healthy ingredients.

Substitution techniques include the following (5,105,332):

- Use cooked dry beans, canned beans, soybeans, or other meat extenders instead of meat.
- Use ground turkey or lean ground beef instead of regular ground beef.
- Use low-fat or fat-free yogurt, mayonnaise, or sour cream instead of regular mayonnaise, sour cream, or creamy salad dressings.
- Use frozen vegetables or low-sodium canned vegetables instead of regular canned vegetables.
- Use frozen fruits or canned fruits packed in juice instead of canned fruits packed in syrup.
- Use nonstick spray or pan liners instead of grease or oil.
- Use seasonings other than salt.
- Use part-skim or low-fat cheese instead of regular cheese.
- Use fat-free, low-fat, soy, or nonfat dry milk instead of whole milk.
- Use vegetable oil instead of shortening, butter, or margarine.

Reduction techniques include the following (5,105,332):

- Use standardized low-fat recipes.
- Use standardized low-sodium recipes.
- Use standardized low-sugar recipes.

Meat preparation techniques include the following (5,105,332):

- Drain fat from browned meat.
- Remove skin from poultry or use skinless poultry.
- Roast, bake, or broil meat rather than frying.
- Roast meat or poultry on a rack so fat will drain.
- Skim fat off warm broth, soup, stew, or gravy.
- Spoon solid fat from chilled meat or poultry broth.

- Trim fat from meat or use lean meat.

Vegetable preparation techniques include the following (5,105,332):

- Boil, mash, roast, or bake potatoes rather than frying or deep frying.
- Prepare vegetables without using butter, margarine, cheese, or creamy sauce.
- Steam, roast, grill, or bake other vegetables such as broccoli, carrots, or green beans.

Nationwide, in 2006, among schools in which school staff members had responsibility for cooking foods for students, the most commonly practiced healthy food preparation methods were using nonstick spray or pan liners instead of grease or oil; draining fat from browned meat; roasting, baking, or broiling meat rather than frying; and steaming or baking other vegetables (excluding potatoes). The least commonly practiced healthy food preparation methods were reducing sugar in recipes or using low-sugar recipes, using low-sodium canned vegetables instead of regular canned vegetables, and using cooked dry beans, canned beans, soy products, or other meat extenders instead of meat (105).

Schools also can use various purchasing techniques to procure healthier options while maintaining food costs. For example, local school districts can form a cooperative (co-op) to improve purchasing power with food distributors. This can increase the availability and reduce cost of healthier foods. Schools also can use USDA Foods (commodities) or ask the school district to consider creating or assigning space for a central warehouse, which allows for storage of large quantities of foods from bulk purchases and USDA Foods shipments. USDA has resources to guide schools on buying food for child nutrition programs, including the Food Buying Guide for Child Nutrition Programs (available at http://www.fns.usda.gov/tn/resources/foodbuyingguide.html) and *Eat Smart--Farm Fresh* (available at http://www.fns.usda.gov/cnd/guidance/farm-to-school-guidance_12-19-2005.pdf). The National Farm to School Network's website also includes resources about buying local foods (available at http://www.farmtoschool.org/publications.php?pt+othe).

Serve foods and beverages that are appealing and presented attractively. Taste tests can be used to determine which healthy options students prefer (333–335). When planning menus and purchasing food items that appeal to students, appearance, texture or consistency (how the food feels in the mouth and how it cuts), flavor, and service temperature (the ideal temperature for serving the food) are important (336). Offering various colorful fruits and vegetables with meals and snacks enhances their nutritional value and appeal. Students drink more milk when it is offered cold and in attractive packaging such as single-serving or portable plastic milk bottles (337). The USDA's Team Nutrition (available at http://teamnutrition.usda.gov), the School Nutrition Association (available at http://www.schoolnutrition.org), and the National Food Service Management Institute (available at http://www.nfsmi.org) offer strategies and technical assistance on serving and presenting appealing foods and beverages for school nutrition programs.

13.5.3.3 ENSURE THAT ALL FOODS AND BEVERAGES SOLD OR SERVED OUTSIDE OF SCHOOL MEAL PROGRAMS ARE NUTRITIOUS AND APPEALING

Competitive foods, which are any foods or beverages sold or served outside of the school meal program, are the principal source of the low-nutrient, energy-dense foods that students consume at school. Unlike school meals, which must meet specified nutrition standards, foods and beverages sold or provided outside of the meal program are largely exempt from federal requirements or standards. The existing federal requirement, last updated in 1985, prohibits the sale of foods of minimal nutritional value (FMNV) during meal periods in areas where reimbursable school meals are served (338,339). FMNV are defined as foods and beverages with <5% of the Recommended Dietary Allowances per serving for eight key nutrients; FMNV include soda, water ices, chewing gum, and certain types of candy, including gum drops, jelly beans, and candy-coated popcorn (340,341). The federal regulations for competitive foods prohibit the sale of FMNV. However, schools can sell these foods and beverages at other locations on the school campus during the entire school day, and other foods and beverages of low nutritional value such as chips, most candy bars, and noncarbonated, high-sugar drinks can be sold anywhere on campus, including the food service area.

The passage of the Healthy, Hunger-Free Kids Act of 2010 requires USDA to develop federal nutrition standards for competitive foods consistent with the *Dietary Guidelines for Americans* (342). These standards will apply to foods and beverages sold on school campus during the school day. In the last decade, a total of 39 states passed a law or policy addressing competitive foods and beverages in schools that was stronger than the current federal requirements. These state laws and policies vary in strength and breadth when compared with the IOM Nutrition Standards for Foods in School (238,343).

Competitive foods are offered in various school-based venues, such as à la carte in the cafeteria, vending machines, school stores and snack bars and concession stands, fundraisers on school grounds, classroom-based activities (e.g., parties and rewards or behavior-management tools), staff and parent meetings, and after-school programs (344,345). In 2006, 33% of elementary schools, 71% of middle schools, and 89% of high schools had a vending machine or a school store, canteen, or snack bar where students could purchase foods or beverages (103). The most commonly available competitive foods are high in sugar, fat, and calories, including high-fat salty snacks, high-fat baked goods, and high-calorie sugar-sweetened beverages, such as soft drinks, sports drinks, and fruit drinks (105,344,346). Some progress has been made in limiting the availability of unhealthy foods in schools. For example, during 2006–2008, across 35 states, the median percentage of schools that allowed students to purchase the following items from vending machines or at the school store, canteen, or snack bar decreased: chocolate candy (from 39% to 21%), other kinds of candy (from 43% to 24%), salty snacks not low in fat (47% to 34%), soda pop (from 62% to 38%), and sports drinks (from 72% to 57%) (347). Consequently, offering competitive foods in vending machines at schools is associated with significantly higher BMI among middle school students (348). Access to sugar-sweetened beverages and low-nutrient, energy-dense foods at school significantly increases student calorie intake from sugar-sweetened beverages per school day. The third School Nutrition Dietary Assessment Study found that sugar-sweetened beverages (not including flavored milk) obtained at school contributed to an additional 29 kcal per school day for middle school students and 46 kcal per school day for high school students. Low-nutrient, energy-dense foods obtained and consumed at school contributed 86 kcal per school day for middle schools students and 111 kcal per school day for high school students. Attending schools without stores or snack bars that sell foods or beverages is estimated to significantly reduce sugar-sweetened beverage consumption by 22 kcal per school day for middle school students and 28 kcal per school day for high school students (349). In addition, restricting access to snack foods is associated with more frequent fruit and vegetable consumption (350).

In a 2001 report to Congress, USDA highlighted four major concerns about competitive foods (351):

1. Many competitive foods and beverages are low in nutrient density and high in fat, sugar, and calories; these products can negatively affect student diets and increase the risk for excess weight gain (352,353).
2. School meal programs are stigmatized when low-income students can receive free or reduced-price meals but only higher-income students can purchase competitive foods and beverages.
3. An increase in the sale of competitive foods and beverages is associated with a decrease in student participation in the reimbursable school meal program, which might affect the viability of the program (354).
4. Students receive inconsistent messages when they are taught about good nutrition and healthy food choices in the classroom but are surrounded by various venues offering primarily less nutritious foods.

Establish strong nutrition standards for competitive foods consistent with the IOM Nutrition Standards for Foods in Schools. Nutrition standards list criteria to help schools determine which foods and beverages should be offered on a school campus. Implementing nutrition standards can involve increasing food and beverage options, such as requiring that schools offer fruits or vegetables at all locations where other foods are available, and limiting options, such as stipulating that schools cannot sell foods with more than a specified number of calories and grams of fat per serving. State and local education agencies can pass nutrition standards that are stronger than the federal requirements limiting the sale of competitive foods.

Implementing nutrition standards can be an effective strategy to improve the nutritional quality of foods offered and purchased in the school setting (355–357), which might affect dietary intake (356). The Healthy, Hunger-Free Kids Act of 2010 requires each school district's local wellness policy to include nutritional guidelines for all foods available on each school campus that promote student health and reduce childhood obesity (358). Schools should implement nutrition standards that provide students with only healthy choices throughout the regular and extended school day and throughout the campus that are consistent with and reinforce positive nutrition education messages received in the classroom. Fruits, vegetables, whole grain products, and fat-free or low-fat dairy products should be offered, whereas foods that do not contain important nutrients; foods that are high in fat, added sugar, or sodium; and sugar-sweetened beverages should be eliminated or limited. Portion sizes should be reasonable for the age of the student (35).

IOM used a rigorous scientific review process to develop the Nutrition Standards for Foods in Schools, which provides guidance on which foods and beverages schools should offer on school campuses (238). The IOM standards recommend that all competitive food offerings be consistent with the *Dietary Guidelines for Americans* and, in particular, help children and adolescents meet the guidelines for consumption of fruits, vegetables, whole grains, and fat-fat or low-fat milk or milk products (238). The IOM standards include 13 standards for foods and beverages sold and available on campus during the school day, after-school activities, evening and community events, and on-campus fundraising. The standards address the nutritive (e.g., calories, saturated fat, sodium, and sugars) and nonnutritive components (e.g., caffeine and nonnutritive sweeteners) of foods and beverages, restrict the marketing of foods and beverages, and prohibit the use of foods and beverages as rewards or punishment. CDC created four audience-specific fact sheets about the IOM standards that can serve as a resource to support the development of strong nutrition standards for foods outside of school meal programs. These fact sheets answer common questions about the IOM standards and provide recommendations for implementation (available at http://www.cdc.gov/Healthyyouth/nutrition/standards.htm).

Schools should systematically track the financial implications of implementing strong nutrition standards. Limited data are available on the impact of changes in nutrition standards in schools on total revenue generated by sales of food and beverages (359). However, mounting evidence suggests that schools can maintain financial stability while offering only foods and beverages that meet strong nutrition standards (268,360–364). Implementing strong nutrition standards can increase school lunch participation, which financially benefits schools (360,361,363). Strategic promotion of healthier food and beverage choices (355) and lowering the price of healthier foods (e.g., fruits, vegetables, and low-fat snacks) in school cafeterias are strategies that can minimize financial risk (272,273). (Additional information is available at http://www.cdc.gov/healthyyouth/nutrition/pdf/financial_implications.pdf .)

Use the contracting process to improve the nutritional quality of competitive foods and beverages. Most secondary school students (67% of middle or junior high schools and 83% of high schools) attend schools that have beverage contracts (365). Schools that adopt strong nutrition standards for competitive foods should revise existing food and beverage contracts so that healthier options are available for students (359). Vending machine contracts that schools establish with food and beverage companies give the companies selling rights in return for cash and noncash benefits or incentive items such as scoreboards, cups, T-shirts, posters, and drink bottles (365). Schools and school districts can cancel, not sign, not renew, or negotiate contracts so that only foods and beverages that meet strong nutrition standards are available to students. For example, some schools have new districtwide vending contracts to centralize purchasing and approval of foods and beverages sold and have placed the management of new contracts under school nutrition departments to ensure better nutritional content of vending machine items (366). The National Policy and Legal Analysis Network to Prevent Childhood Obesity has resources to support schools in using the contracting process to improve the nutritional quality of foods and beverages sold on school property and how to negotiate favorable terms and conditions in vending contracts (available at http://www.nplanonline.org). State departments of education can support schools by providing online nutrition calculators or an updated list of products that meet nutrition standards. Schools can use these tools to ensure that products meet nutrition standards and help select products to include in a vending contract.

Market healthier foods and beverages. Schools can take advantage of marketing strategies to promote the appeal of healthier foods and beverages in various ways. Marketing healthy options might persuade students to purchase healthy foods and beverages. For example, cafeteria taste tests offer students an opportunity to taste the healthier options offered in the cafeteria (355,367). Taste testing provides students an opportunity to inform staff members which healthy food and beverage products they like and dislike (268). Strategies to promote the appeal of fruits and vegetables in schools and influence student purchases of healthy foods and beverages include (268,368–371)

- offering a free fruit and vegetable program;
- having students grow vegetables in a school garden;
- offering vegetables and dip on à la carte lines;
- moving fruits and vegetables to the front of the school meal serving line;
- offering sliced or wedged versions of fruits and vegetables;
- using colorful and imaginative language and images of fruits and vegetables on menus, in hallways, and in the cafeteria;
- collecting suggestions from students and families for meals and snack items that might be offered; and
- improving the lighting in the serving area and placing the salad bar near the cashier rather than away from the main serving area.

Additional strategies for low-cost changes to improve the lunch room environment are available at http://smarterlunchrooms.org.

Schools also can build partnerships to market healthy food choices to students (372). Strategies to present a consistent message for offering healthier foods and beverages throughout the school community include linking the cafeteria with the classroom (e.g., discussing health benefits of specific fruits and vegetables in the classroom and offering these fruits and vegetables in the cafeteria at the same time); building connections with community partners such as supermarkets, restaurants, youth-serving agencies, and local farms or farmers' organizations (e.g., hosting a school market program that works with local vendors to sell fruits and vegetables during the school day in a store managed by students); and connecting with local or regional vendor associations to partner on a healthy foods and beverages promotion campaign (e.g., partnering with the regional dairy association on a healthy milk vending program) (368,373,374). Schools can involve students in leading changes toward healthier competitive foods and beverages. Involving students in the decision-making process can decrease resistance to change. Students can survey and poll their peers, provide valuable input to shape policy, help plan and market changes, and promote the sustainability of healthy eating initiatives. Action for Healthy Kids' Students Taking Charge program (available at http://www.studentstakingcharge.org) and the Alliance for a Healthier Generation's empowerME@school toolkit (available at http://www.empowerme2b.org) are resources that involve students in making changes for healthier food and beverage options at school.

Use fundraising activities and student rewards that support health. Schools should incorporate fundraising activities that use only healthy foods, involve physical activity, or sell nonfood items. In 2006, nearly one in four schools held fundraiser nights at fast-food restaurants, and 54% sold baked goods that were not low in fat (105). Fundraising that involves selling nutritious foods and beverages (e.g., fruits, vegetables, 100% fruit juice, and low-fat or fat-free dairy products) or selling nonfood items such as wrapping paper, candles, or student artwork can support student health. One study found that policies to regulate food used for fundraising were more common in middle schools than in high schools, where the sale of foods high in fat and added sugar remained a prevalent fundraising practice (375). Events that engage the community in physical activity, such as runs, walks, and bicycle rides, also can be used to raise money. Other examples include basketball and golf tournaments, dance-a-thons, and car washes. In addition, as described in guideline 2, schools should use constructive classroom rewards that support student health and do not include food.

13.5.4 GUIDELINE 4. IMPLEMENT A COMPREHENSIVE PHYSICAL ACTIVITY PROGRAM WITH QUALITY PHYSICAL EDUCATION AS THE CORNERSTONE

A substantial percentage of recommended child and adolescent physical activity can be provided through a comprehensive school-based physical activity program. A comprehensive program includes before, during, and after-school physical activity through recess and other physical activity breaks, intramurals and physical activity clubs, interscholastic sports, walk- and bicycle-to-school initiatives, and quality physical education (376,377). Quality physical education serves as the cornerstone of a comprehensive program because it provides the unique opportunity for students to obtain the knowledge and skills needed to establish and maintain physically active lifestyles throughout childhood and adolescence and into adulthood. A quality physical education program: 1) meets the needs of all students, 2) is an enjoyable experience for students, 3) keeps students active for most of physical education class time, 4) teaches self-management as well as movement skills, and 5) emphasizes knowledge and skills that can be used for a lifetime (293,378).

Other physical activity program components (e.g., recess and intramural programs) should complement rather than take the place of physical education by serving as venues for students to explore various physical activities. Recess, classroom activity breaks, intramurals, interscholastic sports, and walking and bicycling to school can provide opportunities to practice and apply the skills taught during physical education (293,379) (Box 4).

13.5.4.1 REQUIRE STUDENTS IN GRADES K–12 TO PARTICIPATE IN DAILY PHYSICAL EDUCATION THAT USES A PLANNED AND SEQUENTIAL CURRICULUM AND INSTRUCTIONAL PRACTICES THAT ARE CONSISTENT WITH NATIONAL OR STATE STANDARDS FOR PHYSICAL EDUCATION

Physical education can increase student participation in physical activity, increase their physical fitness (146,147,380–383), and enhance their knowledge and skills about why and how they should be physically active (380,384).

Require daily physical education for students in grades K–12. Daily physical education for grades K–12 (150 minutes per week for elementary students and 225 minutes per week for secondary students) is recommended by the National Association for Sport and Physical Education (293,379) and the more than 30 collaborating organizations that developed the *Health, Mental Health, and Safety Guidelines for Schools* (215). Daily physical education also is one of the national health objectives of *Healthy People 2020* (10). However, in 2006, only 4% of elementary schools, 8% of middle schools, and 2% of high schools provided daily physical education or the equivalent for the entire school year for all students in the school (144).

Participation in daily physical education is associated with an increased likelihood of participating regularly in moderate to vigorous intensity physical activity (118). Daily quality physical education provides consistent instruction in various motor skills, movement forms, self-assessment and management, physical activities, and fitness activities that are important to become physically active for a lifetime.

All students should take all required physical education courses and no substitutions, waivers, or exemptions should be permitted (385). Schools and school districts should not allow students to be exempted from required physical education for the following reasons: enrollment in other courses, participation in school sports, participation in other school activities, participation in community sport activities, high physical fitness competency test scores, participation in vocational training, or participation in community service activities. Exemptions and waivers deprive students of instruction time that is critical for developing motor, movement, and behavioral skills that are essential for the lifelong maintenance of a physically active lifestyle; furthermore, exemptions and waivers might send the message to students that physical education is not as important as other academic content areas and activities (385). Among the 84% of middle schools and 95% of high schools that required physical education in 2006, 12% of middle schools and 25% of high schools allowed students to be exempted from physical education requirements for participation in school sports. Fourteen percent of these middle schools and 20% of these high schools allowed students to be exempted from physical education for participation in school activities other than sports such as band or chorus (144).

Achieving the recommended 225 minutes per week for physical education can be difficult in the many secondary schools that have block schedules, which feature a fewer number of classes, and these classes last longer than those at schools with different schedules. Therefore, secondary schools with block schedules are recommended to provide 450 minutes of physical education every 10 days. Schools that do not have resources (e.g., facilities and teachers) to offer daily physical education classes can gradually add more time for physical education (i.e., increase physical education from 1 or 2 days per week to at least 3 days per week).

Implement physical education curricula consistent with national or state physical education standards. Physical education curricula provide a framework for delivering age-appropriate instruction. Written curricula should be based on an appropriate sequencing of learning activities, including the following: 1) lessons focused on motor skills, physical activity, and fitness assessments that are age and developmentally appropriate; 2) methods of teaching motor, movement, and behavioral skills that ensure basic skills lead to more advanced skills; and 3) student assessment plans to appropriately monitor and reinforce student learning. Without a physical education curriculum, documenting what should be taught, what has been taught, and whether students are achieving learning objectives or outcomes is difficult.

School districts typically are responsible for identifying and providing schools with a physical education curriculum. However, in 2006, only 55% of school districts provided a curriculum to elementary schools; 58% provided a curriculum to middle schools; and 56% provided a curriculum to high schools (144).

Curricula should be based on the national standards for physical education (293). Based on research and consensus among physical education experts, the national standards provide the framework for identifying student performance expectations for each grade level. The national standards provide guidance for states and school districts that are developing state-level standards, instructional frameworks, and curricula. A total of 71% of states require school districts or schools to follow national or state physical education standards or guidelines, and 81% of districts require schools to do so (144). Among these states and districts, most require or recommend standards or guidelines based on the national standards for physical education (144), which describe what students should know and be able to do as a result of quality physical education.

The national standards emphasize competency in motor skills and movement patterns, movement principles and strategies, regular participation in physical activity, achievement and maintenance of health-related fitness (muscular strength and endurance, cardiorespiratory fitness, flexibility, and body composition), responsible social and personal behavior in physical activity settings, and the value of physical activity for health and enjoyment. Physical education curricula should emphasize knowledge about the physical, social, and mental health benefits of physical activity; components of health-related fitness; the recommended amounts and types of physical activity needed to promote health; the relationship between physical activity and physical fitness (293); principles of exercise; injury prevention; energy expenditure; and social influences on physical activity (386). For children, adolescents, and adults, knowledge about how to be physically active might be more important than knowledge about why physical activity is beneficial (387,388). Thus, physical education curricula also should include the development of safe and effective individualized physical activity plans.

In 2006, CDC released the Physical Education Curriculum Analysis Tool (PECAT) (available at http://www.cdc.gov/healthyyouth/pecat). The PECAT helps school districts conduct clear, complete, and consistent analyses of written physical education curricula based on the national physical education standards. Results from PECAT can help schools enhance an existing curriculum, develop their own curriculum, or select a published curriculum for the delivery of quality physical education in schools (389).

Systems and criteria have been created to identify evidence-based interventions for certain school health topics such as HIV prevention. Such criteria are based on scientific evidence of effectiveness and can help school districts and schools select and approve curricula. No comprehensive system or set of criteria specifically focused on physical education curricula exists. However, the National Cancer Institute does have a system, the Research-Tested Intervention Programs (RTIPs), which includes a scoring process for comprehensive school-based programs focused on healthy eating and physical activity. Many of the programs included within RTIPs have a physical education component, although the curricula are not extensively or separately analyzed. (Additional information available at http://rtips.cancer.gov/rtips/index.do.) In addition, the Task Force on Community Preventive Services reviewed 13 studies that focused on improving physical education through policy, curriculum, and instructional changes. After the review, the task force strongly recommended enhanced school-based physical education as an intervention strategy to increase youth physical activity (378).

Include protocols for student assessment in physical education. A physical education curriculum should include age-appropriate protocols for student assessment (293,379). Student assessment in physical education should be used to determine how well students meet national or state physical education standards, align with the content delivered through instruction, and allow teachers and schools to monitor and reinforce student learning. Assessments have many formats, including demonstration of specific skills (390), knowledge-based testing (386), out-of-school assignments that support learning and practice, assessments of progress in motor skills (391), and establishment of active lifestyles. The National Association for Sport and Physical Education (NASPE) has various resources on student assessments (available at http://www.aahperd.org/naspe/publications/products/pemetrics.cfm and http://www.aahperd.org/naspe/publications/products/assessment.cfm).

Schools may consider conducting fitness testing to provide feedback to students and their parents, teach students how to apply behavioral skills (e.g., self-assessment, goal-setting, decision-making, and self-management), or measure schoolwide fitness levels (392). Fitness testing also can be used to determine student achievement of national or state physical education standards that focus on maintaining a healthy fitness level (293). If fitness assessments are used, students should be taught the skills needed for self-monitoring or self-testing of health-related physical fitness (392–395). Fitness testing should be conducted in a manner that respects and preserves the dignity of all students (e.g., results kept confidential and tests only administered after students are aware of the testing procedures). The results of physical fitness testing should not be used to assign report card grades or be used to assess program effectiveness because the validity of these measurements might vary substantially, and overall fitness and improvements in fitness are influenced by factors (e.g., genetics and physical maturation) that are beyond the control of teachers and students (396,397).

13.5.4.2 PROVIDE A SUBSTANTIAL PERCENTAGE OF EACH STUDENT'S RECOMMENDED DAILY AMOUNT OF PHYSICAL ACTIVITY IN PHYSICAL EDUCATION CLASS

Even if students participate in daily physical education, they might not always be adequately active during class. Schools should adhere to the NASPE recommendations that students engage in moderate to vigorous physical activity for at least 50% of the time they spend in physical education class, one of the most critical outcome measures in determining the quality of a physical education program (398–400). Several observational studies of students' physical activity levels during physical education indicated that students were not moderately to vigorously physically active for at least 50% of class time (383,401,402). Physical education teachers often use too much of their class time for activities related to administrative and management tasks (e.g., taking attendance and making announcements) that do not facilitate moderate to vigorous physical activity (383,403–406).

Implement curricular and instructional practices to increase student physical activity during physical education. After a rigorous review of physical activity intervention research, the Task Force on Community Preventive Services (available at http://www.thecommunityguide.org) recommended enhanced, school-based physical education as an effective strategy for increasing physical activity among students (378). Schools should adopt the enhancements to physical education recommended by the task force that include making physical education classes longer, incorporating fitness activities into physical education classes, and improving curricula and instruction. Curricular and instructional changes that increase the likelihood of keeping students active during the majority of class time include the following:

- modifying traditional game rules to make games more active (146)
- replacing games or activities that are inherently less active (e.g., traditional softball and kickball) with more active options (e.g., soccer)
- spending time in physical education class on aerobic activities that can easily be incorporated into students' lifestyles, such as hopping, skipping, dancing, jumping rope, and aerobic games modified to be noncompetitive

and that do not include eliminating students from the game (e.g., traditional tag and dodge ball) (381,407,408)
- ensuring all students have enough needed equipment such as balls and jump ropes to prevent students from waiting in lines and to allow adequate time for skill practice and participation (382,409,410)
- having students walk or engage in other forms of physical activity, rather than sitting or standing during roll call (146,382,409,410)

13.5.4.3 USE INSTRUCTIONAL STRATEGIES IN PHYSICAL EDUCATION THAT ENHANCE STUDENTS' BEHAVIORAL SKILLS, CONFIDENCE IN THEIR ABILITIES, AND DESIRE TO ADOPT AND MAINTAIN A PHYSICALLY ACTIVE LIFESTYLE

Incorporate instructional strategies to improve students' behavioral skills in physical education and physical activity programs. Behavioral skills such as self-assessment (e.g., assessing current levels of physical activity) and self-monitoring (e.g., tracking activity levels over time), self-management, goal-setting, and decision-making might help students establish and maintain regular involvement in physical activity (380,384,387,411,412). Children and adolescents who believe they have the ability to address barriers and opportunities and lead a physically active life have more motivation for participation in physical activity (413). Therefore, activities or assignments that enable students to identify and address and internal barriers and opportunities for physical activity should be integrated into physical education.

Incorporate instructional strategies in physical education to improve students' confidence in their ability to be physically active and maintain physical activity behaviors. Physical education should help students master and gain confidence in motor, movement, and behavioral skills needed to establish and maintain physically active lifestyles. The development of fundamental motor skills (e.g., running, hopping, and skipping) should be taught to elementary school students (391). As students move into adolescence, lifetime physical activities (e.g., walking, bicycling, tennis, and swimming) that students enjoy and succeed in are important to include in physical education lessons (293,386,387). To master skills and establish self-confidence in their ability, students should be taught skills that are broken down into components ranging from easy to hard (394). Providing students with choices during physical education class might increase students' confidence in their ability to participate in physical activity in general (414–416). For example, allowing students to choose the type or intensity of a specific physical activity might help increase their confidence in their ability to perform the activity in the future; they can progressively add more intensity (412).

Incorporate instructional strategies in physical education and physical activity programs that lead to positive attitudes and perceptions toward physical activity. Influencing students' attitudes toward and perceptions of physical activity might affect their involvement in physical activity outside of physical education class (417,418). Physical education should encourage students to believe that physical activity is important and enjoyable. Increasing students' self-efficacy for engaging in physical activity increases the likelihood of enjoyment and therefore the likelihood of regular participation in physical activity (384,411). Meeting the needs and interests of all students through various activities, emphasizing the many benefits of physical activity, and integrating opportunities to apply newly acquired skills help students develop positive attitudes toward physical activity. Other teaching practices that might increase students' participation in physical activity include enthusiastic role modeling and positive verbal reinforcement for being active (146,383,402).

13.5.4.4 PROVIDE AMPLE OPPORTUNITIES FOR ALL STUDENTS TO ENGAGE IN PHYSICAL ACTIVITY OUTSIDE OF PHYSICAL EDUCATION CLASS

The school setting can offer multiple opportunities for students to enjoy physical activity outside of physical education class and increase daily amounts of physical activity, including (377,419)

- recess periods for unstructured or structured play in elementary schools;
- physical activity breaks;
- after-school and lunch-time intramural and physical activity clubs;
- interscholastic sports; and
- walk- and bicycle-to-school programs.

Require daily recess. All elementary schools should follow the NASPE recommendation that at least one daily 20-minute period of recess be provided to all students (420). In 2006, 67% of elementary schools offered recess 5 days per week for ≥20 minutes on average in all grades (421).

Regularly scheduled recess periods enable children to accumulate a portion of their recommended 60 minutes of daily physical activity (422–424). Recess allows children to apply skills learned in physical education (e.g., motor skill development, decision-making, cooperation, conflict resolution, and negotiation) (420,425). However, recess should not replace physical education or be used to meet time requirements set forth in physical education policies. Participation in recess is associated with academic benefits, such as improving attentiveness, concentration, behavior, and time-on-task in the classroom (280,281,420,426–429).

Schools might try to facilitate increased physical activity during recess by having staff members encourage students to be active; providing students with space, facilities, equipment, and supplies that can make participation in activity appealing; using point-of-decision prompts; and providing structured, organized physical activities (e.g., four-square, active tag, or flag football) for interested students (241,420,424,425,430–432).

Provide physical activity breaks during the school day. Another way to increase physical activity during the school day is to incorporate activity within the classroom. Some schools offer physical activity in the classroom as part of planned lessons that teach mathematics, language arts, and other academic subjects through movement. For example, teachers might read a book aloud while students walk at a moderate pace around the room. The teacher might then ask students to identify the verbs or action words in the book by acting them out through physical activity (433). Such activities contribute to accumulated physical activity during the school day (434). Physical activity within the regular classroom also can enhance on-task classroom behavior of students (433) and establish a school environment that promotes regular physical activity.

Offer students opportunities to participate in intramural physical activity programs during after-school hours. Intramural physical activity programs provide additional opportunities for students to achieve their recommended daily amount of physical activity. Intramural physical activities should provide opportunities for both males and females; meet the needs of students at all levels of skills and physical abilities, particularly those who are not athletically gifted; and reflect student interest (246). In 2006, almost half (48%) of all schools offered intramural programs (144). NASPE has outlined three characteristics of quality intramural programs: 1) students have a choice of activities or participation, 2) every student is given equal opportunity to participate regardless of ability level, and 3) students have the opportunity to be involved with planning and implementing activities (246).

Lifetime physical activities such as walking, running, hiking, swimming, tennis, dancing, and bicycling should be included in intramural programs (246). Partnerships with parents and community-based organizations (e.g., health and wellness facilities such as YMCAs) might increase the availability and quality of intramural programs, as well as the time students spend being active (118,328). Successful program implementation can be influenced by staff training on proper program implementation (435) and coordination with community groups (436).

Offer interscholastic sports. Nationwide, 77% of middle schools and 91% of high schools offered interscholastic sports programs in 2006 (144); in 2009, 58% of high school students reported that they had played on one or more sports teams run by their school or community group (78).

School or community-based sports programs provide structured time for children and adolescents to accumulate minutes of physical activity, establish cooperative and competitive skills, and learn sport-specific and performance-based skills. Evidence indicates that participation in sports is related to higher levels of participation in overall physical activity (437–439). In addition, participation in sports programs has been associated with improved mental health and fewer risky health behaviors (440,441).

Interscholastic sports programs should provide structured, competitive opportunities for students to develop both sport-specific and behavioral skills (260). Although typically limited to students who are athletically gifted, interscholastic sports also provide unique opportunities for applying skills (e.g., sport-specific movements) and behaviors (e.g., self-monitoring and management) taught in physical education.

Implement and promote walk- and bicycle-to-school programs. Walking and bicycling to school has become less common among school-aged children and adolescents. As of 2005, <15% of children and adolescents walked or bicycled to and from school, compared with 41% in 1969 (110). Students who use physically active forms of transportation have higher overall levels of physical activity (442–444) and are more likely to meet physical activity recommendations (445,446).

Federal legislation that provides funding to states to create a Safe Routes to School initiative (110) has enhanced the popularity of walk- and bicycle-to-school programs. Schools making changes to the built environment (e.g., adding sidewalks and crosswalks) have experienced increases in the prevalence of students walking and bicycling to school (447). To support communities with developing and implementing walk- and bicycle-to-school programs, CDC has developed the KidsWalk-to-School guide (available at http://www.cdc.gov/nccdphp/dnpa/kidswalk) (448). The guide provides users with a step-by-step checklist, implementation tools, safety tips, and ideas to make walking to school active and exciting. The National Center for Safe Routes to School provides technical assistance and professional development to states, school districts, and schools on how to develop and implement Safe Routes to School programs (available at http://www.saferoutesinfo.org).

13.5.4.5 ENSURE THAT PHYSICAL EDUCATION AND OTHER PHYSICAL ACTIVITY PROGRAMS MEET THE NEEDS AND INTERESTS OF ALL STUDENTS

All students, regardless of sex, race/ethnicity, health status, or physical or cognitive ability or disability, should have access to physical education and other physical activity programs. Physical education and physical activity programs that overemphasize team sports and do not emphasize lifetime physical activities (e.g., walking, bicycling, and tennis) could exclude potential participants (293,379).

Promote and ensure inclusion of all students. Children and adolescents who are obese or who have physical or cognitive disabilities, chronic diseases (e.g., diabetes or asthma), or low fitness levels might benefit from physical education and physical activity programs to increase physical activity participation, develop motor skills, improve physical fitness, and encourage enjoyment and success (449,450). Nationwide, 62% of schools had students with long-term physical, medical, or cognitive disabilities. Often, students who have disabilities or chronic health conditions are discouraged from participating in physical education class and other forms of physical activity. For example, among the schools that had students with disabilities enrolled, only 59% had students with long-term disabilities participate in required physical education (144). Rather than excluding these children from physical education and activity programs, teachers and program leaders should modify physical education and other school- and community-based programs for these students.

Whether a student with disabilities participates in the general physical education class, works with a teaching assistant in a general physical education class, participates in a separate class with teaching assistants, or receives one-on-one instruction, appropriate modifications should be in place. Such modifications include adapting activities through 1) changes in games to increase participation by students with disabilities; 2) adaptive equipment (e.g., larger or lighter bats, balls in various sizes and textures, or lowered goals or targets) that can be used with ease; 3) adapted instructional strategies such as simplified movement patterns and modified body positions; and 4) frequent rest periods (451). Finally, students with disabilities should have measurable physical education goals and objectives (established by the physical education teacher or other school staff members) included in their IEP. These measurable goals and objectives enable the school or school district to ensure that students' IEP physical education goals and objectives are being met (451).

13.5.5 GUIDELINE 5. IMPLEMENT HEALTH EDUCATION THAT PROVIDES STUDENTS WITH THE KNOWLEDGE, ATTITUDES, SKILLS, AND EXPERIENCES NEEDED FOR HEALTHY EATING AND PHYSICAL ACTIVITY

Health education supports the development of health-related knowledge, skills, and attitudes to increase the likelihood that students engage in healthy behaviors and to avoid or reduce health risks. Health education curricula and instruction should address various health topics, including healthy eating and physical activity, systematically and sequentially to ensure attainment of national and state standards and corresponding learning objectives and outcomes (452,453). Health education curricula should be developmentally appropriate and address physical, mental, emotional, and social dimensions of health to improve health knowledge, attitudes, skills, and behaviors (452,453) (Box 5).

13.5.5.1 REQUIRE HEALTH EDUCATION FROM PREKINDERGARTEN THROUGH GRADE 12

Health education is integral to the primary mission of schools, providing students with the knowledge and skills they need to become successful learners and healthy adults. In 2002, the Joint Committee on Health Education Terminology defined health education as "the development, delivery, and evaluation of planned, sequential, and developmentally appropriate instruction, learning experiences, and other activities designed to protect, promote, and enhance the health literacy, attitudes, skills, and well-being of students, prekindergarten through grade 12" (454). Health education is a fundamental part of an overall school health program. Increasing the number of schools that require health education and teach ways to prevent important health problems, such as those resulting from poor dietary behaviors and lack of physical activity, are national health objectives (objective EMC 4) (10).

Most states and districts require, but devote few hours to, health education and instruction on nutrition and physical activity. Nationwide in 2006, the median number of hours of required instruction on nutrition was 3.4 hours for elementary schools, 4.2 hours for middle schools, and 5.9 for high schools. The median number of hours of required instruction on physical activity was 2.4 hours for elementary schools, 3.1 hours for middle schools, and 4.5 for high schools (455). Schools also require less health education as students progress through school. Almost two thirds (61%) of all schools required health instruction in at least one specific grade, but 34% of schools with 9th-grade students required it in 9th grade, 25% in 10th grade, 12% in 11th grade, and 9% in 12th grade (455).

Nutrition and physical activity topics also can be integrated into other academic disciplines to complement comprehensive health education and physical education programs (456,457). Examples might include biology lessons on energy balance (458) and the physics of body movement, math lessons on nutrient analysis, family and consumer science courses on cooking skills, and language arts lessons analyzing food advertisements (459). Integration of health topics throughout the school curriculum should not replace health education as a course in school; a comprehensive health education curriculum is necessary to enable students to achieve the national and state standards for health education. Schools that rely on integration into other academic areas as the sole means of providing health education might provide less instructional time for health and cover fewer topics than when health education is a separate course.

13.5.5.2 IMPLEMENT A PLANNED AND SEQUENTIAL HEALTH EDUCATION CURRICULUM THAT IS CULTURALLY AND DEVELOPMENTALLY APPROPRIATE, ADDRESSES A CLEAR SET OF BEHAVIORAL OUTCOMES THAT PROMOTE HEALTHY EATING AND PHYSICAL ACTIVITY, AND IS BASED ON NATIONAL STANDARDS

Implement a planned and sequential curriculum that is culturally and developmentally appropriate. Health education curricula should include (453)

- clearly articulated learning outcomes or learning objectives;
- a planned progression of developmentally and culturally appropriate lessons or learning experiences that lead to achieving these objectives;
- continuity between lessons or learning experiences that clearly reinforce the adoption and maintenance of specific health-enhancing behaviors;
- accompanying content or materials that correspond with the sequence of learning events and help teachers and students meet the learning objectives;
- consideration of cultural heritage, family attitudes and customs, and differences in physical activity and diet of students when designing lesson plans; and
- assessment strategies to determine whether students have achieved the desired learning objectives.

Health education should incorporate student assessment strategies that enable students to demonstrate their understanding of primary health concepts and apply health-related skills to real-life situations. Quality health education assessment protocols include criteria for examining student work (such as a rubric) and incorporate multiple measures over time (453,460,461).

A student assessment should help improve and inform teaching practices and promote learning (453,462–464), use multiple sources of information, and provide fair, valid, and reliable information (453,465). The choice of specific assessment methods should be determined by the nature of the learning outcomes being assessed, the purpose of the assessments, and the grade level of the students (466). Assessments that are performance based (rather than based on recall and recognition) enable students to apply knowledge and skills and are well-suited to learning skills such as effective decision-making and interpersonal communication (453,462,467). Performance-based assessments are designed to measure a student's knowledge, ability, skill, and attitude consistently, emphasizing methods other than standardized achievement tests, particularly those using multiple-choice formats (453,465,468,469). Performance-based assessments typically include performance tasks, exhibitions, demonstrations, written or oral responses, journals, and portfolios (465,469). Examples include photo essays, skits, infomercials, public service announcements, and letters to the editor.

Implement a curriculum that addresses a clear set of behavioral outcomes that promote healthy eating and physical activity. Health education that incorporates the topics of healthy eating and physical activity has been shown to improve student dietary behaviors (148,467,470–472) and physical activity participation levels (148,217); reduce sedentary behaviors (159,457,473); and improve serum cholesterol levels (474–476), blood pressure (474,477), and BMI (457,459,474,477). School-based type 2 diabetes prevention programs with health education components have resulted in increased knowledge about the disease (478,479) and improvements in student blood glucose levels for diverse groups of students at high risk for the disease (480–482).

Nutrition education should be part of a comprehensive school health education curriculum. As a result of participation in a K–12 health education curriculum that includes nutrition, students should have the knowledge and skills to do the following (199,200,462,483):

- Eat a variety of whole grain products, fruits and vegetables, and nonfat or low-fat milk or equivalent milk products every day.

- Eat the appropriate amounts from each food group every day.
- Choose foods that provide ample amounts of vitamins and minerals.
- Eat the appropriate amounts of high-fiber foods.
- Drink plenty of water.
- Limit foods and beverages high in added sugar.
- Limit the intake of fat, avoiding foods with saturated and trans fats.
- Eat breakfast every day.
- Eat healthy snacks.
- Eat healthy food when dining out.
- Prepare food in healthy ways.
- Balance caloric intake with caloric expenditure.
- Follow a plan for healthy weight management.
- Support others to eat healthy.

Health education curricula should reinforce the information taught in physical education classes and provide opportunities for students to apply physical activity knowledge and skills. As a result of participation in a K–12 health education curriculum that includes physical activity, students should have the knowledge and skills to be able to do the following (147,462):

- Engage in moderate to vigorous physical activity for at least 60 minutes every day.
- Regularly engage in physical activities that enhance cardiorespiratory endurance, flexibility, muscle endurance, and muscle strength.
- Engage in warm-up and cool-down activities before and after exercise.
- Drink plenty of water before, during, and after physical activity.
- Follow a physical activity plan for healthy weight management.
- Avoid injury during physical activity.
- Support others to be physically active.

Health education should foster positive attitudes toward being a physically active person by emphasizing the benefits and enjoyment of physical activity, supporting students who are physically active, and incorporating self-management techniques (e.g., assessing personal physical activity level and setting goals to be more active) into lessons (484).

Skill-based health education also should include lessons on limiting sedentary screen time (e.g., television, video games, and computer usage). Studies have found that such lessons can reduce television viewing and other screen and media time among students and demonstrate promise in preventing childhood obesity (159,457,473). The Task Force on Community Preventive Services conducted a rigorous review of research and recommended behavioral interventions to reduce screen time among preschool children and school-aged children and adolescents. The seven interventions included in the review focused on establishing classes for building skills, tips, setting goals, and reinforcement techniques, and parent or family support through schools or other organizations providing information on environmental strategies to reduce exposure to and use of televisions, computers, and video games. (Additional details about the review are available at http://www.thecommunityguide.org/obesity/behavioral.html.) Finally, health education curricula should focus on building student skills (e.g., self-monitoring, setting goals, and decision-making) to help decrease television viewing, decrease consumption of high-fat food, increase fruit and vegetable intake, and increase physical activity (457,473).

Implement health education curricula that are consistent with the National Health Education Standards. The National Health Education Standards and performance indicators outline the health-related concepts, skills, and healthy beliefs, values, and norms students need for healthy behaviors (453). These standards provide a foundation for selecting or developing curricular and instructional materials, delivering instruction, and assessing student knowledge, attitudes, skills, and behaviors. Many state boards of education, state departments of education, and local school boards have adopted their own state or local health education standards using the National Health Education Standards as a guide. In 2006, most (72%) states required or encouraged districts or schools to follow health education standards or guidelines based specifically on the national standards, and most districts (66%) required or encouraged the same for schools (455). A national health objective strives to increase the proportion of elementary, middle, and senior high schools that have health education goals or objectives that address the knowledge and skills in the National Health Education Standards (high school, middle school, and elementary school) (objective ECBP 3) (10).

The National Health Education Standards emphasize the development of skills and specify that, as a result of health education, students should be able to 1) understand concepts related to health promotion and disease prevention; 2) analyze the influence of family, peers, culture, media, technology, and other factors on health behaviors; 3) access valid information, products, and services to enhance health; 4) use interpersonal communication skills to enhance health and avoid or reduce health risks; 5) use decision-making skills to enhance health; 6) use goal-setting skills to enhance health; 7) practice health-enhancing behaviors and avoid or reduce health risks; and 8) advocate for personal, family, and community health (453).

CDC's Health Education Curriculum Analysis Tool (HECAT) helps school districts conduct clear, complete, and consistent analyses of written health education curricula based on the National Health Education Standards and research-based characteristics of effectiveness. HECAT addresses a wide range of health topics, including modules on healthy eating and physical activity. Results from HECAT can help schools enhance an existing curriculum, develop their own curriculum, or select a published curriculum that will deliver quality health education (462). The tool is available online at http://www.cdc.gov/HealthyYouth/hecat.

13.5.5.3 USE CURRICULA THAT ARE CONSISTENT WITH SCIENTIFIC EVIDENCE OF EFFECTIVENESS IN HELPING STUDENTS IMPROVE HEALTHY EATING AND PHYSICAL ACTIVITY BEHAVIORS

Health education curricula, regardless of the topic, should reflect the research that emphasizes teaching functional health information (essential concepts), shaping personal values that support healthy behaviors, shaping group norms that value a healthy lifestyle, and developing essential health skills necessary to adopt and maintain health-enhancing behaviors. Similar to physical education, most of the school-based programs included in RTIPs have a health education component; however, the curricula are not extensively or separately analyzed (additional information available at http://rtips.cancer.gov/rtips/index.do). Health education curricula and materials should be based on theories of behavior change and have the following characteristics (453):

- focus on clear health goals and specific behavioral outcomes
- be research-based and theory-driven
- address individual values and group norms that support health-enhancing behaviors

- focus on increasing the personal perception of risk and harmfulness of engaging in specific health risk behaviors as well as reinforcing protective factors
- address social pressures and influences
- build personal competence, social competence, and increase confidence in skills
- provide functional health knowledge that is basic and accurate and directly contributes to health-promoting decisions and behaviors
- use strategies designed to personalize information and engage students
- provide age-appropriate and developmentally appropriate information, learning strategies, teaching methods, and materials
- incorporate learning strategies, teaching methods, and materials that are culturally inclusive
- provide adequate time for instruction and learning
- provide opportunities to reinforce skills and positive health behaviors
- provide opportunities to make positive connections with influential others
- include teacher information and plans for professional development that enhance effectiveness of instruction and student learning

13.5.5.4 USE CLASSROOM INSTRUCTIONAL METHODS AND STRATEGIES THAT ARE INTERACTIVE, ENGAGE ALL STUDENTS, AND ARE RELEVANT TO THEIR DAILY LIVES AND EXPERIENCES

Health education instruction should include the use of active learning strategies that encourage student participation and help develop the concepts, attitudes, and skills needed to make healthy eating choices and be physically active from childhood through adulthood (485). Interactive lessons that include demonstration, modeling, rehearsal, and feedback are more likely to result in positive behavioral changes than a traditional didactic approach (148,482,486,487). The use of goal-setting skills also can be integrated into health education to help students identify personal goals for dietary and physical activity behaviors (488). Adequate professional development should be offered to teachers because these active learning strategies may be unfamiliar to some (182).

Use interactive learning strategies. Students are more likely to adopt healthy eating and physical activity behaviors when

- they learn about these behaviors through enjoyable, participatory activities rather than through lectures (230,488–490);

- lessons emphasize the positive, appealing aspects of physical activity and healthy eating patterns rather than the negative consequences and present the benefits in the context of what is already important to students (491–494); and
- they have repeated opportunities to practice physical activity and healthy eating behaviors that are relevant to their daily lives (485,488,489,495,496).

Use methods and strategies that are developmentally appropriate. Educational strategies should match the different stages of students' cognitive development. For example, nutrition education for younger children should focus on concrete experiences, such as increasing exposure to many healthy foods and building skills in choosing healthy foods (230,490,497). By middle school, students can understand and act on the connection between physical activity, healthy eating behaviors, and their overall health as well as the role these behaviors play in preventing chronic diseases (453,491).

Developmentally appropriate strategies for adolescents include skill development (such as learning a dance or preparing a certain fruit), self-monitoring (such as a diary of physically active and sedentary behaviors or tracking fruit and vegetable consumption), and promotion of regular physical activity and healthy eating (498). Health education for middle and high school students should focus on self-assessment and setting personal goals (498,499). Lessons for older students should emphasize personal responsibility for making healthy and positive choices, decision-making skills for healthy eating and physical activity, analysis of dietary and physical activity behaviors and their influence on chronic disease risk, resisting negative social pressures, and advocating for individual, family, and community health (500–502). HECAT provides concepts and skill examples deemed appropriate for various grade groups (i.e., grades pre-kinderten–2, 3–5, 6–8, and 9–12).

Integrate computer-based instruction into health education. Computer-based instruction on physical activity and healthy eating offers opportunities for self-paced health education (485,495,503,504). Interactive computer programs can help students learn and assess their own physical activity and healthy eating skills (505–507). For example, students can track via computer their daily physical activity for a week and receive a report on how many days they met the physical activity guidelines. Students also can be exposed to interactive computer programs that enable them to track the foods they have eaten over a given period and receive a nutritional analysis.

13.5.6 GUIDELINE 6. PROVIDE STUDENTS WITH HEALTH, MENTAL HEALTH, AND SOCIAL SERVICES TO ADDRESS HEALTHY EATING, PHYSICAL ACTIVITY, AND RELATED CHRONIC DISEASE PREVENTION

Schools are responsible for the physical health, mental health, and safety of students during the school day (215). School health, mental health, and social services staff members can

- teach students the skills they need to live a healthy life;
- identify risky student behaviors and intervene when needed;
- identify and resolve health-care needs that affect educational achievement;
- provide case management for health and mental health issues;
- address behavioral and psychological problems;
- link students and families to community health resources; and
- provide overall leadership for school health programs, including those designed to promote physical activity and healthy eating.

School health, mental health, and social services are accessible to students who have special needs or chronic health conditions and those who do not have health insurance or might not make regular visits to a health-care provider. Qualified professionals such as nurses, physicians, dentists, health educators, and other allied health personnel provide school health services. Professionals such as certified school counselors, psychologists, social workers, and, occasionally, psychiatrists provide mental health and social services (508). Schools can refer students for additional care to community agencies, organizations, or health-care providers not on the school property or to school-based health centers.

School nurses can play a critical role in coordinating student health-care services at the school. When necessary, they coordinate with community health-care providers or school-based health centers providing care to students (509). A national health objective aims to increase the proportion of the U.S. schools that have a nurse-student ratio of at least 1:750 well children (objective ECBP 5) (10). Certain schools might need a higher nurse-student ratio for students who require daily professional nursing services or students with complex health needs (509). In 2006, 45% of all schools had a nurse-student ratio of at least 1:750; 36% of all schools had a full-time school nurse (510).

School nurses should have a minimum of a bachelor's degree in nursing. A certification in the specialty of school nursing is preferred, with a current state license as a registered nurse to be able to serve both as a full-time health-care provider and health educator (509,511,512). School nurses have the knowledge and expertise to address a range of services that includes promotion of healthy eating, physical activity, and weight management (513). Schools also need access to a consulting physician to provide services such as school-based standing orders, consultations and supplementary training for staff members, recommendations for families, review of school health and health services policies and procedures, and communication with and referrals to physicians or other health-care providers (182,215,509). To address mental health concerns, schools might link students to school-based health centers or community-based services or employ mental health and social services staff members.

Because of the range of activities that require the involvement of various professionals, staff members should work collaboratively to coordinate student care and school health, mental health, and social services both within and outside of the school setting (215,509,514–517). The goal of staff collaboration within the school setting should be to provide consistent messages about health behaviors to all students; delegate case management to the staff member with the most appropriate training, competency, and licensure for a particular health issue (215); and coordinate care among health, mental health, and social services staff members when students have physical health conditions that might coexist with mental health problems (Box 6).

13.5.6.1 ASSESS STUDENT NEEDS RELATED TO PHYSICAL ACTIVITY, NUTRITION, AND OBESITY, AND PROVIDE COUNSELING AND OTHER SERVICES TO MEET THOSE NEEDS

Identification, follow-up, and treatment of health and mental health conditions related to diet, physical activity, and weight are important for student health (182,518). School health, mental health, and social services staff members should collaborate with community health-care providers to increase student access to care, coordinate care, and promote evidence-based physical activity and healthy eating initiatives (215). Schools should link students to appropriate services within the local medical community that are staffed by employees with appropriate training and are accessible to all students, including those with low family incomes or without insurance (215). Schools also should identify and link students and their families to community-based health promotion programs that encourage physical activity and healthy eating.

Assess eating and physical activity behaviors of students. School nurses, together with other health, mental health and social services staff members, can assess the healthy eating and physical activity behaviors of students during routine interactions. Information about the number of students in the school who meet diet, physical activity, and weight status recommendations can be used to guide program planning and policy advocacy efforts. Assessment also enables staff members to identify students in need of counseling and referral services. Some student assessment results might reveal signs and symptoms of health risks that require urgent attention, such as hypertension, hunger, use of illegal performance-enhancing drugs, or disordered eating. All school staff members may be given guidance on how to recognize early signs of these risk behaviors and confidentially refer students with diet, physical activity, or mental health concerns to health, mental health, and social services staff members. Students with signs of serious conditions or health risk behaviors should be referred to a primary health-care provider (519).

Following are some of the topics that a health practitioner can address during a rapid dietary assessment. Evidence indicates that these behaviors are associated with energy intake and can be a focus of change if needed (37,38,520):

- frequency of eating fast food or outside the home in restaurants
- usual daily intake of sugar-sweetened beverages and 100% fruit juice
- typical portion sizes
- frequency of eating breakfast
- usual daily intake of foods that are high in energy density
- usual intake of fruits and vegetables

- meal frequency and snacking patterns

Staff members should also refer to the *Dietary Guidelines for Americans* for current recommendations for dietary intakes for children and adolescents (5).

Following are some topics that a health practitioner can address during a rapid physical activity assessment (37,38,520):

- amount of daily physical activity participation (e.g., whether student is physically active for ≥60 minutes per day through free play, time spent outside, physical education, and involvement in organized activities such as school or community recreation programs)
- number of hours per day of television, movies, video game, and computer use (e.g., whether student is viewing >1–2 hours of quality programming per day)
- presence of a television or a computer in student's bedroom
- participation in physical education classes
- amount of physically active discretionary activities, such as walking or bicycling to school, taking stairs, or doing chores

Staff members also should refer to the 2008 Physical Activity Guidelines for Americans (9), the CDC Youth Physical Activity Guidelines Toolkit (available at http://www.cdc.gov/healthyyouth/physicalactivity/guidelines.htm), and AAP policy guidance on screen time (160).

Staff members also might refer to the National Association of School Nurses' SCOPE (School Nurse Childhood Obesity Prevention Education) manual (521) or the AAP's Pediatric Obesity Clinical Decision Support Chart (522). The questions should be age appropriate; students aged <10 years might not be able to answer questions as reliably as older students. Obtaining a more accurate assessment of younger students might require posing questions to parents or caregivers (520).

Schools initiating BMI measurement programs should implement safeguards. In many schools, nurses measure students' height and weight and use the results to determine their BMI status. Data on the percentage of students who are obese and overweight in a school or school district can be useful for program planning, policy advocacy efforts, and evaluation. Some schools send BMI results home to students' families, along with guidance on improving student physical activity and nutrition behaviors.

This process is often called BMI screening. BMI information can help correct parent and student misperceptions about weight status and might motivate families to seek medical care and make healthy lifestyle changes. However, there is not enough evidence to recommend for or against BMI screening programs in schools (518). Research studies have not yet fully assessed the usefulness of school-based BMI screening in preventing and reducing obesity among students; the impact of BMI screening on weight-related knowledge, attitudes, and the behaviors of students and their families; or of any potential harm that might result from such screening (e.g., stigmatizing students or encouraging harmful weight loss practices) (518). In 2007, an expert panel recommended that BMI should be calculated and plotted at least annually at all well-child visits at the primary health-care provider (38). Schools that make the decision to conduct BMI screening should implement safeguards to ensure respect for students' privacy and confidentiality, protect students from potential harm, and increase the likelihood that the program will have a positive impact on promoting a healthy weight. Schools should ensure that appropriate follow-up diagnosis and care are available to students at a community health-care provider. Essential safeguards for and more detailed information about school-based BMI measurement programs are described in CDC's document, Body Mass Index Measurement in Schools (available at http://www.cdc.gov/healthyyouth/obesity/bmi/pdf/BMI_execsumm.pdf) (518).

Counsel students on how to achieve healthy eating and physical activity recommendations. Counseling can begin with motivational interviewing, a nonjudgmental, empathetic, and encouraging approach that allows students to express positive or negative feelings toward healthy eating and physical activity and identify their own reasons and plans for improvement. Motivational interviewing involves staff members asking, informing, advising, and listening about healthy eating and physical activity behaviors. Staff members who provide counseling should have the appropriate training necessary to counsel students about eating healthfully and being active (520). Student assessment results will guide the counseling sessions, and staff members can ask students to identify the behavior they might be interested in changing or that might be easiest to change (37,520). Staff members can further assess students' readiness and motivation to change by asking how important it is to them and how confident they feel about their ability to change. Counseling that involves students' families might have a greater impact on the environmental influences that shape students' diet and physical activity behaviors away from school (37).

Subsequent to assessment and motivational interviewing, staff members can use behavioral strategies, such as goal-setting, positive reinforcement, and self-monitoring, to facilitate changes in students' health behaviors (520). Goal-setting should be a process, incrementally moving toward the desired outcomes (e.g., increase physical activity by 10% per week) (520,523). Staff members should schedule follow-up sessions to assess students' progress toward their goals (520).

Students who are already active and have healthy diets should be encouraged to continue these behaviors. Emphasizing the benefits of healthy eating and regular physical activity and encouraging students to be role models for their peers are ways to reinforce these behaviors (215,498,524).

Students with eating disorders, who are binge eating, or who have other weight concerns might need more specific mental health and social services (519). Obese students, for example, are at increased risk for being teased, bullied, or socially isolated and having low self-esteem and depression (35,282,525–529). Students with weight concerns are at increased risk for unhealthy dieting behaviors (530,531). In addition, students with extreme perceptions of body size (e.g., perceive themselves as very overweight) are at increased risk for suicide ideation and suicide attempts (532). Health, mental health, and social services staff members should be prepared to promote positive body image and body satisfaction; help students overcome barriers to healthy eating and physical activity; help students find social support, cope with teasing, set goals, and make decisions; and refer students who might require primary medical care (518). All staff members should be aware of early signs and symptoms of mental health problems that might become evident during physical activity, dietary, and weight assessments (519).

Manage the physical activity and nutritional needs of students with chronic health conditions. Diet and physical activity are critical to the management of many chronic health conditions, such as asthma, diabetes, obesity, and food allergies. Health, mental health, and social services staff members should be attentive to students with these conditions to ensure they are meeting healthy eating and activity recommendations (533–535).

Health services staff members, in partnership with medical providers and families, play a key role in developing and coordinating the implementation of individualized health plans established for students with chronic health conditions (509,533,534,536,537) and encouraging them to participate fully in structured and unstructured physical activity, regardless of ability, unless medically contraindicated. Health, mental health, and social services staff members can collaborate with students' families and health-care providers to maximize student participation, provide modified activities when appropriate, and eliminate barriers to student participation. Families and health-care providers should notify schools about dietary restrictions or modifications and schedules for meals and snacks related to the condition (519). Health, mental health, and social services staff members can request written permission from families to exchange confidential health information with students' health-care providers (515). Trained school health staff members can collaborate with students' primary health-care providers to ensure monitoring of vital signs and compliance with treatment program and to address students' health issues in a confidential and sensitive manner (519). These efforts ensure that students who require ongoing management for chronic health conditions will receive continuous care and monitoring at school. This network is important to facilitate quick notification to all parties when a change is observed in the students' health status or when there is a revision to the health management plan (538).

If a student has a medical provider–prescribed weight management plan, then health, mental health, and social services staff members can communicate with the student's health-care provider to discuss their role in monitoring implementation and assisting the student with compliance. Unless specified otherwise, the goal of the weight management strategy should be weight maintenance versus weight loss. To ensure appropriate and safe oversight, the health, mental health, and social services staff member coordinating care with the student's health-care provider needs to have training in pediatric weight management or behavioral counseling (539). The *Expert Committee Recommendations Regarding the Prevention, Assessment, and Treatment of Child and Adolescent Overweight and Obesity* include detailed guidance on assessment, counseling, and management for health-care workers providing care for overweight and obese young persons (37,38,520,539).

13.5.6.1 ENSURE STUDENTS HAVE ACCESS TO NEEDED HEALTH, MENTAL HEALTH, AND SOCIAL SERVICES

Health, mental health, and social services staff members serve as liaisons between school staff members, students, families, community programs, and health-care providers (515). Community resources can address health, mental health, and social service gaps that the school might not have the resources or expertise to address adequately. In addition, this collaborative approach keeps the community informed about school-based healthy eating and physical activity initiatives and keeps school staff members aware of community-based services (520). Health, mental health, and social services staff members should seek out partnerships and serve on community health coalitions (515). Coordination of services might increase student and family participation in community-based healthy eating, physical activity, and obesity prevention programs (540–542).

Refer students to community-based health-care providers and healthy eating and physical activity services. School health personnel should establish systematic processes and criteria for referring students to primary health-care providers (215). Students with signs of disordered eating or diet-related health conditions (e.g., sudden weight loss, eating disorders, or obesity) should be referred to a primary health-care provider for diagnosis and, if needed, establishment of management or treatment plans. For example, students classified as obese or overweight after BMI screening require further medical examination to determine whether the student in fact has excess body fat or other conditions related to obesity (e.g., diabetes or prediabetes, high blood cholesterol and triglyceride levels, or early pubertal maturation) (543–545).

Health, mental health, and social services staff members play an important role in developing and marketing a referral system for students and families (215,498,513,535). To establish a referral system, health, mental health, and social services staff members should identify health-care services and school- or community-based programs that encourage healthy eating and physical activity and address obesity and eating disorders. These services include school-linked health clinics, local health departments, universities, medical schools, outside health-care providers (e.g., private physicians and dentists, hospitals, psychologists and other mental health workers, pediatric weight management clinics, community health clinics, and managed care organizations), and community-based nutrition and physical activity providers and services (e.g., dieticians, recreational programs, and cooking classes).

The list of referral services should be based on the health needs of the student population, barriers to health care in the community, past student use of community services, and current community culture. Health, mental health, and social services staff members can assess which services are available at the school and which require outside referral (182). The list should include services that are accessible to all students, including those with low family incomes or without health insurance or transportation. If feasible, arrangements can be made to bring community-based services to the school. With a comprehensive referral system in place, health, mental health, and social services staff members are able to respond to requests from families seeking guidance and increase access to care among students (546).

13.5.6.2 PROVIDE LEADERSHIP IN ADVOCACY AND COORDINATION OF EFFECTIVE SCHOOL PHYSICAL ACTIVITY AND NUTRITION POLICIES AND PRACTICES

Health, mental health, and social services staff members can take an active role in implementing coordinated school health practices and be highly involved in the school health council (513,515). Staff members can work through the school health council to establish policies and practices that promote the school health agenda.

In addition to providing care directly to students, school nurses can coordinate school health, mental health, and social services staff member efforts to advocate for a healthy school environment; increase student and staff member knowledge and promote healthy behaviors through health education; lead efforts to assess, develop, and evaluate health policies, practices, and programs; and serve as a liaison between teachers and families regarding student health needs (515,519,542,547–549).

Advocate on behalf of students to create a healthy, safe, and supportive school environment that allows students to make healthy dietary and physical activity choices both in and out of school. School health advocacy raises awareness about the importance of health behaviors and can increase school and community support for instruction, programs, policies, and environmental changes that support healthy eating and physical activity (550). Effective advocacy requires collaboration within the school setting and in the broader community. Health, mental health, and social services staff members are ideally situated to engage community health-care providers and organizations in supporting healthy eating and physical activity policies and practices within schools (540,541,551).

Health, mental health, and social services staff members can advocate for schools to develop strong policies and practices that help students achieve healthy eating and physical activity recommendations (515,520,552–554). Advocacy efforts should promote a safe and supportive environment for all students, regardless of athletic ability, weight status, special needs, or chronic health condition (515). For example, they can support adoption of a universal bullying prevention program to address disrespectful behavior and prevent bullying of students with chronic health conditions or weight issues and all other students (518). Health, mental health, and social services staff members can work with physical education and health education teachers, nutrition service staff members, principals, and other school staff members to establish a healthy environment and consistently promote healthy eating and physical activity messages and activities throughout the school setting (542,550,555).

13.5.7 GUIDELINE 7. PARTNER WITH FAMILIES AND COMMUNITY MEMBERS IN THE DEVELOPMENT AND IMPLEMENTATION OF HEALTHY EATING AND PHYSICAL ACTIVITY POLICIES, PRACTICES, AND PROGRAMS

Families and community members (including community organizations) contribute to the academic success of students and are key stakeholders in healthy eating and physical activity policies and practices in schools (556–558). Partnerships among schools, families, and community members can enhance student learning, promote consistent messages about healthy behaviors, increase resources, and engage, guide, and motivate students to eat healthfully and be active (557,559). These three sectors of society influence the growth and development of children and adolescents and share the responsibility for nurturing them into healthy and productive adults (557,559).

Families shape the context of children's everyday social and physical environments; they control the availability of food and influence eating and activity practices (560–562). Although evaluations of the effects of family involvement in school and community-based health interventions have been inconclusive (largely because of variability in study design and inadequate family participation) (334,472,479,563–577), certain findings are worth noting. Family involvement in health can increase their children's knowledge and attitudes about healthy lifestyles (569), influence behavior change (570,575,576,578–581), and provide social support for being healthy (573). Studies that have assessed strategies to prevent and treat childhood obesity or promote physical activity and healthy eating have demonstrated more success when focusing on both the family and the child rather than the child alone (571,578,579,582).

Community partners, including individual persons, agencies, and organizations, can offer multiple resources for healthy eating and physical activity initiatives at schools (e.g., sharing health services) (556,559), provide funding, provide guidance on specific health topics, and provide volunteer support (447,559,583,584). Partners might include businesses, health departments, community health educators, health-care providers, health-care organizations, parks and recreation departments, universities and educational institutions, transportation authorities and other government agencies, faith-based organizations, senior citizen organizations, cultural institutions, local foundations, national service and volunteer organizations, local chefs, and other community volunteers (556).

To develop successful and meaningful partnerships, all partners involved should demonstrate a commitment to student health and communicate intent and expectations about their level of involvement and respective roles in making decisions. Schools should provide a respectful and welcoming climate to families and outside organizations, and the school principal should fully support outside involvement (556) (Box 7).

13.5.7.1 ENCOURAGE COMMUNICATION AMONG SCHOOLS, FAMILIES, AND COMMUNITY MEMBERS TO PROMOTE ADOPTION OF HEALTHY EATING AND PHYSICAL ACTIVITY BEHAVIORS AMONG STUDENTS

Communicate frequently and use various dissemination methods. Schools should communicate with families and community members frequently to emphasize that they are a valuable asset in student learning, health, and well-being (556,585). Schools that communicate with families and community members about healthy eating and physical activity initiatives create a greater understanding of school activities, which might increase support and participation in school policies and practices from students and their families (188,557). Lines of communication should be open for feedback from families and other community members (586,587). Schools can work with families and community members to design needs assessments to gather information on the types of communication that families and community members would like to receive and identify resources offered within the community (588). Examples of topics that schools might address with families and community members include the following:

- school healthy eating and physical activity policies (e.g., types of food allowed at school celebrations and the length of recess provided to students)
- how to provide input on policies, curricula, and programs that are being considered for adoption
- how to participate in the school health council
- nutrition and physical activity instruction in health education
- physical education instruction, including student fitness and physical activity assessment results
- opportunities for physical activity in the school (e.g., physical activity clubs, intramural sports, and interscholastic athletics)
- how to access school physical activity facilities after school hours
- what is being offered by the school nutrition services program (e.g., school breakfast program, school lunch program, menus for school meals, and nutrient analysis of school meals)
- strategies for healthy cooking at home
- school events related to physical activity and healthy eating (e.g., open houses, athletic events, and cooking workshops)
- tips on how to be physically active with children

- community resources on physical activity (e.g., parks and recreation departments), healthy eating (e.g., cooking classes, and food banks), and weight management
- opportunities to volunteer and be involved

Informational or promotional flyers, newsletters, telephone calls, conversations at school, communication via e-mail or websites, and media coverage can be used for communication with families and community members (587,589,590). Local media outlets provide an opportunity to disseminate school messages and remind families and community members to engage in healthy behaviors (589,590).

13.5.7.2 INVOLVE FAMILIES AND COMMUNITY MEMBERS ON THE SCHOOL HEALTH COUNCIL

To participate in planning of and decision-making about school health policies and practices, families and community members should be members of the school health council. All groups invested in school health, including families and community members, and those who will be affected by policies or programs should have representation on the school health council (194,586,591,592). In 2006, among the 73% of school districts that had a district school health council, 89% included community members, 76% included families of students, 51% included local health-care providers, 50% included representatives from the local health department, 40% included representatives from local social service agencies, and 26% included representatives from local health organizations (e.g., the local Red Cross chapter) (593).

The school health council should identify strategies for establishing partnerships with families and community members. The school health action plan should include goals that specifically address establishing partnerships with families and community members. To help inform the action plan, the school health council can assess the status of family and community partnerships at their school through formal questionnaires, telephone interviews, surveys, or the CDC School Health Index (199,200,556).

Families and community members should be invited to provide input on the planning and implementation of healthy eating and physical activity policies, programs, and practices. Their input will help create partnerships that appropriately blend into the community's culture, resulting in greater awareness and buy-in from students and families (557,584,586,587,591,594). Persons already active in work groups, projects, or campaigns (e.g., parent-teacher associations [PTAs]) might help recruit other interested participants through announcements, telephone trees, and reminders when families are at the school (585). Families and community members can identify potential challenges to implementation of policies, programs, and practices (588), as well as identify community supporters such as cultural or political leaders critical to the success of the initiative (589,592,594).

13.5.7.3 DEVELOP AND IMPLEMENT STRATEGIES FOR MOTIVATING FAMILIES TO PARTICIPATE IN SCHOOL-BASED PROGRAMS AND ACTIVITIES THAT PROMOTE HEALTHY EATING AND PHYSICAL ACTIVITY

In 2006, 56% of required health education classes and 31% of physical education courses incorporated homework or projects that involved family members (593). Schools and districts can provide professional development instruction for teachers on engaging families in student learning and school health program activities. In 2006, only 33% of required physical education classes or courses and 41% of required health education classes or courses had a teacher who had received instruction in the past 2 years on encouraging family and community involvement (593).

Formats for involving families include family homework assignments, healthy eating and physical activity newsletters (334,472,479,564, 566,567,569–572), family nights focused on health promotion (564,572, 574,577), and Internet-based programs (563). However, to have an effect on children's health knowledge, attitudes, and behaviors, schools must strive to achieve high levels of parent participation and provide parents with multiple opportunities to participate and engage in activities (569).

Provide various formats for involving families and offer frequent opportunities for participation. When a school offers a family activity confined to only one format, the activity is often not successful at attracting high levels of participation (563,564,566,569,570,572,577). Use of multiple formats provides families with options and the ability to choose activities that are interesting and fit their schedule (574,575,588). For example, the purposes of family homework assignments and activity newsletters are to reinforce health and physical education coursework at school, facilitate communication with families about healthy eating and physical activity initiatives at school and within the community, and increase family knowledge of healthy behaviors (e.g., healthy meal preparation and physical family activities) (334,472,479,564,566,567,569–572,574). Although only a few studies have demonstrated that homework activities and newsletters improve student knowledge of and attitudes toward healthy behaviors (566,570) or affect behaviors (569,595), distributing homework and newsletters to families more frequently might increase their effects (569,570).

Family nights are designed to attract families to the school to engage them in health education and promotion activities. This type of event might include skill-building workshops for families on preparing healthy meals or physical activity stations to participate in active games (564,572,574,577). However, participation in family nights is typically low (564,572,577). Internet-based programs might include interactive online activities such as prompts to be physically active or eat a nutritious snack, weight and behavioral assessments, goal-setting, tracking progress toward achieving health goals, and suggestions for overcoming barriers. Internet-based interventions are appealing because parents and children can participate in the program at a convenient time; however, an evaluation of one study found low participation, possibly because of the time required (563).

Two substantial barriers to family participation in school-based programs and activities are scheduling conflicts and lack of transportation. One technique to overcome these barriers is to link health promotion initiatives to activities that already involve family members (580), such as PTA meetings, parent-teacher conferences, tutoring programs, interscholastic sports, and school plays. Schools might consider providing transportation to and offering child care during events (558).

13.5.7.4 ACCESS COMMUNITY RESOURCES TO HELP PROVIDE HEALTHY EATING AND PHYSICAL ACTIVITY OPPORTUNITIES FOR STUDENTS

School collaborations with community resources can link students and their families to programs and services that the school is unable to provide independently. Partnerships are beneficial because they conserve resources; reach a wide audience; accomplish objectives of multiple organizations, including schools; increase credibility; improve information sharing; make use of a range of expertise; and foster coordination across sectors of society (596). Schools can leverage community resources to offer health promotion activities and events, purchase equipment and safety gear, pay for staff training, create safer environments for play (e.g., safe school yards) and physically active transportation to school (e.g., traffic interventions), attract awareness about healthy lifestyle behaviors, repeat consistent health messages, increase support for school initiatives to promote healthy eating and physical activity, and ensure sustainable funding (447,583,589,597,598). Schools also can interact with state and local agriculture through farm-to-school programs. These programs provide local produce, promote and support locally based agriculture, and often connect farmers and students with visits to farms and visits from farmers to the classroom, enabling students to learn how and where food is produced (599). Schools also can work with the community to address barriers to healthy eating and physical activity, such as areas that lack access to affordable foods needed for a healthy diet (i.e., food deserts) and a lack of safe places to be active. For example, schools might address food deserts by ensuring that healthy options are offered or available for purchase at all school-sponsored activities (on and off campus) (600). Partnerships between schools and local government can create joint-use agreements to use school facilities to host farmers' markets, plant community gardens, or allow public access to school facilities, fitness centers, gymnasiums, or running tracks (601).

Involve staff members from universities, hospitals, health centers, and other health organizations in school initiatives on healthy eating and physical activity. Health professionals outside of the school can advise on health education curricula and contribute to lessons and presentations specific to nutrition and physical activity; conduct health screenings; provide expertise on nutrition and physical activity at health fairs, family or teacher workshops, and for health services; and initiate walking and other physical activity initiatives (592,602). In 2006, 26% of schools reported working with a local hospital, and 25% reported collaborating with a college or university on school health program activities related to health education (593). University faculty members and students in the health field can provide programmatic and evaluation assistance to schools while gaining practical experience (603).

Recruit parent, family, and community volunteers to assist with healthy eating and physical activity initiatives. Parents, other family members, and community members can volunteer their time and skills to support school initiatives and help provide necessary assistance and supervision. For example, families and other community members can supervise school physical activity facilities after regular school hours, allowing for community access to safe and supervised facilities. Volunteers have been shown to be an important component for sustaining programs, even when limited funding is available (447,584,592). Schools can offer cost-effective incentives to compensate for volunteers' time (e.g., raffles, door prizes, grocery coupons, T-shirts, childcare, gift cards, discounted trip tickets, transportation tickets, or gas cards) (604,605). Parents can relate to volunteers who are also parents, and this networking can be a useful tool for sustaining participation in volunteer programs (587). Volunteer groups also can recruit from existing parent networks (such as the PTA) in the school or community.

Link to out-of-school programs that promote healthy eating and physical activity. Out-of-school programs (e.g., after school programs and parks and recreation programs) offer additional opportunities to reinforce health promotion messages taught in schools and can engage students in healthy eating and physical activity (606). Such programs can provide health-related experiences that are complementary to the school's curriculum (e.g., opportunities for physical activity, cooking lessons, promoting healthy snacks, farm trips) (589). Offering transportation to and from these programs might increase student participation (574,607).

13.5.7.5 DEMONSTRATE CULTURAL AWARENESS IN HEALTHY EATING AND PHYSICAL ACTIVITY PRACTICES THROUGHOUT THE SCHOOL

Customize activities and communication to reflect the culture of the community. Activities should reflect both the social and environmental aspects of a community (291,560). Engaging members from all cultural or language groups represented in the community can foster stronger partnerships among students, families, and community members (589,594,608). Policy and program information that is shared with family and community members should be culturally appropriate and translated as needed, with the goal of respecting diverse backgrounds and beliefs (609).

Surveying the interests and understanding the culture of families in the community can help schools offer diverse physical activity initiatives that are feasible and aligned with community interests (588,597,607). Local markets can provide information about the healthy foods available in the community. Schools should use this information to promote healthy diets and recipes that are feasible for students and their families to incorporate into their lifestyle (573). Other factors that can enhance family and community relationships include training of all school staff members in family engagement and hiring staff members and volunteers who reflect the culture of the community (587).

13.5.8 GUIDELINE 8. PROVIDE A SCHOOL EMPLOYEE WELLNESS PROGRAM THAT INCLUDES HEALTHY EATING AND PHYSICAL ACTIVITY SERVICES FOR ALL SCHOOL STAFF MEMBERS

Nearly 6 million persons work in schools in the United States (610). Implementing and sustaining an employee wellness program has the potential to improve staff productivity, decrease employee absenteeism, and decrease employee health-care costs (611,612). In addition, employee wellness programs can increase employee morale and improve worker retention and recruitment of new employees (613,614). Conversely, employee health risks (e.g., high blood pressure and high cholesterol levels) and lack of participation in worksite fitness and wellness programs are related to higher rates of employee absenteeism (615). School employee wellness programs that include healthy eating and physical activity components can increase teacher morale and improve general well-being and perceived ability to handle job stress (616–618). A national health objective strives to increase the proportion of worksites that offer an employee health promotion program (objective ECBP 8) (10).

Because employee wellness programs might increase healthy eating and physical activity among staff members, these staff members would model positive health behaviors for students (619,620). For example, school staff members can have a substantial influence on tobacco-free environments in schools (621–623). Students who see teachers smoking during a smoking ban are less likely to adhere to the tobacco-free environment rules (623). Furthermore, school staff members are more likely to abstain from use of tobacco on school grounds when they believe that they influence the students' behavior (621).

School employee wellness programs typically include health screenings to identify chronic disease risk factors such as high blood pressure or high cholesterol, health education classes, organizational policies that support worksite wellness, and employee assistance programs (624). In 2006, 16% of schools offered physical activity and fitness counseling for school staff members, 17% offered nutrition education, and 17% offered weight management services (624).

School employee wellness programs for healthy eating and physical activity could include the following components: information and educational activities (e.g., lectures, written materials, and educational software), behavioral strategies (e.g., individual and group behavior counseling, skill-building activities, and rewards or reinforcement), and policy and environmental strategies (e.g., increased access to healthy foods and on-site opportunities for physical activity). *School Employee Wellness: A Guide for Protecting the Assets of our Nation's Schools*, from Directors of Health Promotion and Education, is a step-by-step guide for implementing school employee wellness programs (625) (Box 8).

13.5.8.1 GATHER DATA AND INFORMATION TO DETERMINE THE NUTRITION AND PHYSICAL ACTIVITY NEEDS OF SCHOOL STAFF MEMBERS AND ASSESS THE AVAILABILITY OF EXISTING SCHOOL EMPLOYEE WELLNESS ACTIVITIES AND RESOURCES

A school employee wellness program should be supported by an environment and a culture that are conducive to health (618,626–628). Members of a school employee wellness committee should review organizational policies, programs, strengths, and barriers to identify priorities for nutrition and physical activity (192,620).

Determine employee health-related costs. In conjunction with district-level human resources, risk management, and employee benefits staff members, school employee wellness committees can identify critical data related to school employee well-being, such as health insurance costs, workers' compensation claims, absenteeism rates (includes costs of substitute teachers), and employee turnover rates. Analyzing reasons for absenteeism and health insurance claims can assist in identifying health conditions that could be addressed through school employee wellness programs (625). Analyzing workers' compensation claims might identify needs for improved worksite safety programs that include physical activity.

Assess the status of school employee wellness activities, and identify the nutrition and physical activity interests and needs of school employees. Assessing the current status of school employee wellness activities provides a starting point for planning future programming (625). The CDC School Health Index provides a series of items to assess current policies, programs, and practices for school employee wellness. The School Health Index helps schools identify strengths and weaknesses of various components of health promotion for staff members, including health screenings, stress management programs, physical activity and fitness programs, and healthy eating and weight management programs. The School Health Index also includes guidance to develop a plan for improvement (199,200). The Community Healthy Living Index (CHILI), developed by the YMCA, is another option for assessing the status of school employee wellness policies and practices (available at www.ymca.net/communityhealthylivingindex/community_healthy_living_index.html). This index contains a series of five assessments that focus on healthy eating and physical activity policies and environmental change strategies in workplaces, schools, and other settings.

Input from school staff members is essential when determining their nutrition and physical activity needs and developing program activities that either influence or affect them personally (192,628,629). Using a confidential employee survey is one method for collecting such information. Schools also might consider conducting confidential health screenings for conditions such as high cholesterol or high blood pressure, as well as assessments of employees' eating and physical activity behaviors (625). Focus groups and structured interviews also can be used, and direct observations of the school environment can help identify characteristics that influence health-related behaviors (e.g., healthy foods and beverages and bicycle racks) (630,631). In addition, schools that establish and sustain school employee wellness programs generally encourage staff members to request activities, classes, and information that are most important for them personally (619,620,632).

13.5.8.2 ENCOURAGE ADMINISTRATIVE SUPPORT FOR AND STAFF INVOLVEMENT IN SCHOOL EMPLOYEE WELLNESS

Sharing information with school administrators about the benefits of employee wellness programs and the interests and needs of school staff members can increase their support and resource allocation for such programs (628,629).

Obtain administrative support for school employee wellness programs that include healthy eating and physical activity. Administrative support is essential for a school employee wellness program to be viable and sustainable. Administrative support should come from the district superintendent, the principal, and other decision-makers, such as managers or counselors from employee assistance programs, human resource officers, and chief financial officers who oversee annual budgets for school districts. To foster administrator support, schools might consider the following methods (625):

- Provide a rationale and demonstrate a need for the program by providing local information and data, such as employee absenteeism rates and reasons for absenteeism.
- Recommend that school administrators attend school wellness conferences offered within their state or by the state education agency.

- Highlight another school or district employee wellness program that has resulted in multiple benefits.
- Develop and deliver a presentation that identifies the need for and benefits of a school employee wellness program in the context of coordinated school health.

Establish a school employee wellness committee, and identify a leader for the committee. An existing committee, such as the school health council or health insurance advisory committee, should have the necessary foundation and components to lead the process of developing a school employee wellness program (628). Members of a school employee wellness committee can include (625)

- representatives of the people the program will affect, such as bargaining units (e.g., unions), teachers, teacher aides, custodians and maintenance staff members, bus drivers, technology staff members, secretaries, and school nutrition employees;
- representatives from health education, physical education, health services, nutrition services, and mental health and social services;
- an administrator from the school who will communicate with the school board or superintendent or both;
- managers of human resources, employee assistance programs, workers' compensation, benefits, and facilities;
- behavioral change specialists; and
- community representatives from health departments, health care, recreation and fitness centers, businesses, and nonprofit organizations.

The school employee wellness leader can be the school health coordinator or an employee who is committed to offering quality programs for all school staff members. Providing an additional stipend or ensuring that school employee wellness responsibilities are written into a leader's job description might increase the likelihood of sustaining programmatic activities. Such responsibilities can include (625)

- coordinating the development, implementation, and evaluation of the program;
- representing school employee wellness on the school health council;
- communicating regularly with administration about the program;
- reporting annually to the school board;
- convening and participating in regularly scheduled meetings of the committee;
- arranging trainings and staff development opportunities;

- communicating with school employees using multiple methods such as e-mail, websites, printed materials, and announcements;
- identifying resources for and scheduling activities;
- developing relationships with community partners; and
- developing and administering the school employee wellness program budget.

13.5.8.3 DEVELOP, IMPLEMENT, AND EVALUATE HEALTHY EATING AND PHYSICAL ACTIVITY PROGRAMS FOR ALL SCHOOL EMPLOYEES

Establish broad goals and specific objectives for healthy eating and physical activity programs for school employees. A comprehensive school employee wellness program includes goals, objectives, and activities for promoting healthy eating and physical activity. Goals should be realistic and written as broad statements, such as, "increase the proportion of school employees that meet the national physical activity guidelines." Objectives indicate what will be done to achieve the goals; they should be specific, measurable, achievable, relevant, and time sensitive. For example, a physical activity objective might be, "By May 2012, physical activity classes will have been offered once per week for all staff members throughout the entire school year." Various activities to help achieve the objectives and goals should be planned. (e.g., a walking club that meets 1 day per week and is led by a staff member).

Implement activities to promote healthy eating and physical activity that emphasize informational, behavioral skill, and policy and environmental approaches. After a rigorous review of worksite health promotion intervention research, the Task Force on Community Preventive Services recommended worksite obesity prevention and control interventions as an effective method of losing weight. The programs evaluated included at least one of the following components: informational, behavioral, policy, or environmental strategies. Educational activities might include lectures, written materials, and educational software (378,633). Behavioral strategies might include individual or group behavioral counseling, skill-building activities, rewards or reinforcement, and inclusion of social support. Policy and environmental strategies should aim to make sustainable organizational changes, such as improving access to healthy foods, providing more on-site opportunities for physical activities, and point-of-decision prompts that encourage use of stairwells (378,633).

Comprehensive environmental, policy, and organizational approaches might result in positive behavior change among school employees. These approaches can include education, employee and peer support for physical activity, physical activity breaks during staff meetings (634,635), ongoing incentives for behavior change, access to safe facilities and nutritious foods, and systematic reminders for healthy eating (636–639). Use of a pedometer-based physical activity program allows employees to determine their current amount of activity, set goals for improvement, and monitor personal progress (636,639).

Evaluate and adapt the school employee wellness program. School employee wellness programs should be evaluated to determine whether objectives have been met, whether employees are satisfied, and what can be done to improve the program. Data and information can be gathered about the process of implementing program strategies and policies. The evaluation also can be used to determine the effects of the program. Questions to consider for assessing the impact include (625) the following:

- Have the dietary and physical activity behaviors of employees improved?
- Have health risks such as high cholesterol, overweight or obesity, or high blood pressure decreased?
- Has there been a change in absenteeism?
- Do employees feel that their nutrition and physical activity needs have been met?
- Has there been a noticeable financial effect through reduced health-care costs or other health-related data?

13.5.9 GUIDELINE 9. EMPLOY QUALIFIED PERSONS, AND PROVIDE PROFESSIONAL DEVELOPMENT OPPORTUNITIES FOR PHYSICAL EDUCATION, HEALTH EDUCATION, NUTRITION SERVICES, AND HEALTH, MENTAL HEALTH, AND SOCIAL SERVICES STAFF MEMBERS, AS WELL AS STAFF MEMBERS WHO SUPERVISE RECESS, CAFETERIA TIME, AND OUT-OF-SCHOOL–TIME PROGRAMS

School staff members who teach physical education or health education, lead nutrition services programs, and implement health, mental health, and social services require certification or specialized training or both (640–642). Providing certified and qualified staff members with regular professional development opportunities enables them to improve current skills and acquire new ones (402,641,643–646). In addition, staff members who supervise recess, cafeteria time, and out-of-school–time programs can be much more effective if they receive ongoing professional development opportunities. National, state, and local education and health agencies; institutions of higher education; and national and state professional organizations should collaborate to provide professional development opportunities to school health staff members (Box 9).

13.5.9.1 REQUIRE THE HIRING OF PHYSICAL EDUCATION TEACHERS, HEALTH EDUCATION TEACHERS, AND NUTRITION SERVICES STAFF MEMBERS WHO ARE CERTIFIED AND APPROPRIATELY PREPARED TO DELIVER QUALITY INSTRUCTION, PROGRAMS, AND PRACTICES

Require the hiring of certified physical education teachers to teach physical education in grades K–12. Schools should develop and adopt policies that require certified physical education teachers, rather than teachers who are certified to teach other subject areas, to teach physical education in grades K–12 to ensure that students receive quality instruction. Certified physical education teachers teach longer lessons, spend more time developing motor and movement skills, impart more knowledge, and provide more moderate and vigorous physical activity than do classroom teachers with little or no specialized training in physical education (146,383,401,641). NASPE has established and recommends the National Standards for Beginning Physical Education Teachers, which outlines the areas in which a highly qualified physical education teacher entering the school system should have expertise, including content knowledge, child and adolescent growth and development, diversity in learning, classroom management and student motivation, communication, planning and instruction, student assessment, reflection, use of technology, and collaboration (647). NASPE has produced guidelines for elementary, middle, and high school physical education, which state that physical education should be taught by a qualified teacher with a degree in physical education (for the appropriate grade level) and a current state license to teach physical education (647–650).

State and district policies are supportive of hiring qualified physical education teachers. For example, in 2006, all states offered at least one type of certification, licensure, or endorsement to teach physical education (144). Many states and districts required newly hired staff members to be certified, licensed, or endorsed by the state to teach physical education. Specifically, 69% of states and 84% of districts had a policy stating that newly hired elementary school physical education teachers be certified, licensed, or endorsed by the state to teach physical education; 88% of states and 87% of districts had such a policy at the middle school level, and 90% of states and 93% of districts had such a policy at the high school level (144).

Require the hiring of certified health education teachers to teach health education in grades K–12. Classroom health education teachers who receive specialized training on health education topics have been shown to effectively implement health education programs (217,651–653). Certified health education teachers should have the knowledge and skills outlined and recommended in the American Association for Health Education's standards for health education teacher preparation programs. Skills include the ability to assess individual and community health needs; plan, implement, and evaluate health education programs; coordinate health education programs and services; act as a resource person for health education; and communicate health and health education needs, concerns, and resources (654).

A national health objective strives to increase the proportion of schools that require newly hired staff members who teach required health education to be certified, licensed, or endorsed by the state in health education (objective EMC 4.2) (10). In 2006, 68% of teachers of elementary school classes covering required health instruction and 67% of teachers of required health education courses in middle and high schools were certified, licensed, or endorsed by the state to teach health education at the appropriate grade level (455). In 2006, 94% of all states offered some type of certification, licensure, or endorsement to teach health education (455). A national health objective also strives to increase the proportion of schools that require newly hired staff members who teach required health education to have undergraduate or graduate training in health education (objective EMC 4.1) (10). In 2006, 21% of states and 42% of districts had a policy stating that newly hired staff members who teach health education at the elementary school level will be certified, licensed, or endorsed by the state to teach health education. In contrast, 72% of states and 70% of districts had this policy at the middle school level, and 79% of states and 83% of districts had this policy at the high school level (455).

Through the certified health education specialist (CHES) program, health education teachers also have the opportunity to gain additional expertise and improve their qualifications. The CHES examination is a competency-based test that measures the possession, application, and interpretation of knowledge related to health education (655). In 2006, 16% of states and 35% of districts had a policy stating that newly hired staff members who teach health education at the middle school level will be CHESs, and 18% of states and 41% of districts had such a policy at the high school level (455).

Require the hiring of qualified nutrition service directors, managers, and staff. Schools should require a minimum level of education and certification for school nutrition professionals to maintain specialized occupational knowledge and expertise. Competencies for school nutrition professionals involve a distinct and complex set of knowledge and skill requirements, such as

- maintaining integrity with federal, state, and local regulations (e.g., use of USDA Foods);
- ensuring that all meals served meet current nutritional standards (e.g., the *Dietary Guidelines for Americans* and meal pattern requirements), including those for children with special needs;
- establishing a leadership role in nutrition education as part of the overall school education program;
- providing a food-safe environment that protects the health and well-being of all school children (e.g., applies principles of the hazard analysis and critical control point system, foodborne illness prevention, and food biosecurity);
- operating effective administrative, procurement, and other financial management protocols to ensure quality food production and distribution;
- implementing a marketing plan for program promotion and creating interest in school meals; and
- managing the school nutrition program staff members according to all federal, state, and local employment regulations, including leadership of professional development opportunities (656,657).

To support such demanding job requirements, school nutrition directors should have, at minimum, a bachelor's degree in a nutrition-related field or food-service management, a dietetics degree, or a certification or credentialing in nutrition services from either the School Nutrition Association or a state program (299). A primary challenge for schools is increasing the professional qualifications of nutrition services staff members to have the skills needed to provide nutritious and appealing school meals that comply with the *Dietary Guidelines for Americans* and to consistently offer students healthy food and beverage options (658).

State- and district-level education agencies and boards can influence local school practices by establishing professional preparation and certification requirements in addition to offering professional preparation and development opportunities. Nationwide in 2006, 27% of states offered certification, licensure, or endorsement for district nutrition services directors, and 22% of states offered this to school nutrition services managers. Only 16% of all districts required a newly hired school nutrition services manager to be certified, licensed, or endorsed by the state (105). Most districts (57%) required only a high school diploma or its equivalent for newly hired district nutrition services directors; 24% of districts did not have any minimum level of education for newly hired district nutrition services directors; 74% of districts required only a high school diploma or its equivalent for newly hired school nutrition services managers; and 22% of districts did not have any minimum level of education for newly hired school nutrition services staff members. In 2006, only 41% of district-level nutrition services directors and 45% of school-level nutrition services managers reported having an undergraduate degree (105).

13.5.9.2 PROVIDE SCHOOL STAFF MEMBERS WITH ANNUAL PROFESSIONAL DEVELOPMENT OPPORTUNITIES TO DELIVER QUALITY PHYSICAL EDUCATION, HEALTH EDUCATION, AND NUTRITION SERVICES

Physical education teachers, health education teachers, and nutrition services staff members should receive regular professional development to improve their knowledge, skills, and competencies and be current on the most effective and innovative teaching and programmatic strategies. Quality professional development delivered in group settings, one-on-one, or through communications technology should improve staff knowledge, enable effective implementation of skills and strategies in schools, and positively affect the behaviors of students (659). The National Staff Development Council has developed and recommends the use of standards for professional development that include context standards (e.g., establishment of adult learning communities, improving leadership, and garnering resources), process standards (e.g., using student data to determine staff learning priorities, preparing school staff members to apply research to decision-making, and using learning strategies appropriate to intended goals), and content standards (e.g., preparing school staff members to understand and appreciate all students, create safe environments, and deepen educators' content knowledge and skills) (659).

Comprehensive professional development programs should 1) be based on staff level of knowledge, experience, and needs; 2) model behavior change techniques; 3) provide opportunities to practice; 4) involve multiple sessions so that teachers can practice in classrooms and report on their experiences; and 5) provide opportunities for teachers to share their experiences with peers during posttraining sessions (640,644,659–662).

Provide annual professional development opportunities for physical education teachers. Professional development should help physical education teachers provide instruction that meets the interests and skill levels of all students. Physical education teachers should have professional development opportunities that teach concepts of quality physical education instruction, such as how to improve teaching methods, administer fitness tests and assess student performance, encourage family involvement in physical activity, incorporate national or state standards into the curriculum, conduct fitness education, use fitness-oriented technology, and increase active time during physical education class (145,641,644,663).

Professional development can enhance teachers' instructional strategies for increasing student physical activity during physical education classes and can enable teachers to develop lesson plans that emphasize student skill development and improve students' enjoyment of being physically active (383,644,663,664). Professional development also might influence physical education teachers' personal attitudes and beliefs toward physical activity and fitness (643,645).

In 2006, 78% of all states and 91% of all districts provided funding for staff development or offered professional development for physical education teachers on at least one physical education topic (e.g., administering or using fitness tests, student assessment, chronic health conditions, and injury prevention) during the 2 years before the study (144). In 2006, physical education teachers from 88% of required physical education classes or courses received professional development on at least one physical education topic. Teachers from at least half of required physical education classes or courses received professional development on injury prevention and first aid, teaching individual or paired activities or sports, teaching movement skills and concepts, and teaching team or group activities or sports. The professional development topics that physical education teachers most reported wanting were teaching methods to promote inclusion and active participation of overweight children, chronic health conditions, using physical activity monitoring devices, helping students develop individualized physical activity plans, and encouraging family involvement in physical activity (144). Understanding the differences between what teachers want and what they receive is important to identify any gaps in professional development topics and plan for future trainings or workshops.

NASPE provides various professional development opportunities for physical education teachers. For example, NASPE's Program Improvement in Physical Education (PIPEline) workshop series delivers standards-based training for grades K–12 physical education teachers. Topics covered in PIPEline workshops include instructional practices, assessment strategies, curriculum development, technology integration, and dance instruction in physical education. (Additional information is available at http://www.aahperd.org/naspe.)

Provide annual professional development opportunities for health education teachers. Health education teachers should receive professional development to effectively teach students about foods and nutrients, physical activity, and their connections to health, obesity, and other chronic diseases; to provide students with the knowledge and skills they need to select physical activities they enjoy and healthy foods to prepare; to help students assess their own physical activity and eating habits and plan for change;

to identify valid sources of nutrition and physical activity information; to acquire advocacy skills for improving nutrition and physical activity environments; and to facilitate students' ability to identify and correct nutrition and physical activity misconceptions (462,640,644,660,661,665).

Professional development also should provide health education teachers with the necessary skills to use innovative, nonlecture techniques, such as active learning strategies, for developing students' knowledge, attitudes, and skills for engaging in healthy eating and physical activity. Strategies that are enjoyable and participatory, emphasize the benefits of healthy eating and physical activity, or provide exposure to new foods and activities are more likely to contribute to student adoption of healthy behaviors (457,473,666–668).

Professional development for health education is associated with successful implementation of the classroom curriculum (217) and contributes to the implementation of innovative health education methods and techniques (669). Health education teachers who receive topic-specific professional development include more instruction on health topics within their lessons than teachers who do not receive topic-specific professional development (670).

A national health objective strives to increase the proportion of required health education classes or courses with a teacher who has had professional development related to teaching personal and social skills for behavior change within the past 2 years (objective EMC 4.4) (10). In 2006, 88% of states provided funding for or offered professional development on nutrition and dietary behavior, and 82% of states provided funding for or offered professional development on physical activity and fitness during the 2 years before the study. During the same time, 65% of districts provided funding for or offered professional development on nutrition and dietary behavior, an increase from 43% in 2000; and 75% of all districts provided funding for or offered professional development on physical activity and fitness, an increase from 43% in 2000 (455). In addition, approximately half of all districts provided professional development for health education teachers on the following teaching methods: encouraging family or community involvement, teaching skills for behavior change, teaching students with long-term disabilities, using classroom management techniques, and using interactive teaching methods (455). Organizations such as the Rocky Mountain Center's

Professional Development Partnership and the Education Development Center (available at http://www.edc.org) provide professional development opportunities that can help schools enhance the delivery of health education curriculum and instruction.

Provide annual professional development opportunities for nutrition services staff members. School nutrition services staff members should receive professional development on topics that support improving the overall school nutrition environment, including healthy food preparation methods; implementing the *Dietary Guidelines for Americans* in school meals (e.g., ensuring that school meals have appealing fruits, vegetables, whole grains, and low-fat or fat-free milk products); competitive food policies; increasing the percentage of students participating in school meals; making school meals more appealing to increase student participation in meal programs; menu planning for healthy meals; preparing fresh fruits and vegetables; food safety; using the cafeteria for nutrition education; offering an array of healthy and culturally appropriate foods and beverages; and reinforcing classroom lessons on healthy food choices in the cafeteria (105,299,671,672). Staff training to implement changes within the school meal program can lead to a reduction in calories from total fat, saturated fat, and sodium (673). In addition, professional development for nutrition services staff members should also address how to positively influence student food choices at the point of purchase (642).

In 2006, two thirds or more of nutrition services managers received professional development on food safety, healthy food preparation methods, personal safety for nutrition services staff members, using hazard analysis and critical control points, selecting and ordering food, and implementing the *Dietary Guidelines for Americans* in school meals during the 2 years before the study. The professional development topics that nutrition service managers reported wanting most were making school meals more appealing, food biosecurity, menu planning for healthy meals, increasing student participation in school meals programs, procedures for food-related emergencies, and using the cafeteria for nutrition education (105). Professional development formats most preferred by nutrition services personnel include hands-on workshops, use of demonstrations, and skill-building workshops with active involvement of participants (672).

The USDA Food and Nutrition Service provides strategies for purchasing, preparing, and serving meals aligned with the Dietary Guidelines for Americans, including practical tips to update menus and recipes, and suggestions for making changes to help students develop a taste for new menu items (available at http://www.fns.usda.gov/tn/Resources/dgfactsheet_hsm.html). Training opportunities on the provision of healthy school meals are available through the USDA Team Nutrition initiative and the National Food Service Management Institute (available at http://www.fns.usda.gov/tn; http://www.nfsmi.org). The School Nutrition Association also provides its members with professional development training opportunities and certifications in school nutrition (available at http://www.schoolnutrition.org/CareerEducation.aspx).

13.5.9.3 PROVIDE ANNUAL PROFESSIONAL DEVELOPMENT OPPORTUNITIES FOR SCHOOL HEALTH, MENTAL HEALTH, AND SOCIAL SERVICES STAFF MEMBERS AND STAFF MEMBERS WHO LEAD OR SUPERVISE OUT-OF-SCHOOL–TIME PROGRAMS, RECESS, AND CAFETERIA TIME

School health, mental health, and social services staff members and staff members who lead or supervise out-of-school–time programs, recess, and cafeteria time (including staff members from partner organizations such as the YMCA or parks and recreation department) should receive professional development to obtain the skills needed to lead effective programs and educate students on healthy behaviors (674). Lack of trained staff is a barrier to implementing safe, organized and effective programs, instruction, and services.

Provide annual professional development opportunities to school health, mental health, and social services staff members. School health, mental health, and social services staff members need preservice and in-service professional development in promoting healthy eating and physical activity and providing healthy eating and physical activity assessment, counseling, and referral. This includes assessing student nutrition, physical activity, and weight status and identifying potential nutrition-related and physical activity-related problems such as eating disorders. Health, mental health, and social services staff members should be equipped with skills to either refer appropriately or assist students with nutrition-related, physical activity–related, or weight-related health problems (675,676). In 2006, approximately 43% of school districts provided funding for or offered professional development for health services staff members to provide nutrition and dietary behavior counseling; and 41% of districts provided funding for or offered professional development for physical activity and fitness counseling during the 2 years before the study (510). In addition, in 2006, 35% of school districts provided funding for or offered professional development for mental health and social services staff members on nutrition and dietary behavior counseling, and 36% of districts provided funding for or offered professional development on physical activity and fitness counseling during the 2 years before the study (677).

For schools implementing BMI measurement programs, health, mental health, and social services staff members must have the appropriate training to obtain accurate and reliable results, ensure privacy and confidentiality, and minimize the potential for stigmatization. Measurements are more likely to be accurate when they are made by trained professionals (518).

Provide annual professional development opportunities to staff members who lead or supervise healthy eating and physical activity programs during out-of-school time. Preservice and in-service professional development should help school staff members, coaches, community volunteers, and staff members from partner organizations such as parks and recreation departments plan and implement out-of-school–time healthy eating and physical activity programs that meet a range of student needs and interests. Out-of-school–time programs serving meals or snacks to students need to ensure the provision of nutritious food to give students the energy and nourishment needed to benefit fully from the educational, enrichment, and physical activities being offered. Staff members who work in programs focusing on healthy eating, physical activity, or both in nonschool settings should be adequately trained in providing healthy and nourishing snacks and beverages to participants. Quality professional development should be provided for leaders of out-of-school–time programs to assist them in educating children and adolescents on the importance of making sound decisions about healthy eating and physical activity (678).

School staff members, coaches, and community volunteers who lead intramural activities and physical activity clubs during out-of-school time should be trained to place less emphasis on competition and more emphasis on having fun and developing skills. Volunteer coaches who work with beginning athletes in schools should have the level 1 coaching competency delineated by NASPE (259) and other professional organizations that provide coaching certification. Like other athletic coaches, volunteer coaches should receive professional development on how to provide experiences for students that emphasize enjoyment, participation, skill development, building confidence, and self-knowledge and also promote healthy behaviors (e.g., healthy eating and adequate fluid replacement). Injury prevention, first aid, cardiopulmonary resuscitation, and precautions against contamination by bloodborne pathogens are other professional development areas for coaches (679,680).

Provide annual professional development opportunities for staff members who lead or supervise recess and cafeteria time. Teachers, school staff members, community volunteers, and staff members from local partner organizations (e.g., local YMCA or parks and recreation departments) who lead or supervise recess should be appropriately trained to provide active supervision, promote physical activity during recess, minimize conflict among students, and maximize cooperation among students. Providing students with various activity choices might maximize physically active time during recess, and working with students to resolve conflict might lead to positive peer interaction during recess and within classrooms.

School staff members supervising cafeteria time should model healthy habits and use appropriate supervisory techniques for managing the school cafeteria. For example, staff members might emphasize good nutrition and healthy eating habits, speak well of the school nutrition program, support social aspects of the meal program (e.g., enjoyment of pleasant conversation, good table manners, and responsible student behavior), and maintain safe, orderly, and pleasant eating environments.

13.6 CONCLUSION

These guidelines were developed through an extensive review of the scientific literature focused on school-based healthy eating and physical activity interventions. Although the scientific interventions highlight what schools can do to address these health behaviors, information is lacking about certain specific intervention strategies that have a long-term effect. For example, the Task Force on Community Preventive Services reported insufficient evidence for school-based nutrition programs and for obesity prevention and control programs in schools. The expert statements and input gathered and reviewed for this report helped contribute to the development of the guidelines and their corresponding strategies. More research could contribute to the strength of these recommendations. Overall, these guidelines provide a comprehensive framework for schools to address healthy eating and physical activity. However, all of these guidelines are not appropriate for every school. Some schools might already be implementing the majority of the guidelines, and other schools might choose to implement only certain guidelines. Prioritizing needs and identifying resources to help implement the guidelines is an important step toward sustaining healthy eating and physical activity policies and practices in schools.

CDC will increase state, territorial, tribal, and local education and health agency awareness of these guidelines through training sessions, conference presentations, webinars, Listservs, and other methods. The findings in this report will help CDC prioritize interventions for school health policies and practices and to identify and develop tools that will assist schools with implementing various components of the guidelines.

Implementing and sustaining school-based healthy eating and physical activity policies and practices will make a substantial contribution toward a healthy future for children and adolescents in the United States. The childhood obesity epidemic and the chronic diseases associated with poor dietary habits and physical inactivity are not likely to be reversed without a strong contribution from schools. Improving and intensifying efforts to promote healthy eating and physical activity is entirely consistent with the fundamental mission of schools: educating young persons to become healthy, productive citizens who can make meaningful contributions to society. School-based policies and practices should be part of coordinated school health programs and reach students from kindergarten through secondary school; prekindergarten programs might also be able to apply these guidelines in their settings. School, district, and state education and health leaders, community leaders, and families can commit to implementing and sustaining healthy eating and physical activity programs within the schools.

REFERENCES

1. US Department of Health and Human Services. The Surgeon General's call to action to prevent and decrease overweight and obesity. Rockville, MD: US Department of Health and Human Services, Public Health Service, Office of the Surgeon General; 2001.
2. Lichtenstein AH, Appel LJ, Brands M, et al. Diet and lifestyle recommendations revision 2006: a scientific statement from the American Heart Association Nutrition Committee. Circulation 2006;114:84–96.
3. Dietary Guidelines Advisory Committee. Report of the Dietary Guidelines Advisory Committee on the dietary guidelines for Americans, 2010, to the Secretary of Agriculture and the Secretary of Health and Human Services. Washington, DC: US Department of Agriculture, Agricultural Research Service; 2010.
4. Physical Activity Guidelines Advisory Committee. Physical Activity Guidelines Advisory committee report, 2008. Washington, DC: US Department of Health and Human Services; 2008.
5. US Department of Agriculture, US Department of Health and Human Services. Dietary guidelines for Americans, 2010. 7th ed. Washington, DC: US Government Printing Office; 2010.
6. Ogden CL, Carroll MD, Curtin LR, Lamb MM, Flegal KM. Prevalence of high body mass index in U.S. children and adolescents, 2007–2008. JAMA 2010;303:242–9.
7. Daniels S, Arnett D, Eckel R, et al. Overweight in children and adolescents: pathophysiology, consequences, prevention, and treatment. Circulation 2005;111:1999–2012.
8. US Department of Health and Human Services, Public Health Service, Office of the Surgeon General. The Surgeon General's vision for a healthy and fit nation. Washington, DC: US Department of Health and Human Services; 2010.
9. US Department of Health and Human Services. Physical activity guidelines for Americans, 2008. Washington, DC: US Department of Health and Human Services; 2008.
10. US Department of Health and Human Services. Healthy people 2020. Washington, DC: US Department of Health and Human Services; 2010. Available at http://www.healthypeople.gov/2020. Accessed August 18, 2011.

11. CDC. Guidelines for school health programs to promote lifelong healthy eating. MMWR 1996;45(No. RR-9) .
12. CDC. Guidelines for school and community programs to promote lifelong physical activity among young people. MMWR 1997;46(No. RR-6) .
13. Green LW. From research to "best practices" in other settings and populations. Am J Health Behav 2001;25:165–78.
14. US Department of Health and Human Services. Physical activity and health: a report of the Surgeon General. Atlanta, GA: CDC; 1996.
15. US Department of Health and Human Services, US Department of Agriculture. Dietary guidelines for Americans, 2005. 6th ed. Washington, DC: US Government Printing Office; 2005.
16. Williams CL, Hayman LL, Daniels SR, et al. Cardiovascular health in childhood: a statement for health professionals from the Committee on Atherosclerosis, Hypertension, and Obesity in the Young (AHOY) of the Council on Cardiovascular Disease in the Young, American Heart Association. Circulation 2002;106:146–60.
17. Kushi LH, Byers T, Doyle C, et al. American Cancer Society guidelines on nutrition and physical activity for cancer prevention: reducing the risk of cancer with healthy food choices and physical activity. CA Cancer J Clin 2006;56:254–81.
18. Xu J, Kochanek KD, Murphy SL, Tejada-Vera B. Deaths: final data for 2007. Natl Vital Stat Rep 2010;58.
19. Mensah GA, Mokdad AH, Ford ES, Greenlund K, Croft J. State of disparities in cardiovascular health in the United States. Circulation 2005;111:1233–41.
20. Thompson PD, Buchner D, Pina IL, et al. Exercise and physical activity in the prevention and treatment of atherosclerotic cardiovascular disease: a statement from the Council on Clinical Cardiology (subcommittee on exercise, rehabilitation, and prevention) and the Council on Nutrition, Physical Activity, and Metabolism (subcommittee on physical activity). Circulation 2003;107:3109–16.
21. Brown L, Rosner B, Willett WW, Sacks FM. Cholesterol-lowering effects of dietary fiber: a meta-analysis. Am J Clin Nutr 1999;69:3042.
22. Ostchega Y, Carroll M, Prineas RJ, McDowell MA, Louis T, Tilert T. Trends of elevated blood pressure among children and adolescents: data from the National Health and Nutrition Examination Survey 1988–2006. Am J Hypertens 2009;22:59–67.
23. Freedman DS, Mei Z, Srinivasan SR, Berenson GS, Dietz WH. Cardiovascular risk factors and excess adiposity among overweight children and adolescents: the Bogalusa Heart Study. J Pediatr 2007;150:12–7.
24. US Cancer Statistics Working Group. United States cancer statistics: 1999–2007 Incidence and mortality web-based report. Atlanta, GA: CDC, National Cancer Institute; 2010.
25. American Cancer Society. Nutrition and cancer. American Cancer Society; 2007. Available at http://www.cancer.org/downloads/PRO/nutrition.pdf . Accessed June 28, 2011.
26. CDC. National diabetes fact sheet: national estimates and general information on diabetes and prediabetes in the United States, 2011. Atlanta, GA: CDC; 2011.
27. Fox CS, Coady S, Sorlie PD, et al. Trends in cardiovascular complications of diabetes. JAMA 2004;292:2495–9.

28. Hu FB, Stampfer MJ, Solomon CG, et al. The impact of diabetes mellitus on mortality from all causes and coronary heart disease in women: 20 years of follow-up. Arch Intern Med 2001;161:1717–23.
29. US Department of Health and Human Services, National Diabetes Education Program. Overview of diabetes in children and adolescents: a fact sheet from the National Diabetes Education Program. Bethesda, MD: National Diabetes Education Program; 2006. Available at http://ndep.nih.gov/diabetes/pubs/Youth_FactSheet.pdf . Accessed June 28, 2011.
30. SEARCH for Diabetes in Youth Study Group. The burden of diabetes mellitus among US youth: prevalence estimates from the SEARCH for diabetes in youth study. Pediatrics 2006;118:1510–8.
31. American Diabetes Association. Type 2 diabetes in children and adolescents. Pediatrics 2000;105:671–80.
32. Pavkov ME, Hanson RL, Knowler WC, Bennett PH, Krakoff J, Nelson RG. Changing patterns of type 2 diabetes incidence among Pima Indians. Diabetes Care 2007;30:1758–63.
33. Dabelea D, Bell RA, D'Agostino RB Jr, et al. Incidence of diabetes in youth in the United States. JAMA 2007;297:2716–24.
34. Li C, Ford ES, Zhao G, Mokdad AH. Prevalence of pre-diabetes and its association with clustering of cardiometabolic risk factors and hyperinsulinemia among U.S. adolescents: NHANES 2005–2006. Diabetes Care 2009;32:342–7.
35. Institute of Medicine. Preventing childhood obesity: health in the balance. Washington, DC: The National Academies Press; 2004.
36. National Institutes of Health, National Heart, Lung, and Blood Institute. Disease and conditions index: What are overweight and obesity? Bethesda, MD: National Institutes of Health; 2010. Available at http://www.nhlbi.nih.gov/health/dci/Diseases/obe/obe_whatare.html. Accessed June 28, 2011.
37. Krebs NF, Himes JH, Jacobson D, Nicklas TA, Guilday P, Styne D. Assessment of child and adolescent overweight and obesity. Pediatrics 2007;120:S193–228.
38. Barlow SE; Expert Committee. Expert committee recommendations regarding the prevention, assessment, and treatment of child and adolescent overweight and obesity: summary report. Pediatrics 2007;120:S164–192.
39. Hedley AA, Ogden CL, Johnson C, Caroll M, Curtin L, Flegal K. Prevalence of overweight and obesity among U.S. children, adolescents, and adults, 1999–2002. JAMA 2004;291:28407–50
40. Ogden CL, Flegal KM, Carroll MD, Johnson CL. Prevalence and trends in overweight among U.S. children and adolescents, 1999–2000. JAMA 2002;288:1728–32.
41. Ogden CL, Carroll MD, Curtin LR, McDowell MA, Tabak CJ, Flegal KM. Prevalence of overweight and obesity in the United States, 1999–2004. JAMA 2006;295:1549–55.
42. Freedman DS, Kettel Khan L, Serdula MK, Ogden CL, Dietz WH. Racial and ethnic differences in secular trends for childhood BMI, weight, and height. Obes Res 2006;14:301–8.
43. Anderson SE, Whitaker RC. Prevalence of obesity among U.S. preschool children in different racial and ethnic groups. Arch Pediatr Adolesc Med 2009;163:344–8.

44. Miech RA, Kumanyika SK, Stettler N, Link BG, Phelan JC, Chang VW. Trends in the association of poverty with overweight among U.S. adolescents, 1971–2004. JAMA 2006;295:2385–93.
45. Dietz WH. Overweight in childhood and adolescence. N Engl J Med 2004;350:855–7.
46. Guo SS, Chumlea WC. Tracking of body mass index in children in relation to overweight in adulthood. Am J Clin Nutr 1999;70:S145–8.
47. Freedman DS, Kettel L, Serdula MK, Dietz WH, Srinivasan SR, Berenson GS. The relation of childhood BMI to adult adiposity: the Bogalusa Heart Study. Pediatrics 2005;115:22–7.
48. Freedman D, Wang J, Thornton JC, et al. Classification of body fatness by body mass index-for-age categories among children. Arch Pediatr Adolesc Med 2009;163:805–11.
49. Freedman DS, Khan LK, Dietz WH, Srinivasan SA, Berenson GS. Relationship of childhood obesity to coronary heart disease risk factors in adulthood: the Bogalusa Heart Study. Pediatrics 2001;108:712–8.
50. Daniels SR. The consequences of childhood overweight and obesity. Future Child 2006;16:47–67.
51. Olshansky J, Passaro D, Hershow R, et al. A potential decline in life expectancy in the United States in the 21st century. N Engl J Med 2005;352:1138–45.
52. Grundy SM, Cleeman JI, Daniels SR, et al. Diagnosis and management of the metabolic syndrome: an American Heart Association/National Heart, Lung, and Blood Institute scientific statement. Circulation 2005;112:2735–52.
53. Ford ES, Giles WH, Mokdad AH. Increasing prevalence of the metabolic syndrome among U.S. adults. Diabetes Care 2004;27:2444–9.
54. Johnson WD, Kroom JJM, Greenway FL, Bouchard C, Ryan D, Katzmarzyk PT. Prevalence of risk factors for metabolic syndrome in adolescents. Arch Pediatr Adolesc Med 2010;163:371–7.
55. Cook S, Weitzman M, Auinger P, Nguyen M, Dietz WH. Prevalence of a metabolic syndrome phenotype in adolescents: findings from the Third National Health and Nutrition Examination Survey. Arch Pediatr Adolesc Med 2003;157:821–7.
56. US Department of Health and Human Services. Bone health and osteoporosis: A report of the Surgeon General. Washington, DC; 2004.
57. National Osteoporosis Foundation. Boning up on osteoporosis: a guide to prevention and treatment. Washington, DC: National Osteoporosis Foundation; 2003.
58. Taylor G, Theiss P, Mirch MC, et al. Orthopedic complications of overweight in children and adolescents. Pediatrics 2006;1172167–74.
59. Nord M, Andrews M, Carlson S. Household food security in the United States, 2008. ERR-83. Washington, DC: Economic Research Service; United States Department of Agriculture; 2009.
60. Cook J, Frank D. Food security, poverty, and human development in the United States. Ann N Y Acad Sci 2008;1136:193–09.
61. Kaiser LL, Townsend MS. Food insecurity among U.S. children: Implications for nutrition and health. Top Clin Nutr 2005;20:313–20.
62. Alaimo K, Olson CM, Frongillo EA. Food insufficiency and American school-aged children's cognitive, academic and psychosocial developments. Pediatrics 2001;108:44–53.

63. Kleinman RE, Murphy JM, Little M, Pagano J, Wehler CA, Regal K et al. Hunger in children in the United States: potential behavioral and emotional correlates. Pediatrics 1998;101:1–6.
64. Murphy JM, Wehler CA, Pagano M, Little M, Kleinman R, Jellinek MS. Relationship between hunger and psychosocial functioning in low-income American children. J Am Acad Child Adolesc Psychiatry 1998;37:163–70.
65. Murphy JM, Pagano MR, Nachmani J, Sperling P, Kane S, Kleinman RR. The relationship of school breakfast to psychosocial and academic functioning. Arch Pediatr Adolesc Med 1998;152:899–107.
66. Fuller B, Caspary G, Kagan SL, et al. Does maternal employment influence poor children's social development? Early Child Res Q 2002;17:470–97.
67. Casey PH, Szeto KL, Robbins JM, et al. Child health related quality of life and household food security. Arch Pediatr Adolesc Med 2005;195:51–6.
68. Ralston K, Newman C, Clauson A, Guthrie J, Busby J. The National School Lunch Program, background, issues, and trends. ERR-61. Washington, DC: US Department of Agriculture, Economic Research Service; 2008.
69. CDC. Iron deficiency—United States, 1999–2000. MMWR 2002;51:897–9.
70. CDC. Recommendations to prevent and control iron deficiency in the United States. MMWR 1998;47(No. RR-3) .
71. US Department of Health and Human Services. Healthy people 2010: with understanding and improving health and objectives for improving health (2nd ed in 2 vols). Washington, DC: US Government Printing Office; 2000.
72. Grantham-McGregor S, Ani C. A review of studies on the effect of iron deficiency on cognitive development in children. J Nutr 2001;131: S64–66.
73. Taras HL. Nutrition and student performance at school. J Sch Health 2005;75:199–213.
74. Cogswell ME, Looker AC, Pfeiffer CM, et al. Assessment of iron deficiency in U.S. preschool children and nonpregnant females of childbearing age: National Health and Nutrition Examination Survey 2003–2006. Am J Clin Nutr 2009;89:1334–42.
75. Nead KG, Halterman JS, Kaczorowski JM, Auinger P, Weitzman M. Overweight children and adolescents: a risk group for iron deficiency. Pediatrics 2004;114:104–8.
76. American Psychiatric Association Task Force on DSM-IV. Diagnostic and statistical manual of mental disorders: DMI-IV. Washington, DC: American Psychiatric Association; 1994.
77. American Psychiatric Association. Practice guideline for the treatment of patients with eating disorders, 3rd ed. Arlington, VA: American Psychiatric Association; 2006.
78. CDC. Youth risk behavior surveillance—United States, 2009. MMWR 2010;59(No. SS-5) .
79. Harris EC, Barraclough B. Excess mortality of mental disorder. Br J Psychiatry 1998;173:11–53.
80. US Department of Health and Human Services. Oral health in America: a report of the Surgeon General—executive summary. Washington, DC: US Department of Health and Human Services, National Institute of Dental and Craniofacial Research, National Institutes of Health; 2000.
81. Marshall TA, Levy SM, Broffitt BA, et al. Dental caries and beverage consumption in young children. Pediatrics 2003;112:e184–91.

82. Marshall TA, Eichenberger-Gilmore JM, Broffitt BA, Warren JJ, Levy SM. Dental caries and childhood obesity: roles of diet and socioeconomic status. Community Dent Oral Epidemiol 2007;35:449–58.
83. US Department of Agriculture, Agricultural Research Service. What we eat in America, NHANES 2007–2008. Snacks: distribution of snack occasions. Washington, DC: US Department of Agriculture; 2010. Available at http://www.ars.usda.gov/SP2UserFiles/Place/12355000/pdf/0708/Table_30_DSO_RAC_07.pdf . Accessed June 28, 2011.
84. Briefel RR., Johnson CL. Secular trends in dietary intake in the United States. Ann Rev Nutr 2004;24:401–31.
85. Sacks FM, Svetkey LP, Vollmer VM, et al. Effects of blood pressure on reduced dietary sodium and the Dietary Approaches to Stop Hypertension (DASH) diet. DASH-Sodium Collaborative Research Group. N Engl J Med 2001;344:3–10.
86. Reedy J, Krebs-Smith SM. Dietary sources of energy, solid fats, and added sugars among children and adolescents in the United States. J Am Diet Assoc 2010;110:1477–84.
87. Forshee RA, Anderson PA, Storey ML. Changes in calcium intake and association with beverage consumption and demographics: comparing data from CSFII 1994–1996, 1998 and NHANES 1999–2002. J Am Coll Nutr 2006;25:108–16.
88. CDC. Trends in intake of energy and macronutrients--United States, 1971–2000. MMWR 2004;53:80–2.
89. Enns CW, Mickle SJ, Goldman JD. Trends in food and nutrient intakes by children in the United States. Fam Econ Nutr Rev 2002;14:56–68.
90. Troiano RP, Briefel RR, Carroll MD, Bialostosky K. Energy and fat intakes of children and adolescents in the United States: data from the National Health and Nutrition Examination Surveys. Am J Clin Nutr 2000;72:S1343–53.
91. Enns CW, Mickle SJ, Goldman JD. Trends in food and nutrient intakes by adolescents in the United States. Fam Econ Nutr Rev 2003;15:15–27.
92. Larson NI, Story M, Wall M, Neumark-Sztainer D. Calcium and dairy intakes of adolescents are associated with their home environment, taste preferences, personal health beliefs, and meal patterns. J Am Diet Assoc 2006;106:1816–24.
93. Harnack L, Walter SA, Jacobs DJ. Dietary intake and food sources of whole grains among U.S. children and adolescents: data from the 1994–1996 continuing survey of food intakes by individuals. J Am Diet Assoc 2003;103:1015–9.
94. Neumark-Sztainer D, Wall M, Perry C, Story M. Correlates of fruit and vegetable intake among adolescents. Findings from Project EAT. Prev Med 2003;37:198–208.
95. Zabinski MF, Daly T, Norman GJ, et al. Psychosocial correlates of fruit, vegetable, and dietary fat intake among adolescent boys and girls. J Am Diet Assoc 2006;106:814–21.
96. Larson NI, Neumark-Sztainer D, Hannan P, Story M. Family meals during adolescence are associated with higher diet quality and healthful meal patterns during young adulthood. J Am Diet Assoc 2007;107:1502–10.
97. Van der Horst K, Oenema A, Ferreira I, et al. A systematic review of environmental correlates of obesity-related dietary behaviors in youth. Health Educ Res 2007;22:203–26.

98. Story M, Neumark-Sztainer D, French S. Individual and environmental influences on adolescent eating behaviors. J Am Diet Assoc 2002;102:S40–51.
99. Baker EA, Schootman M, Barnidge E, Kelly C. The role of race and poverty in access to foods that enable individuals to adhere to the dietary guidelines. Prev Chronic Dis 2006;3:A76.
100. Zenk SN, Schulz AJ, Israel BA, James SA, Bao S, Wilson ML. Neighborhood racial composition, neighborhood poverty, and the spatial accessibility of supermarkets in metropolitan Detroit. Am J Public Health 2005;95:660–7.
101. Larson NI, Story M, Nelson MC. Neighborhood environments: disparities in access to healthy foods in the U.S. Am J Prev Med 2009;36:74–81.
102. Powell LM, Slater S, Mirtcheva D, Yanjun B, Chaloupka FJ. Food store availability and neighborhood characteristics in the United States. Prev Med 2007;44:189–95.
103. Bowman SA, Gortmaker SL, Ebbeling CB, Pereira MA, Ludwig DS. Effects of fast-food consumption on energy intake and diet quality among children in a national household survey. Pediatrics 2004;113:112–8.
104. Paeratakul S, Ferdinand DP, Champagne CM, Ryan DH, Bray GA. Fast-food consumption among U.S. adults and children: dietary and nutrient intake profile. J Am Diet Assoc 2003;103:1332–8.
105. O'Toole T, Anderson S, Miller C, Guthrie J. Nutrition services and foods and beverages available at school: results from the school health policies and programs study 2006. J Sch Health 2007;77:500–21.
106. Fox MK, Gordon AR, Nogales R, Wilson A. Availability and consumption of competitive foods in U.S. public schools. J Am Diet Assoc 2009;109:S57–66.
107. Institute of Medicine. Food marketing to children and youth: threat or opportunity? Washington, DC: Institute of Medicine; 2006.
108. Federal Trade Commission. Marketing food to children and adolescents: A review of industry expenditures, activities, and self regulation. Washington, DC, Federal Trade Commission; 2008.
109. CDC. Physical activity levels among children aged 9–13 years—United States, 2002. MMWR 2003;52:785–8.
110. US Department of Transportation Federal Highway Administration. Conference Report on H.R. 3, Safe, Accountable, Flexible, Efficient Transportation Equity Act: A Legacy for Users (SAFETEA-LU). Washington, DC: US Department of Transportation; 2005.
111. Carlson SA, Densmore D, Fulton JE, Yore MM, Kohl HW. Differences in physical activity prevalence and trends from 3 U.S. surveillance systems: NHIS, NHANES, and BRFSS. J Phys Act Health 2009;6:S18–27.
112. Sallis JF, Prochaska JJ, Taylor WC. A review of correlates of physical activity of children and adolescents. Med Sci Sport Exer 2000;32:963–75.
113. Lindquist CH, Reynolds KD, Goran MI. Sociocultural determinants of physical activity among children. Prev Med 1999;29:305–12.
114. Pate RR, Trost SG, Felton GM, Ward DS, Dowda M, Saunders R. Correlates of physical activity behavior in rural youth. Res Q Exerc Sport 1997;68:241–8.
115. Robbins LB, Pis MB, Pender NJ, Kazanis AS. Physical activity self-definition among adolescents. Res Theory Nurs Pract 2004;18:317–30.

116. Walton J, Hoerr S, Heine L, Frost S, Roisen D, Berkimer M. Physical activity and stages of change in fifth and sixth graders. J Sch Health 1999;69:285–9.
117. Sallis JF. Determinants of physical activity behavior in children. In: Pate R, Hohn R, eds. Health and fitness through physical education. Champaign, IL: Human Kinetics; 1994:31–43.
118. Gordon-Larsen P, McMurray RG, Popkin BM. Determinants of adolescent physical activity and inactivity patterns. Pediatrics 2000;105:83-91. Epub June 1, 2000. Available at http://pediatrics.aappublications.org/content/105/6/e83.abstract. Accessed July 1, 2011.
119. CDC. Trends in leisure-time physical inactivity by age, sex, and race/ethnicity--United States, 1994–2004. MMWR 2005;54:991–4.
120. Robbins LB, Pender NJ, Kazanis AS. Barriers to physical activity perceived by adolescent girls. J Midwifery Womens Health 2003;48:206–12.
121. Haverly K, Davison KK. Personal fulfillment motivates adolescents to be physically active. Arch Pediatr Adolesc Med 2005;159:1115–20.
122. Van der Horst K, Paw MJ, Twisk JW, van Mechelen W. A brief review on correlates of physical activity and sedentariness in youth. Med Sci Sport Exer 2007;39:1241–50.
123. Trost SG, Pate RR, Ward DS, Saunders R, Riner W. Correlates of objectively measured physical activity in preadolescent youth. Am J Prev Med 1999;17:120–6.
124. Baker CW, Little TD, Brownell KD. Predicting adolescent eating and activity behaviors: the role of social norms and personal agency. Health Psychol 2003;22:189–98.
125. Frenn M. Determinants of physical activity and low-fat diet among low income African American and Hispanic middle school students. Public Health Nurs 2005;22:89–97.
126. Motl R, Dishman R, Saunders R, Dowda M, Pate R. Perceptions of physical and social environment variables and self-efficacy as correlates of self-reported physical activity among adolescent girls. J Pediatr Psychol 2007;32:6–12.
127. Springer AE, Kelder SH, Hoelscher DM. Social support, physical activity and sedentary behavior among 6th-grade girls: a cross-sectional study. Int J Behav Nutr Phys Act 2006;3:8–18.
128. Voorhees CC, Murray D, Welk G, et al. The role of peer social network factors and physical activity in adolescent girls. Am J Health Behav 2005;29:183–90.
129. Vu MB, Murrie D, Gonzalez V, Jobe JB. Listening to girls and boys talk about girls' physical activity behaviors. Health Educ Behav 2006;33:81–96.
130. Gustafson SL, Rhodes RE. Parental correlates of physical activity in children and early adolescents. Sports Med 2006;36:79–97.
131. Sallis JF, Prochaska JJ, Taylor WC, Hill JO, Geraci JC. Correlates of physical activity in a national sample of girls and boys in grades 4 through 12. Health Psychol 1999;18:410–5.
132. Strauss RS, Rodzilsky D, Burack G, Colin M. Psychosocial correlates of physical activity in healthy children. Arch Pediatr Adolesc Med 2001;155:897–902.
133. Dowda M, Dishman R, Pfeiffer KA, Pate R. Family support for physical activity in girls from 8th to 12th grade in South Carolina. Prev Med 2006;44:153–9.
134. Heitzler CD, Martin SL, Duke J, Huhman M. Correlates of physical activity in a national sample of children aged 9–13 years. Prev Med 2006;42:254–60.

135. Trost S, Sallis J, Pate R, Freedson P, Taylor W, Dowda M. Evaluating a model of parental influence on youth physical activity. Am J Prev Med 2003;25:277–82.
136. Gomez JE, Johnson BA, Selva M, Sallis JF. Violent crime and outdoor physical activity among inner-city youth. Prev Med 2004;39:876–81.
137. Romero AJ, Robinson TN, Kraemer HC, et al. Are perceived neighborhood hazards a barrier to physical activity in children? Arch Pediatr Adolesc Med 2001;155:1143–8.
138. Ferreira I, Van der Horst K, Wendel-Vos W, Kremers S, Van Lenthe FJ, Brug J. Environmental correlates of physical activity in youth—a review and update. Obes Rev 2006;8:129–54.
139. Mota J, Almeida M, Santos R, Ribeiro JC, Santos MP. Association of perceived environmental characteristics and participation in organized and non-organized physical activities in adolescents. Pediatr Exerc Sci 2009;21:233–9.
140. Carver A, Timperio A, Crawford D. Playing it safe: The influence of neighborhood safety on children's physical activity—a review. Health & Place 2008; 14:217-27.
141. Davison KK, Lawson CT. Do attributes of the physical environment influence children's physical activity? A review of the literature. Int J Behav Nutr Phys Act 2006;3:1–17.
142. Cohen L, Davis R, Lee V, Valdovinos E. Addressing the intersection: Preventing violence and promoting healthy eating and active living. Oakland, CA: Prevention Institute; 2010. Available at http://www.preventioninstitute.org/component/jlibrary/article/id-267/127.html. Accessed July 1, 2011.
143. CDC. Barriers to children walking to or from school—United States, 2004. MMWR 2005:949–52.
144. Lee SM, Burgeson CR, Fulton JE, Spain CG. Physical education and physical activity: results from the school health policies and programs study 2006. J Sch Health 2007;77:435–63.
145. McKenzie TL, Sallis JF, Prochaska JJ, Conway TL, Marshall SJ, Rosengard P. Evaluation of a two-year middle-school physical education intervention: M-SPAN. Med Sci Sports Exerc 2004;36:1382–8.
146. Sallis JF, McKenzie TL, Alcaraz JE, Kolody B, Faucette N, Hovell MF. The effects of a 2-year physical education program (SPARK) on physical activity and fitness in elementary school students. Sports, Play, and Active Recreation for Kids. Am J Public Health 1997;87:1328–34.
147. Luepker RV, Perry CL, McKinlay SM, et al. Outcomes of a field trial to improve children's dietary patterns and physical activity. The Child and Adolescent Trial for Cardiovascular Health. JAMA 1996;275:768–76.
148. Nader P, Stone E, Lytle L, et al. Three-year maintenance of improved diet and physical activity: the CATCH cohort. Child and Adolescent Trial for Cardiovascular Health. Arch Pediatr Adolesc Med 1999;153:695–704.
149. Pate R, Ward D, Saunders R, Felton G, Dishman R, Dowda M. Promotion of physical activity among high-school girls: a randomized controlled trial. Am J Public Health 2005;95:1582–7.
150. Andersen RE, Crespo CJ, Bartlett S, Cheskin L, Pratt M. Relationship of physical activity and television watching with body weight and level of fatness among children: results from the Third National Health and Nutrition Examination Survey. JAMA 1998;279:938–42.

151. Coon KA, Tucker KL. Television and children's consumption patterns. A review of the literature. Minerva Pediatr 2002;54:423–36.
152. Crespo C, Smit E, Troiano RP, Bartlett S, Macera C, Andersen R. Television watching, energy intake, and obesity in U.S. children: results from the third National Health and Nutrition Examination Survey, 1988–1994. Arch Pediatr Adolesc Med 2001;155:360–5.
153. Gortmaker SL, Must A, Sobol AM, Peterson K, Colditz GA, Dietz WH. Television viewing as a cause of increasing obesity among children in the United States, 1986–1990. Arch Pediatr Adolesc Med 1996;150:356–62.
154. Hancox RJ, Milne BJ, Poulton R. Association between child and adolescent TV viewing and adult health: a longitudinal birth cohort study. Lancet 2004;364:257–62.
155. Lowry R, Wechsler H, Galuska DA, Fulton JE, Kann L. Television viewing and its associations with overweight, sedentary lifestyle, and insufficient consumption of fruits and vegetables among U.S. high school students: differences by race, ethnicity, and gender. J Sch Health 2002;72:413–21.
156. Utter J, Scragg R, Schaaf D. Associations between television viewing and consumption of commonly advertised foods among New Zealand children and young adolescents. Pub Health Nutr 2006;9:606–12.
157. Viner RM, Cole TJ. Television viewing in early childhood predicts adult body mass index. J Pediatr 2005;147:429–35.
158. Epstein LH, Roemmich JN, Robinson JL, et al. A randomized trial of the effects of reducing television viewing and computer use on body mass index in young children. Arch Pediatr Adolesc Med 2008;162:239–45.
159. Robinson TN. Reducing children's television viewing to prevent obesity: a randomized controlled trial. JAMA 1999;282:1561–7.
160. American Academy of Pediatrics, Committee on Public Education. American Academy of Pediatrics: children, adolescents, and television. Pediatrics 2001;107:423–6.
161. Rideout VJ, Foehr UG, Roberts DF. Generation M: media in the lives of 8- to 18-year-olds. Menlo Park, CA: The Henry J. Kaiser Family Foundation; 2010.
162. Adachi-mejia AM, Longacre MC, Gibson JJ, Beach ML, Titus-Ernstoff LT, Dalton MA. Children with a TV in their bedroom at higher risk for being overweight. Int J Obes 2007;31:644–51.
163. Christakis DA, Ebel BE, Rivara FP, Zimmerman FJ. Television, video, and computer game usage in children under 11 years of age. J Pediatr 2004;145:652–6.
164. Dennison BA, Erb TA, Jenkins PL. Television viewing and television in bedroom associated with overweight risk among low-income preschool children. Pediatrics 2002;109:1028–35.
165. Matheson DM, Killen JD, Wang Y, Varady A, Robinson TN. Children's food consumption during television viewing. Am J Clin Nutr 2004;79:1088–94.
166. Delmas C, Platat C, Schweitzer B, Wagner A, Oujaa M, Simon C. Association between television in bedroom and adiposity throughout adolescence. Obesity Res 2007;15:2495–503.
167. Saelens BM, Sallis JF, Nader PR, Broyles SL, Berry CC, Taras HL. Home environmental influences on children's television watching from early to middle childhood. J Dev Behav Pediatr 2002;23:127–32.

168. Grimm GC, Harnack L, Story M. Factors associated with soft drink consumption in school-aged children. J Am Diet Assoc 2004;104:1244–9.
169. Wiecha JL, Peterson KE, Ludwig DS, Kim J, Sobol A, Gortmaker SL. When children eat what they watch. Arch Pediatr Adolesc Med 2006;160:436–42.
170. American Academy of Pediatrics, Committee on Communications. Children, adolescents, and advertising. Pediatrics 2006;118:2563–9.
171. Coon KA, Goldberg J, Rogers BL, Tucker KL. Relationships between use of television during meals and children's food consumption patterns. Pediatrics 2001;107:E7. Epub January 1. 2001. Available at http://pediatrics.aappublications.org/content/107/1/e7.full. Accessed July 1, 2011.
172. Salmon J, Campbell KJ, Crawford DA. Television viewing habits associated with obesity risk factors: a survey of Melbourne schoolchildren. Med J Aust 2006;184:64-7.
173. Taveras EM, Sandora TJ, Shih M, Ross-Degnan D, Goldmann DA, Gillman MW. The association of television and video viewing with fast food intake by preschool-age children. Obesity Res 2006;14:2034–41.
174. Boynton-Jarrett R, Thomas T, Peterson K, Wiecha J, Sobol A, Gortmaker S. Impact of television viewing patterns on fruit and vegetable consumption among adolescents. Pediatrics 2003;112:1321–6.
175. National Center for Education Statistics. Digest of education statistics: 2004. Washington, DC: National Center for Education Statistics; 2005. Available at http://nces.ed.gov/programs/digest/2004menu_tables.asp. Accessed July 1, 2011.
176. US Department of Education, Institute of Education Sciences. Educational indicators, indicator 24: time in formal instruction. Washington, DC: US Department of Education; 2010. Available at http://nces.ed.gov/pubs/eiip/eiipid24.asp. Accessed July 1, 2011.
177. Dewey JD. Reviewing the relationship between school factors and substance use for elementary, middle, and high school students. J Prim Prev 1999;19:177–225.
178. Dunkle MC, Nash MA. Beyond the health room. Washington, DC: Council of Chief State School Officers, Resource Center on Educational Equity; 1991. Available at http://www.eric.ed.gov/PDFS/ED340681.pdf . Accessed July 1, 2011.
179. Mandell DJ, Hill SL, Carter L, Brandon RN. The impact of substance use and violence/delinquency on academic achievement for groups of middle and high school students in Washington. Seattle, WA: Washington Kids Count, Human Services Policy Center, Evans School of Public Affairs, University of Washington; 2002. Available at http://www.preventionworksinseattle.org/uploads/Impact%20of%20Substance%20Abuse%20on%20Academic%20Achievement.pdf . Accessed July 1, 2011.
180. Shephard R. Habitual physical activity and academic performance. Nutr Rev 1996;54:S32–36.
181. Kolbe LJ. Education reform and the goals of modern school health programs. The State Education Standard 2002;3:4–11. Epub 2002. Available at http://wvde.state.wv.us/healthyschools/documents/Education_Reform.pdf . Accessed July 1, 2011.
182. Allensworth D, Lawson E, Nicholson L, Wyche J, eds; Institute of Medicine. Schools and health: our nation's investment. Washington, DC: The National Academies Press; 1997.

183. Kleinman R, Hall S, Green H, et al. Diet, breakfast, and academic performance in children. Ann Nutr Metab 2002;46(Suppl 1):S24–30.
184. Widenhorn-Muller K, Hill K, Klenk J, Wiland U. Influence on having breakfast on cognitive performance and mood in 13- to 20-year old high school students: Results of a crossover trial. Pediatrics 2008;122:279–84.
185. Rampersaud GC, Pereira MA, Girard BL, Adams J, Metzl JD. Breakfast habits, nutritional status, body weight, and academic performance in children and adolescents. J Am Diet Assoc 2005;105:743–60.
186. Hoyland A, Dye L, Lawton CL. A systematic review of the effect of breakfast on the cognitive performance of children and adolescents. Nutr Res Rev 2009;22:220–43.
187. CDC. The association between school-based physical activity, including physical education, and academic performance. Atlanta, GA: US Department of Health and Human Services; 2010. Available at http://www.cdc.gov/healthyyouth/health_and_academics/pdf/pa-pe_paper.pdf . Accessed July 1, 2011.
188. Marx E, Wooley FS, Northrop D. Health is academic. New York, NY: Teachers College Press; 1998.
189. Fetro JV. Implementing coordinated school health programs in local schools. In: Marx E, Wooley SF, Northrop D, eds. Health is academic. New York, NY: Teachers College Press; 1998:15–42.
190. Cho H, Nadow M. Understanding barriers to implementing quality lunch and nutrition education. J Community Health 2004;29:421–35.
191. Pateman B, Irvin LH, Shoji L, Serna K. Building school health programs through public health initiatives: the first three years of the Healthy Hawaii Initiative partnership for school health. Prev Chronic Dis 2004;1:A10–6.
192. Valois RF, Hoyle TB. Formative evaluation results from the Mariner Project: a coordinated school health pilot program. J Sch Health 2000;70:95–103.
193. Jones SE, Fisher C, Greene BZ, Hertz MF, Pritzl J. Healthy and safe school environment, part 1: Results from the School Health Policies and Programs Study 2006. J Sch Health 2007;77:522–43.
194. American Cancer Society. Improving school health: a guide to school health councils. Atlanta, GA: American Cancer Society; 1999.
195. Shirer K. Promoting healthy youth, schools, and communities: a guide to community-school health councils. Atlanta, GA: American Cancer Society; 2003.
196. American Cancer Society. Improving school health: a guide to the role of the school health coordinator. Atlanta, GA: American Cancer Society; 1999.
197. Winnail S, Dorman S, Stevenson B. Training leaders for school health programs: the National School Health Coordinator Leadership Institute. J Sch Health 2004;74:79–84.
198. Resnicow K, Allensworth D. Conducting a comprehensive school health program. J Sch Health 1996;66:59–63.
199. CDC. School health index: a self-assessment and planning guide. Middle school/high school version. Atlanta, GA: US Department of Health and Human Services; 2005. Available at http://www.cdc.gov/HealthyYouth/shi/pdf/MiddleHigh.pdf . Accessed at July 1, 2011.
200. CDC. School health index: a self-assessment and planning guide. Elementary school version. Atlanta, GA: US Department of Health and Human Services; 2005. Available at http://www.cdc.gov/HealthyYouth/shi/pdf/Elementary.pdf . Accessed July 1, 2011.

201. Austin S, Fung T, Cohen-Bearak A, Wardle K, Cheung LWY. Facilitating change in school health: a qualitative study of schools' experiences using the school health index. Prev Chronic Dis 2006;3:A35–42.
202. Staten LK, Teufel-Shone NI, Steinfelt VE, et al. The school health index as an impetus for change. Prev Chronic Dis 2006;2:A19–28.
203. Pearlman DN, Dowling E, Bayuk C, Cullinen K, Thatcher AK. From concept to practice: using the school health index to create healthy school environments in Rhode Island elementary schools. Prev Chronic Dis 2005;2 (Spec Issue):A09–A25.
204. Bogden JF. Fit, healthy, and ready to learn: a school health policy guide. Part 1: physical activity, healthy eating, and tobacco-use prevention. Alexandria, VA: National Association of State Boards of Education; 2000.
205. Child Nutrition and WIC Reauthorization Act of 2004, 118 Stat. 729, Sect. 101-502, 108th Cong. (June 30, 2004).
206. Chriqui JF, Schneider L, Chaloupka FJ, Ide K, Pugach O. Local wellness policies: assessing school district strategies for improving children's health 2006–07 and 2007–08. Chicago, IL: Bridging the Gap Program, University of Illinois at Chicago; 2009.
207. Richard B. Russell National School Lunch Act, 42 U.S.C.A. Sect. 1758(b) (2011).
208. US Department of Agriculture. Team nutrition: local wellness policy. Washington, DC: US Department of Agriculture, Food and Nutrition Service; 2004. Available at www.fns.usda.gov/tn/healthy/wellnesspolicy.html. Accessed July 15, 2011.
209. Action for Healthy Kids. Wellness policy development tool. Action for Healthy Kids; 2005. Available at: www.actionforhealthykids.org/resources_wp.php. Accessed July, 15, 2011.
210. California Project LEAN, The Center for Weight and Health, University of California Berkeley. Policy in action: a guide to implementing your local school wellness policy. Sacramento, CA: California Project LEAN; 2006. Available at http://www.californiaprojectlean.org/doc.asp?id=168. Accessed July 15, 2011.
211. McKenna M.L. Issues in implementing school nutrition policies. Can J Diet Pract Res 2003;64:208-13.
212. CDC. Framework for program evaluation in public health. MMWR 1999;48:1–40 .
213. CDC. Physical activity evaluation handbook. Atlanta, GA: CDC; 2002.
214. Muraskin L. Understanding evaluation: the way to better prevention programs. Washington, DC: US Department of Education; 1993.
215. Taras H, Duncan P, Luckenbill D, Robinson J, Wheeler L, Wooley S. Health, mental health, and safety guidelines for schools; 2004. Available at http://www.nationalguidelines.org. Accessed July 15, 2011.
216. Allensworth D. Improving the health of youth through a coordinated school health programme. Promot Educ 1997;4:42–7.
217. Hoelscher D, Feldman H, Johnson C, et al. School-based health education programs can be maintained over time: results from the CATCH institutionalization study. Prev Med 2004;38:594–606.
218. Lytle LA, Ward J, Nader PR, Pedersen S, Williston BJ. Maintenance of a health promotion program in elementary schools: results from the CATCH-ON study key informant interviews. Health Educ Beh 2003;30:503–18.

219. California Department of Education, Advisory Committee on Nutrition Implementation Strategies. School nutrition by design. Sacramento, CA: California Department of Education; 2006.
220. US Department of Agriculture. Guidance for school food authorities: developing a school food safety program based on the process approach to HACCP principles. 4–79. Washington, DC: US Department of Agriculture; 2005.
221. National Food Service Management Institute. Serving it safe. 2nd ed. University, MS: National Food Service Management Institute; 2002.
222. US Department of Agriculture. Changing the scene: improving the school nutrition environment. Alexandria, VA: US Department of Agriculture; 2000.
223. National Coalition for Food Safe Schools. The food-safe schools action guide. Washington, DC: US Department of Health and Human Services; 2005.
224. Conklin MT, Lambert LG, Anderson JB. How long does it take students to eat lunch? A summary of three studies. J Child Nutr Manag 2002;26:1–6.
225. Bergman EA, Beurgel NS, Englund TF, Femrite A. The relationship of meal and recess schedules to plate waste in elementary schools. J Child Nutr Manag 2004.
226. Tanaka C, Richards KL, Takeuchi LS, Otani M, Maddock J. Modifying the recess before lunch program: a pilot study in Kaneohe elementary school. California J Health Promot 2005;3:1–7.
227. Graham H, Beall DL, Lussier M, McLaughlin P, Zidenberg-Cherr S. Use of school gardens in academic instruction. J Nutr Educ Behav 2005;37:147–51.
228. Morris JL, Zidenberg-Cherr S. Garden-enhanced nutrition curriculum improves fourth-grade school children's knowledge of nutrition and preferences for some vegetables. J Am Diet Assoc 2002;102:91–3.
229. Murphy JM. Education for sustainability: findings from the evaluation study of the edible schoolyard. Berkeley, CA: Center for Ecoliteracy; 2003.
230. McAlleese JD, Rankin LL. Garden-based nutrition education affects fruit and vegetable consumption in sixth-grade adolescents. J Am Diet Assoc 2007;107:662–5.
231. Parmer SM, Salisbury-Glennon J, Shannon D, Struempler B. School-gardens: an experiential learning approach for a nutrition education program to increase fruit and vegetable consumption among second-grade students. J Nutr Educ Behav 2009;41:212–7.
232. US Department of Agriculture, Food and Nutrition Service. 2002 Farm Bill, section-by-section summary of provisions affecting child nutrition programs section 4304. Washington, DC: US Department of Agriculture, Food and Nutrition Service; 2008. Available at http://lobby.la.psu.edu/_107th/123_Farm_Bill/Agency_Activities/US_Department_of_Agriculture/USDA_Farm_Bill_Summary_Child_Nutrition_Programs.htm. Accessed July 15, 2011.
233. Richard B. Russell National School Lunch Act, 42 U.S.C.A. Sect. 1758(j) (2011).
234. Harmon A. Farm to school: an introduction for food service professionals, food educators, parents and community leaders. Los Angeles, CA: National Farm to School Program, Center for Food and Justice, Urban and Environmental Policy Institute; 2003. Available at http://www.foodroutes.org/eflyers/FarmtoSchoolGuide.pdf . Accessed July 15, 2011.
235. Robinson-Obrien R, Story M, Heim S. Impact of garden-based youth nutrition intervention programs: a review. J Am Diet Assoc 2009;109:273–80.

236. Ozer EJ. The effects of school gardens on students and schools: conceptualization and considerations for maximizing healthy development. Health Educ Behav 2007;34:846–63.
237. 42 USCA, 1758(a)(5). 2011.
238. Institute of Medicine. Nutrition standards for foods in schools: leading the way toward healthier youth. Washington DC: Institute of Medicine of the National Academies; 2007.
239. Kaushik A, Mullee MA, Bryant TN, Hill CM. A study of the association between children's access to drinking water in primary schools and their fluid intake: can water be 'cool' in school? Child: Care, Health & Development 2007;33:409–15.
240. Muckelbauer R, Libuda L, Clausen K, Toschke AM, Reinehr T, Kersting M. Promotion and provision of drinking water in schools for overweight prevention: randomized, controlled cluster trial. Pediatrics 2009;123:e661–3667.
241. Wechsler H, Devereaux RS, Davis M, Collins J. Using the school environment to promote physical activity and healthy eating. Prev Med 2000;31(Suppl):S121–137.
242. Sallis JF, Conway TL, Prochaska JJ, McKenzie TL, Marshall SJ, Brown M. The association of school environments with youth physical activity. Am J Public Health 2001;91:618–20.
243. US Consumer Product Safety Commission. Public playground safety handbook. Washington, DC: US Government Printing Office; 2010. Available at http://www.cpsc.gov/cpscpub/pubs/325.pdf. Accessed July 15, 2011.
244. Olsen HM, Hudson SD, Thompson D. Developing a playground injury prevention plan. J Sch Nurs 2008;24:131–7.
245. Hart JE, Ritson RJ. Liability and safety in physical education and sport. 2nd ed. Reston, VA: National Association for Sport and Physical Education; 2002.
246. National Association for Sport and Physical Education. Guidelines for after-school physical activity and intramural sport programs: a position paper of the National Intramural Sports Council. Reston, VA: National Association for Sport and Physical Education; 2001. Available at http://www.ncpublicschools.org/docs/curriculum/healthfulliving/resources/instructional/intramural-guidelines.pdf. Accessed July 15, 2011.
247. Children's Safety Network at Education Development Center Inc. Injuries in the school environment: a resource guide. 2nd ed. Newton, MA: Education Development Center Inc; 1997.
248. US Department of Education, National Center for Education Statistics, National Forum on Education Statistics; Szuba T, Young R, School Facilities Maintenance Task Force, eds. Planning guide for maintaining school facilities. Washington, DC: National Center for Education Statistics; 2003. Available at http://nces.ed.gov/pubs2003/2003347.pdf. Accessed August 19, 2011.
249. Janda DH, Bir C, Wild B, Olson S, Hensinger RN. Goal post injuries in soccer. A laboratory and field testing analysis of a preventive intervention. Am J Sports Med 1995;23:340–4.
250. Janda DH, Bir C, Kedroske B. A comparison of standard vs. breakaway bases: an analysis of a preventative intervention for softball and baseball foot and ankle injuries. Foot Ankle Int 2001;10:810–6.

251. Janda DH. The prevention of baseball and softball injuries. Clin Orthop Relat Res 2003;409:20–8.
252. Heck JF, Clarke KS, Peterson TR, Torg JS, Weis MP. National Athletic Trainers' Association position statement: head-down contact and spearing in tackle football. J Athl Train 2004;39:101–11.
253. Jones NP. Eye injury in sport. Sports Med 1989;7:163–81.
254. Jambor T, Palmer SD. Playground safety manual. Birmingham, AL: Alabama Chapter of the American Academy of Pediatrics; 1991.
255. CDC. Promising practice in chronic disease prevention: a public health framework for action. Atlanta, GA: US Department of Health and Human Services; 2003.
256. Veigel JD, Pleacher MD. Injury prevention in youth sports. Curr Sports Med Rep 2008;7:348–52.
257. McKeag DB, Moeller JL. Preparticipation screening. In: McKeag DB, Moeller JL, eds. ACSM's primary care sports medicine. 2nd ed. Philadelphia, PA: Lippincott Williams & Wilkins; 2007:55–80.
258. Demorest RA, Landry GL. Training issues in elite young athletes. Curr Sports Med Rep 2004;3:167–72.
259. National Association for Sport and Physical Education. National standards for athletic coaches. Reston, VA: National Association for Sport and Physical Education; 2006.
260. National Association for Sport and Physical Education. Eight domains of coaching competencies. Reston, VA: National Association for Sport and Physical Education; 2006.
261. Saluja G, Marshall SW, Gilchrist J, Schroeder T. Sports and recreational injuries. In: Liller K, ed. Injury prevention for children and adolescents: integration of research, practice, and advocacy. 1st ed. Washington, DC: American Public Health Association; 2006:233–60.
262. Schwebe DC. Safety on the playground: mechanisms through which adult supervision might prevent playground injury. J Clin Psychol Med S 2006;13:135–43.
263. National Program for Playground Safety. S.A.F.E. playground supervision kit. Cedar Falls, IA: National Program for Playground Safety; 2002.
264. Evenson KR, McGinn AP. Availability of school physical activity facilities to the public in four U.S. communities. Am J Health Promot 2004;18:243–50.
265. Farley TA, Meriweather RA, Baker ET, Watkins LT, Johnson CC, Webber LS. Safe places to promote physical activity in inner-city children: results from a pilot study of an environmental intervention. Am J Public Health 2007;97:1625–31.
266. Spengler JO, Young SJ, Linton LS. Schools as a community resource for physical activity: legal considerations for decision makers. Am J Health Promot 2007;21:390–6.
267. Choy LB, McGurk MD, Tamashiro R, Nett B, Maddock JE. Increasing access to places for physical activity through a joint use agreement: a case study in urban Honolulu. Prev Chronic Dis 2008;5.
268. Food and Nutrition Service, US Department of Agriculture; CDC, US Department of Health and Human Services; US Department of Education. Making it happen: school nutrition success stories. Alexandria, VA: US Department of Agriculture; 2005.
269. French SA. Pricing effects on food choices. J Nutr 2003;133:S841–3.

270. Shannon C, Story M, Fulkerson JA, French SA. Factors in the school cafeteria influencing food choices by high school students. J Sch Health 2002;72:229–34.
271. French SA, Wechsler H. School-based research and initiatives: fruit and vegetable environment, policy, and pricing workshop. Prev Med 2004;39(Suppl 2):S101–107.
272. French SA, Story M, Jeffery RW, et al. Pricing strategy to promote fruit and vegetable purchase in high school cafeterias. J Am Diet Assoc 1997;97:1008–10.
273. French SA, Jeffery RW, Story M, et al. Pricing and promotion effects on low-fat vending snack purchases: the CHIPS study. Am J Public Health 2001;91:112–7.
274. Hannan P, French SA, Story M, Fulkerson JA. A pricing strategy to promote sales of lower fat foods in high school cafeterias: acceptability and sensitivity analysis. Am J Health Promot 2002;17:1–6.
275. Baxter SD. Are elementary schools teaching our children to prefer candy but not vegetables? J Sch Health 1998;68:111–3.
276. Birch LL. Development of food preferences. Annu Rev Nutr 1999;19:41–62.
277. Fisher J, Birch L. Restricting access to palatable foods affects children's behavioral response, food selection, and intake. Am J Clin Nutr 1999;69:1264–72.
278. Puhl RM, Schwartz MB. If you are good you can have a cookie: How memories of childhood food rules link to adult eating behaviors. Eat Behav 2003;4:283–93.
279. National Association for Sport and Physical Education. What constitutes a quality physical education program? Reston, VA: National Association for Sport and Physical Education; 2003.
280. Jarrett OS, Maxwell DM, Dickerson C, Hoge P, Davies G, Yetley A. Impact of recess on classroom behavior: group effects and individual differences. J Educ Res 1998;92:121–6.
281. Pellegrini AD, Davis PD. Relations between children's playground and classroom behaviour. Br J Educ Psychol 1993;63:89–95.
282. Eisenberg ME, Neumark-Sztainer D, Story M. Associations of weight-based teasing and emotional well-being among adolescents. Arch Pediatr Adolesc Med 2003;157:733–8.
283. Michigan Department of Education. The role of Michigan schools in promoting healthy weight: a consensus paper. Lansing, MI: Michigan Department of Education; 2001. Available at http://www.michigan.gov/documents/healthyweight_13649_7.pdf . Accessed July 15, 2011.
284. National Association for Sport and Physical Education. Position on dodgeball in physical education. Reston, VA: National Association for Sport and Physical Education; 2004.
285. Discrimination Prohibited, 7 C.F.R. Sect. 15.3 (2011).
286. US Department of Agriculture, Food and Nutrition Service. Accommodating children with special dietary needs in the school nutrition programs: guidance for school food service staff. Alexandria, VA: US Department of Agriculture; 2001.
287. Wilson TK, Bogden JF. Fit, healthy, and ready to learn, part III: policies related to asthma, school health services, and healthy environments. Alexandria, VA: National Association of State Boards of Education; 2005.
288. Block ME, Garcia C. Including students with disabilities in regular physical education. Block ME, Garcia C, eds. Reston, VA: National Association for Sport and Physical Education, American Association for Active Lifestyle and Fitness; 1995

289. American Dietetic Association. Position of the American Dietetic Association: individual-, family-, school-, and community-based interventions for pediatric overweight. J Am Diet Assoc 2006;106:925–45.
290. Durstine JL, Pinter P, Franklin BA, Morgan D, Pitetti KH, Roberts SO. Physical activity for the chronically ill and disabled. Sports Med 2000;30:207–19.
291. Flynn MA, McNeil DA, Maloff B, et al. Reducing obesity and related chronic disease risk in children and youth: a synthesis of evidence with 'best practice' recommendations. Obes Rev 2006;7:7–66.
292. Fulton JE, Garg M, Galuska DA, Rattay KT, Caspersen CJ. Public health and clinical recommendations for physical activity and physical fitness: Special focus on overweight youth. Sports Med 2004;34:581–99.
293. National Association for Sport and Physical Education. Moving into the future: national standards for physical education. 2nd ed. Reston, VA: National Association for Sport and Physical Education; 2004.
294. National Asthma Education and Prevention Program. Students with chronic illnesses: guidance for families, schools, and students. J Sch Health 2003;73:131–2.
295. Oude Luttikhuis H, Baur L, Jansen H, et al. Interventions for treating obesity in children. CD001872. Cochrane Database Systematic Review; 2003.
296. National Asthma Education and Prevention Program. Breathing difficulties related to physical activity for students with asthma: exercise-induced asthma. Bethesda, MD: National Asthma Education and Prevention Program; National Heart, Lung, and Blood Institute; 2005.
297. National Heart Lung and Blood Institute. Expert panel report 3: guidelines for the diagnosis and management of asthma. 08-4051. Bethesda, MD: National Institutes of Health, US Department of Health and Human Services; 2007.
298. American Dietetic Association. Position of the American Dietetic Association: local support for nutrition integrity in schools. J Am Diet Assoc 2006;106:122–3.
299. American Dietetic Association; Society for Nutrition Education; American School Food Service Association. Position of the American Dietetic Association, Society for Nutrition Education, and American School Food Service Association. Nutrition services: an essential component of comprehensive school health programs. J Nutr Educ Behav 2003;35:57–67.
300. Birch LL, Fisher JO. Development of eating behaviors among children and adolescents. Pediatrics 1998;101:539–49.
301. Perry CL, Bishop DB, Taylor GL, et al. A randomized school trial of environmental strategies to encourage fruit and vegetable consumption among children. Health Educ Behav 2004;31:65–76.
302. Gordon AR, Cohen R, Crepinsek MK, Fox MK, Hall J, Zeidman E. The Third School Nutrition Dietary Assessment Study: background and study design. J Am Diet Assoc 2009;109(Suppl 2):S20–30.
303. United States Department of Agriculture. National School Lunch Program: participation and lunches served. Washington, DC: US Department of Agriculture; 2011. Available at http://www.fns.usda.gov/pd/slsummar.htm. Accessed July 15, 2011.
304. US Department of Agriculture. School breakfast program participation and meals served. United States Department of Agriculture; 2011. Available at http://www.fns.usda.gov/pd/sbsummar.htm. Accessed July 15, 2011.

305. Briefel RR, Wilson A, Gleason P. Consumption of low-nutrient, energy-dense foods and beverages at school, home, and other locations among school lunch participants and nonparticipants. J Am Diet Assoc 2009;109(Suppl 2):S79–90.
306. Condon EM, Crepinsek MK, Fox MK. School meals: types of foods offered to and consumed by children at lunch and breakfast. J Am Diet Assoc 2009;109(Suppl 2):S67–78.
307. Gordon AR, Crepinsek MK, Briefel RR, Clark MA, Fox MK. The third school nutrition dietary assessment study: summary and implications. J Am Diet Assoc 2009;109(Suppl 1):S129–135.
308. Clark MA, Fox MK. Nutritional quality of the diets of U.S. public school children and the role of the school meals program. J Am Diet Assoc 2009;109(Suppl 2):S44–56.
309. Gleason PM, Dodd AH. School breakfast program but not school lunch program participation is associated with lower body mass index. J Am Diet Assoc 2009;109(Suppl 2):S118–28.
310. Murphy JM, Pagano M, bishop SJ. Impact of a universally-free, in-classroom school breakfast program on achievement: results from the Abell Foundation's Baltimore Breakfast Challenge Program. Boston, MA: Massachusetts General Hospital; 2001.
311. Murphy JM, Drake JE, Weineke KM. Academics and breakfast connection pilot: final report on New York's Classroom Breakfast Project. Albany, NY: Nutrition Consortium of New York; 2005.
312. Powell CA, Walker SP, Chang SM, Grantham-McGregor SM. Nutrition and education: a randomized trial of the effects of breakfast in rural primary school children. Am J Clin Nutr 1998;68:873–9.
313. Meyers A, Sampson A, Weitzman M, Rogers B, Kayne H. School breakfast program and school performance. Am J Dis Child 1989;143:1234–9.
314. US Department of Agriculture, Food and Nutrition Service; Gordon A, Fox MK, Clark M, et al, eds. School Nutrition Dietary Assessment Study—III, vol II: student participation and dietary intakes. CN-07-SNDA-III. Alexandria, VA: US Department of Agriculture; 2007.
315. Bernstein LS, McLaughlin JE, Crepins MK, Daft IM. Evaluation of the school breakfast program pilot project: final report. Alexandria, VA: US Department of Agriculture; 2004.
316. Determining Eligibility for Free and Reduced Price Meals and Free Milk in Schools, 7 C.F.R. Sect. 245 (2011).
317. Kennedy E, Davis C. U.S. Department of Agriculture school breakfast program. Am J Clin Nutr 1998;67(Suppl):S798–803.
318. Healthy, Hunger-Free Kids Act of 2010. PL 111-296, 201. 12-13-2010. 124 Stat 3183.
319. Institute of Medicine. School meals: building blocks for healthy children. Washington, DC: The National Academies Press; 2010.
320. Richard B. Russell National School Lunch Act, 42 U.S.C.A. Sect. 1758(h) (2011).
321. Crepinsek MK, Gordon AR, McKinney PM, Condon EM, Wilson A. Meals offered and served in U.S. public schools: do they meet nutrient standards? J Am Diet Assoc 2009;109(Suppl 1):S31–43.
322. US Department of Agriculture, Food and Nutrition Service. A menu planner for healthy school meals. Washington, DC: US Department of Agriculture; 1998

323. US Government Accountability Office. School meal programs: revenue and expense information from selected states. GAO-03-569. Washington, DC: US Government Accountability Office; 2003.
324. Mississippi Department of Education, Office of Healthy School and Child Nutrition Programs. Nutrition integrity in Mississippi schools, replacing kitchen fryers with combination oven steamers: six steps to success. Mississippi Department of Education, Office of Healthy Schools and Child Nutrition Programs; 2008.
325. Roberts SM, Pobocik RS, Deek R, Besfrove A, Prostine BA. A qualitative study of junior high school principals' and school food service directors' experiences with the Texas school nutrition policy. J Nutr Educ Behav 2009;41:293–9.
326. Brown DM. Prevalence of food production systems in school foodservice. J Am Diet Assoc 2005;105:1261–5.
327. Lambert LG, Raidl M, Carr DH, Safaii S, Tidwell DK. School nutrition directors' and teachers' perceptions of the advantages, disadvantages, and barriers to participation in the school breakfast program. J Child Nutr Manag 2007;31.
328. Sallis JF, McKenzie TL, Conway TL, et al. Environmental interventions for eating and physical activity: a randomized controlled trial in middle schools. Am J Prev Med 2003;24:209–17.
329. US Department of Agriculture. School lunch and breakfast cost study—II, final report. Washington, DC: US Department of Agriculture; 2008.
330. Wagner B, Senauer B, Runge CF. An empirical analysis of and policy recommendations to improve the nutritional quality of school meals. Rev Agric Econ 2007;29:672–88.
331. Almanza B. Equipment purchasing and facility design for school nutrition programs. R-131-08 (GY05). University, MS: University of Mississippi, National Food Service Management Institute; 2009.
332. US Department of Agriculture. The road to SMI success—a guide for school foodservice directors. Washington, DC: US Department of Agriculture; 2007.
333. O'Neil CE, Nicklas TA. Gimme 5: an innovative, school-based nutrition intervention for high school students. J Am Diet Assoc 2002;102(Suppl 3):S93–6.
334. Story M, Mays Warren R, Bishop D, et al. 5-a-day power plus: process evaluation of a multicomponent elementary school program to increase fruit and vegetable consumption. Health Educ Behav 2000;27:187–200.
335. Zive MM, Pelletier RL, Sallis JF, Elder JP. An environmental intervention to improve a la carte foods at middle schools. J Am Diet Assoc 2002;102(Suppl 3):S76–8.
336. National Food Service Management Institute. Culinary techniques for healthy school meals. 2nd ed. University, MS: National Food Service Management Institute; 2009.
337. Gorski-Berry DM. Wrapping it all up: the value of packaging. J Dairy Sci 1999;82:2257–8.
338. National School Lunch Program, Competitive Food Services, 7 C.F.R. Sect. 210.11 (2011).
339. School Breakfast Program, Competitive Food Services, 7 C.F.R. Sect. 220.12 (2011).
340. National School Lunch Program, Categories of Foods of Minimal Nutritional Value, 7 C.F.R. Sect. 210 App. B (2011).
341. School Breakfast Program, Categories of Foods of Minimal Nutritional Value, 7 C.F.R. Sect. 220 App. B (2011).

342. Child Nutrition Act of 1966, 42 U.S.C.A. Sect. 1779(b) (2011).
343. CDC. Competitive foods and beverages in U.S. schools--a state policy analysis, October 2010. Atlanta, GA, CDC; In press 2011.
344. US Government Accountability Office. School meal programs: competitive foods are widely available and generate substantial revenues for schools. GAO-050563. Washington, DC: US Government Accountability Office; 2005.
345. Abraham SM, Chattopadhvav M, Montgomery M, Steiger DM, Daft B. The School Meals Initiative Implementation Study--third year report. Nutrition Assistance Program Report Series CN02-SMI3. Alexandria, VA: US Department of Agriculture, Food and Nutrition Service, Office of Analysis, Nutrition and Evaluation; 2002.
346. CDC. Competitive foods and beverages available for purchase in secondary schools--selected sites, United States, 2006. MMWR 2008;57:935–38.
347. Brener ND, McManus T, Foti K, et al. School health profiles 2008: characteristics of health programs among secondary schools. Atlanta, GA: CDC; 2009.
348. Fox MK, Dodd AH, Wilson A, Gleason PM. Association between school food environment and practices and body mass index of U.S. public school children. J Am Diet Assoc 2009;109(Suppl 2):S108–17.
349. Briefel RR, Crepinsek MK, Cabili C, Wilson A, Gleason PM. School food environments and practices affect dietary behaviors of U.S. public school children. J Am Diet Assoc 2009;109(Suppl 2):S91–107.
350. Gonzalez W, Jones SJ, Frongillo EA. Restricting snacks in U.S. elementary schools is associated with higher frequency of fruit and vegetable consumption. J Nutr 2009;139:142–4.
351. US Department of Agriculture. Foods sold in competition with USDA meal programs: a report to Congress. Washington, DC: US Department of Agriculture; 2001.
352. Kubik M, Lytle L, Hannan P, Perry C, Story M. The association of the school food environment with dietary behaviors of young adolescents. Am J Public Health 2003;93:1168–73.
353. Kubik M, Lytle L, Story M. Schoolwide food practices are associated with body mass index in middle school students. Arch Pediatr Adolesc Med 2005;159:1111–4.
354. US Department of Agriculture, Food and Nutrition Service; Fox MK, Crepinsek MK, Connor P, Battaglia M, eds. School nutrition dietary assessment study--II: summary of findings. Alexandria, VA: US Department of Agriculture; 2001.
355. French SA, Story M, Fulkerson JA, Hannan P. An environmental intervention to promote lower-fat food choices in secondary schools: outcomes of the TACOS Study. Am J Public Health 2004;94:1507–12.
356. Jones SJ, Gonzalez W, Frongillo EA. Policies that restrict sweetened beverage availability may reduce consumption in elementary-school children. Pub Health Nutr 2009;13:589–95.
357. Snelling AM, Kennard T. The impact of nutrition standards on competitive food offerings and purchasing behaviors of high school students. J Sch Health 2009;79:541–6.
358. Richard B. Russell National School Lunch Act, 42 U.S.C.A. Sect. 1758(b)(2) (2011).
359. Wharton CM, Long M, Schwartz MB. Changing nutrition standards in schools: the emerging impact on school revenue. J Sch Health 2008;78:245–51.

360. Wojcicki J, Heyman MB. Healthier choices and increased participation in a middle school lunch program: effects of nutrition policy changes in San Francisco. Am J Public Health 2006;96:1542–7.
361. Center for Weight and Health, University of California, Berkeley. Pilot implementation of SB 19 in California middle and high schools: report on accomplishments, impact, and lessons learned. Berkeley, CA: University of California, Berkeley; 2005.
362. West Virginia University, Robert C. Byrd Health Sciences Center, Health Research Center. West Virginia Healthy Lifestyles Act: year one evaluation report. Morgantown, WV: West Virginia University; 2009.
363. Connecticut State Department of Education. Summary data report on Connecticut's healthy snack pilot. Hartford, CT: Connecticut State Department of Education; 2006.
364. Brown DM, Tammineni SK. Managing sales of beverages in schools to preserve profits and improve children's nutrition intake in 15 Mississippi schools. J Am Diet Assoc 2009;109:2036–42.
365. Johnston LD, Delvaux K, O'Malley PM. Soft drink availability, contracts, and revenues in American secondary schools. Am J Prev Med 2007;33(Suppl 4):S209–225.
366. Greves MH, Rivara F. Report card on school snack food policies among the United States' largest school districts in 2004–2005: room for improvement. Int J Behav Nutr Phys Act 2006;3:1.
367. Fulkerson JA, French SA, Story M, Nelson H, Hannan PJ. Promotions to increase lower-fat food choices among students in secondary schools: description of outcomes of TACOS (Trying Alternative Cafeteria Options in Schools). Public Health Nutr 2004;7:665–74.
368. Cullen KW, Thompson VJ, Watson K, Nicklas T. Marketing fruits and vegetables to middle school students: formative assessment results. J Child Nutr Manag 2005;29.
369. Davis EM, Cullen KW, Watson KB, Konarik M, Radcliffe J. A fresh fruit and vegetable program improves high school students' consumption of fresh produce. J Am Diet Assoc 2009;109:1227–31.
370. Food and Nutrition Service. Fruits and vegetables galore: helping kids eat more. Washington, DC: US Department of Agriculture; 2004.
371. Just DR, Mancino L, Wansink B. Could behavioral economics help improve diet quality for nutrition assistance program participants? Washington, DC: US Department of Agriculture; 2007.
372. US Department of Agriculture, Food and Nutrition Service. Fruit and vegetable program handbook. Washington, DC: US Department of Agriculture; 2008.
373. The Food Trust. Food Trust healthy food toolkit. Philadelphia, PA: The Food Trust; Available at http://www.thefoodtrust.org/php/programs/comp.school.nutrition.php. Accessed July 15, 2011.
374. Nemours Health and Prevention Services. Planting the seeds for healthy schools: building effective district wellness policies. Jacksonville, FL: Nemours Health and Prevention Services; 2008.
375. Kubik M, Lytle L, Farbakhsh K, Moe S, Samuelson A. Food use in middle and high school fundraising: Does policy support healthful practice? Results from a survey of Minnesota school principals. J Am Diet Assoc 2009;109:1215–19.
376. National Association for Sport and Physical Education. Is it physical education or physical activity?: understanding the difference. Reston, VA: National Association

for Sport and Physical Education; 2005. Available at http://www.aahperd.org/naspe/publications/teachingTools/PAvsPE.cfm. Accessed July 15, 2011.
377. National Association for Sport and Physical Education. Comprehensive school physical activity programs. Reston, VA: National Association for Sport and Physical Education; 2008. Available at http://www.aahperd.org/naspe/standards/upload/Comprehensive-School-Physical-Activity-Programs-2008.pdf. Accessed July 15, 2011.
378. Kahn EB, Ramsey LT, Brownson RC, et al. The effectiveness of interventions to increase physical activity. A systematic review. Am J Prev Med 2002;22(Suppl 4):S73–107.
379. National Association for Sport and Physical Education. Physical education is critical to a complete education. Reston, VA: National Association for Sport and Physical Education; 2001. Available at http://www.aahperd.org/naspe/standards/upload/Physical-Education-is-Critical-to-a-Complete-Education-2001.pdf . Accessed July 15, 2011.
380. Trudeau F, Shephard RJ. Contribution of school programmes to physical activity levels and attitudes in children and adults. Sports Med 2005;35:89–105.
381. Donnelly JE, Jacobsen DJ, Whatley JE, et al. Nutrition and physical activity program to attenuate obesity and promote physical and metabolic fitness in elementary school children. Obes Res 1996;4:229–43.
382. McKenzie TL, Nader PR, Strikmiller PK, et al. School physical education: effect of the Child and Adolescent Trial for Cardiovascular Health. Prev Med 1996;25:423–31.
383. McKenzie TL, Marshall SJ, Sallis JF, Conway TL. Student activity levels, lesson context, and teacher behavior during middle school physical education. Res Q Exerc Sport 2000;71:249–59.
384. Dishman RK, Motl RW, Saunders R, et al. Enjoyment mediates effects of a school-based physical-activity intervention. Med Sci Sports Exerc 2005;37:478–87.
385. National Association for Sport and Physical Education. Opposing substitution and waiver/exemptions for required physical education. Reston, VA: National Association for Sport and Physical Education; 2006. Available at http://www.aahperd.org/naspe/standards/upload/Opposing-Substition-Waiver-Exemptions-for-Required-PE-2006.pdf. Accessed July 15, 2011.
386. Ayers SF. High school students' physical education conceptual knowledge. Res Q Exerc Sport 2004;75:272–87.
387. Dale D, Corbin CB. Physical activity participation of high school graduates following exposure to conceptual or traditional physical education. Res Q Exerc Sport 2000;71:61–8.
388. Fardy PS, White RE, Haltiwanger-Schmitz K, et al. Coronary disease risk factor reduction and behavior modification in minority adolescents: the PATH program. J Adolesc Health 1996;18:247–53.
389. CDC. Physical education curriculum analysis tool. Atlanta, GA: US Department of Health and Human Services; 2006. Available at http://www.cdc.gov/healthyyouth/pecat/pdf/PECAT.pdf. Accessed July 15, 2011.
390. Pellett TL, Blakemore CL. Comparisons of teaching presentation and development of content: implications for effectiveness of teaching. Percept Mot Skills 1997;85:963–72.

391. Karabourniotis D, Evaggelinou C, Tzetzis G, Kourtessis T. Curriculum enrichment with self-testing activities in development of fundamental movement skills of first-grade children in Greece. Percept Mot Skills 2002;94:1259–70.
392. Ernst M, Beighle A, Corbin CB, Pangrazi R. Appropriate and inappropriate uses of Fitnessgram: A commentary. J Phys Act Health 2006;3(Suppl 2):S90–100.
393. Twisk JW, Kemper HC, van Mechelen W. The relationship between physical fitness and physical activity during adolescence and cardiovascular disease risk factors at adult age. The Amsterdam Growth and Health Longitudinal Study (AGAHLS). Int J Sports Med 2002;23(Suppl 1):S8–14.
394. Pangrazi R. Dynamic physical education for elementary school students. 15th ed. London, England: Benjamin Cummings; 2006.
395. Whitehead JR, Eklund RC, Williams AC. Using skinfold calipers while teaching body fatness-related concepts: cognitive and affective outcomes. J Sci Med Sport 2003;6:461–76.
396. Bouchard C, Daw EW, Rice T, et al. Familial resemblance for V02max in the sedentary state: the HERITAGE family study. Med Sci Sports Exerc 1998;30:252–8.
397. Bouchard C, An P, Rice T, et al. Familial aggregation of V02max response to exercise training: results from the HERITAGE family study. J Appl Physiol 1999;87:1003–8.
398. National Association for Sport and Physical Education. Appropriate instructional practice guidelines for elementary school physical education. 3rd ed. Reston, VA: National Association for Sport and Physical Education; 2009. Available at http://www.cahperd.org/cms-assets/documents/ToolKit/NASPE_ApprroPrac/5287-207931.elementaryappropractpdf . Accessed July 15, 2011.
399. National Association for Sport and Physical Education. Appropriate instructional practice guidelines for middle school physical education. 3rd ed. Reston, VA: National Association for Sport and Physical Education; 2009. Available at http://www.cahperd.org/cms-assets/documents/ToolKit/NASPE_ApprroPrac/5289-666992.msappropracpdf . Accessed July 15, 2011.
400. National Association for Sport and Physical Education. Appropriate instructional practices for high school physical education. 3rd ed. Reston, VA: National Association for Sport and Physical Education; 2009. Available at http://www.cahperd.org/cms-assets/documents/ToolKit/NASPE_ApprroPrac/5288-573262.hsappropracpdf. Accessed July 15, 2011.
401. McKenzie TL, Feldman H, Woods SE, et al. Children's activity levels and lesson context during third-grade physical education. Res Q Exerc Sport 1995;66:184–93.
402. McKenzie T, Stone E, Feldman H, et al. Effects of the CATCH physical education intervention: teacher type and lesson location. Am J Prev Med 2001;21:101–9.
403. Fairclough S, Stratton G. Physical education makes you fit and healthy. Physical education's contribution to young people's physical activity levels. Health Educ Res 2005;20:14–23.
404. Scruggs PW, Beveridge SK, Eisenman PA, Watson DL, Shultz BB, Ransdell LB. Quantifying physical activity via pedometry in elementary physical education. Med Sci Sports Exerc 2003;35:1065–71.
405. Simons-Morton BG, Taylor WC, Snider SA, Huang IW, Fulton JE. Observed levels of elementary and middle school children's physical activity during physical education classes. Prev Med 1994;23:437–41.

406. van Beurden E, Barnett LM, Zask A, Dietrich UC, Brooks LO, Beard J. Can we skill and activate children through primary school physical education lessons? "Move it groove it"—a collaborative health promotion intervention. Prev Med 2003;36:493–501.
407. Baquet G, Berthoin S, Van PE. Are intensified physical education sessions able to elicit heart rate at a sufficient level to promote aerobic fitness in adolescents? Res Q Exerc Sport 2002;73:282–8.
408. Simons-Morton BG, Parcel G, Baranowski T, Forthofer R, O'Hara N. Promoting physical activity and a healthful diet among children: results of a school-based intervention study. Am J Public Health 1991;81:986–91.
409. Manios Y, Moschandreas J, Hatzis C, Kafatos A. Evaluation of a health and nutrition education program in primary school children of Crete over a three-year period. Prev Med 1999;28:149–59.
410. Vandongen R, Jenner DA, Thompson C, et al. A controlled evaluation of a fitness and nutrition intervention program on cardiovascular health in 10- to 12-year-old children. Prev Med 1995;24:9–22.
411. Dishman RK. Self-management strategies mediate self-efficacy and physical activity. Am J Prev Med 2005;29:10–8.
412. Shimon JM, Petlichkoff LM. Impact of pedometer use and self-regulation strategies on junior high school physical education students' daily step counts. J Phys Act Health 2009;6:178–84.
413. Motl RW, Dishman RK, Ward DS, et al. Comparison of barriers self-efficacy and perceived behavioral control for explaining physical activity across 1 year among adolescent girls. Health Psychol 2005;24:106–11.
414. Xiang P, Lee A. The development of self-perceptions of ability and achievement goals and their relations in physical education. Res Q Exerc Sport 1998;69:231–41.
415. Xiang P, McBride R, Guan J. Children's motivation in elementary physical education: a longitudinal study. Res Q Exerc Sport 2004;75:71–80.
416. Chase MA. Children's self-efficacy, motivational intentions, and attributions in physical education and sport. Res Q Exerc Sport 2001;72:47–54.
417. Papacharisis V, Goudas M. Perceptions about exercise and intrinsic motivation of students attending a health-related physical education program. Percept Mot Skills 2003;97:689–96.
418. Daley AJ, Buchana J. Aerobic dance and physical self-perceptions in female adolescents: some implications for physical education. Res Q Exerc Sport 1999;70:196–200.
419. Jago R, Baranowski T. Non-curricular approaches for increasing physical activity in youth: a review. Prev Med 2004;39:157–63.
420. National Association for Sport and Physical Education. Recess for elementary school students. Reston, VA: National Association for Sport and Physical Education; 2006. Available at http://www.aahperd.org/naspe/standards/upload/Recess-for-Elementary-School-Students-2006.pdf . Accessed July 15, 2011.
421. CDC. School health policies and programs study 2006 [unpublished data]. Atlanta, GA: US Department of Health and Human Services, CDC; 2009.
422. Ridgers ND, Stratton G, Fairclough SJ. Physical activity levels of children during school playtime. Sports Med 2006;36:359–71.

423. Ridgers ND, Stratton G, Fairclough SJ. Assessing physical activity during recess using accelerometry. Prev Med 2005;41:102–7.
424. Zask A, van Beurden E, Barnett L, Brooks LO, Dietrich UC. Active school playgrounds–-myth or reality? Results of the "move it groove it" project. Prev Med 2001;33:402–8.
425. Burdette HL, Whitaker RC. Resurrecting free play in young children: looking beyond fitness and fatness to attention, affiliation, and affect. Arch Pediatr Adolesc Med 2005;159:46–50.
426. Sluckin A. Growing up in the playground: the social development of children. London, England: Routledge & Kegan Paul; 1981.
427. Barros RM, Silver EJ, Stein RE. School recess and group classroom behavior. Pediatr 2009;123:431–6.
428. Caterino MC, Polak ED. Effects of two types of activity on the performance of second-, third-, and fourth-grade students on a test of concentration. Percept Mot Skills 1999;89:245–8.
429. Pelligrini AD, Kato K, Blatchford P, Baines E. A short-term longitudinal study of children's playground games across the first year of school: implications for social competence and adjustment to school. Am Educ Res J 2002;39:991–1015.
430. Stratton G, Mullan E. The effect of multicolor playground markings on children's physical activity level during recess. Prev Med 2005;41:828–33.
431. Verstraete SJ, Cardon GM, De Clercq DL, De Bourdeaudhuij IM. Increasing children's physical activity levels during recess periods in elementary schools: the effects of providing game equipment. Eur J Pub Health 2006;23:1–5.
432. Robert Wood Johnson Foundation. Recess rules: why the undervalued playtime may be America's best investment for healthy kids and healthy schools. Princeton, NJ: Robert Wood Johnson Foundation; 2007. Available at http://www.rwjf.org/files/research/sports4kidsrecessreport.pdf . Accessed July 15, 2011.
433. Mahar MT, Murphy SK, Rowe DA, Golden J, Shields A, Raedeke TD. Effects of a classroom-based program on physical activity and on-task behavior. Medicine and science in sports and exercise 2006;38:2086–94.
434. Stewart JA, Dennison DA, Kohl HW, Doyle JA. Exercise level and energy expenditure in the TAKE 10! in-class physical activity program. J Sch Health 2004;74:397–400.
435. Kelder S, Hoelscher DM, Barroso CS, Walker JL, Cribb P, Hu S. The CATCH Kids Club: a pilot after-school study for improving elementary students' nutrition and physical activity. Public Health Nutr 2005;8:133–40.
436. Hellison D. Physical activity programs for underserved youth. J Sci Med Sport 2000;3:238–42.
437. Harrison PA, Gopalakrishnan N. Differences in behavior, psychological factors, and environmental factors associated with participation in school sports and other activities in adolescence. J Sch Health 2003;73:113–20.
438. Vilhjalmsson R, Kristjansdottir G. Gender differences in physical activity in older children and adolescents: the central role of organized sport. Soc Sci Med 2003;56:363–74.
439. Katzmarzyk PT, Malina R. Contribution of organized sports participation to estimated daily energy expenditure in youth. Pediatr Exerc Sci 2000;13:378–85.

440. Pate R, Trost S, Levin S, Dowda M. Sports participation and health-related behaviors among U.S. youth. Arch Pediatr Adolesc Med 2000;154:904–11.
441. Seefeldt V, Ewing ME. Youth sports in America. The President's Council on Physical Fitness and Sports Research Digest 1997;2:1–12.
442. Cooper AR, Page AS, Foster LJ, Qahwaji D. Commuting to school: are children who walk more physically active? Am J Prev Med 2003;25:273–6.
443. Cooper AR. Physical activity levels of children who walk, cycle, or are driven to school. Am J Prev Med 2005;29:179–84.
444. Tudor-Locke C, Neff LJ, Ainsworth BE, Addy CL, Popkin BM. Omission of active commuting to school and the prevalence of children's health-related physical activity levels: the Russian Longitudinal Monitoring Study. Child Care Health Dev 2002;28:507–12.
445. Alexander LM, Inchley J, Todd J, Currie D, Cooper AR, Currie C. The broader impact of walking to school among adolescents: seven day accelerometry based study. BMJ 2005;331:1061–2.
446. Sirard J, Riner WJ, McIver K, Pate R. Physical activity and active commuting to elementary school. Med Sci Sports Exerc 2005;37:2062–9.
447. Staunton CE, Hubsmith D, Kallins W. Promoting safe walking and bicycling to school: the Marin County success story. Am J Public Health 2003;93:1431–4.
448. CDC. Kids walk-to-school. A guide to promote walking to school. Atlanta, GA: US Department of Health and Human Services; 2006. Available at http://www.cdc.gov/nccdphp/dnpa/kidswalk/pdf/kidswalk.pdf . Accessed July 15, 2011.
449. Block ME, Klavina A, Flint W. Including students with severe, multiple disabilities in general physical education. JOPERD 2007;78:29–32.
450. Klavina A, Block ME. The effect of peer tutoring on interaction behaviors in inclusive physical education. Adapt Phys Activ Q 2008;25:132–58.
451. National Consortium for Physical Education and Recreation for Individuals with Disabilities. Adapted physical education national standards. 2nd ed. Champaign, IL: Human Kinetics; 2006.
452. Lohrmann DK, Wooley SF. Comprehensive school health education. In: Marx E, Wooley SF, eds. Health is academic. New York, NY: Teachers College Press; 1998:43–66.
453. Joint Committee on National Health Education Standards. National health education standards: achieving excellence. 2nd ed. Atlanta, GA: American Cancer Society; 2007.
454. Gold RS, Miner KR; 2000 Joint Committee on Health Education and Promotion Terminology. Report of the 2000 Joint Committee on Health Education and Promotion Terminology. J Sch Health 2002;72:3–7.
455. Kann L, Telljohann SK, Wooley S. Health education: results from the School Health Policies and Programs Study 2006. J Sch Health 2007;77:408–34.
456. Briggs M, Safaii S, Beall DL; American Dietetic Association; Society for Nutrition Education; American School Food Service Association. Position of the American Dietetic Association, Society for Nutrition Education, and American School Food Service Association—Nutrition services: an essential component of comprehensive school health programs. J Am Diet Assoc 2003;103:505–14.

457. Gortmaker SL, Peterson K, Wiecha J, et al. Reducing obesity via a school-based interdisciplinary intervention among youth: Planet Health. Arch Pediatr Adolesc Med 1999;153:409–18.
458. Moreno NP, Denk JP, Roberts JK, Tharp BZ, Bost M, Thompson WA. An approach to improving science knowledge about energy balance and nutrition among elementary- and middle-school students. Cell Biol Educ 2004;3:122–30.
459. Doak CM, Visscher TL, Renders CM, Seidell JC. The prevention of overweight and obesity in children and adolescents: a review of interventions and programmes. Obes Rev 2006;7:111–36.
460. Resnicow K, Davis M, Smith M, et al. How best to measure implementation of school health curricula: a comparison of three measures. Health Educ Res 1998;13:239–50.
461. Tomkins KO, Kamal KM, Chapman D. The West Virginia Health Education Assessment Project. J Sch Health 2005;75:193–8.
462. CDC. Health Education Curriculum Analysis Tool (HECAT). Atlanta, GA: US Department of Health and Human Services, CDC; 2007. Available at http://www.cdc.gov/healthyyouth/hecat/index.htm. Accessed July 15, 2011.
463. Popham WJ. Transformative assessment. Alexandria, VA: Association for Supervision and Curriculum Development; 2008.
464. Popham WJ. Instruction that measures up. Alexandria, VA: Association for Supervision and Curriculum Development; 2009.
465. Wiggins G, McTighe J. Understanding by design. 2nd ed. Alexandria VA: Association for Curriculum Development; 2005.
466. Marzano RJ, Pickering D, McTighe J. Assessing outcomes: performance assessment using dimensions of learning. Alexandria, VA: Association for Supervision and Curriculum Development; 1993.
467. Baranowski T. Gimme 5 fruit, juice, and vegetables for fun and health: outcome evaluation. Health Education & Behavior 2000;27:96–111.
468. Van Reusen K, Robinson J. Standards-based assessment in school health education. Education 1996;116:528–34.
469. Council of Chief State School Officers. State Collaborative on Assessment and Student Standards. Health Education Assessment Project (HEAP)—technical report. Washington, DC: Council of Chief State School Officers; 2000.
470. Lytle LA, Stone EJ, Nichaman MZ, et al. Changes in nutrient intakes of elementary school children following a school-based intervention: results from the CATCH Study. Prev Med 1996;25:465–77.
471. Nicklas TA, Johnson CC, Myers L, Farris RP, Cunningham A. Outcomes of a high school program to increase fruit and vegetable consumption: Gimme 5—a fresh nutrition concept for students. J Sch Health 1998;68:248–53.
472. Perry CL, Bishop DB, Taylor G, et al. Changing fruit and vegetable consumption among children: the 5-a-Day Power Plus program in St. Paul, Minnesota. Am J Public Health 1998;88:603–9.
473. Gortmaker SL, Cheung LW, Peterson KE, et al. Impact of a school-based interdisciplinary intervention on diet and physical activity among urban primary school children: eat well and keep moving. Arch Pediatr Adolesc Med 1999;153:975–83.

474. Harrell JS, Gansky SA, McMurray RG, Bangdiwala SI, Frauman AC, Bradley CB. School-based interventions improve heart health in children with multiple cardiovascular disease risk factors. Pediatrics 1998;102:371–80.
475. Manios Y, Kafatos A, Preventive Medicine and Nutrition Clinic University of Create Research Team. Health and nutrition education in primary schools in Crete: 10 years follow-up of serum lipids, physical activity and macronutrient intake. Br J Nutr 2006;95:568–75.
476. Kafatos I, Manios Y, Moschandreas J, Kafatos A. Health and nutrition education program in primary schools of Crete: changes in blood pressure over 10 years. Eur J Clin Nutr 2007;61:837–45.
477. Burke V, Thompson C, Taggart AC, et al. Differences in response to nutrition and fitness education programmes in relation to baseline levels of cardiovascular risk in 10- to 12-year-old children. J Hum Hypertens 1996;10(Suppl 3):S99–106.
478. Holcomb JD, Lira J, Kingery PM, Smith DW, Lane D, Goodway J. Evaluation of Jump Into Action: a program to reduce the risk of non-insulin dependent diabetes mellitus in school children on the Texas-Mexico border. J Sch Health 1998;68:282–8.
479. Trevino RP, Pugh JA, Hernandez AE, Menchaca VD, Ramirez RR, Mendoza M. Bienestar: a diabetes risk-factor prevention program. J Sch Health 1998;68:62–7.
480. Ritenbaugh C, Teufel-Shone NI, Aickin MG, et al. A lifestyle intervention improves plasma insulin levels among Native American high school youth. Prev Med 2003;36:309–19.
481. Shaw-Perry M, Horner C, Trevino RP, Sosa ET, Hernandez I, Bhardwaj A. NEEMA: A school-based diabetes risk prevention program designed for African-American Children. J Natl Med Assoc 2007;99:368–75.
482. Trevino RP, Yin Z, Hernandez A, Hale DE, Garcia OA, Mobley C. Impact of the bienestar school-based diabetes mellitus prevention program on fasting capillary glucose levels. Arch Pediatr Adolesc Med 2004;158:911–7.
483. Stang J, Taft Bayerl C, Flatt M, Associations Committee Positions Workgroup. Position of the American Dietetic Association: child and adolescent food and nutrition programs. J Am Diet Assoc 2006;106:1467–75.
484. Marcoux MF, Sallis JF, McKenzie TL, Marshall S, Armstrong CA, Goggin K. Process evaluation of a physical activity self-management program for children: SPARK. Psych Health 1999;14:659–77.
485. Allensworth DD. The research base for innovative practices in school health education at the secondary level. J Sch Health 1994;64:180–7.
486. Zahner L, Puder JJ, Roth R, et al. A school-based physical activity program to improve health and fitness in children aged 6–13 years ("Kinder-Sportstudie KISS"): study design of a randomized controlled trial. BMC Public Health 2006;6:147–59.
487. Bandura A. Social learning theory. Englewood Cliffs, NJ: Prentice Hall; 1997.
488. Shilts MS, Horowitz M, Townsend MS. Guided goal setting: effectiveness in a dietary and physical activity intervention with low-income adolescents. Int J Adolesc Med Health 2009;21:111–22.
489. Anderson AS, Porteous LE, Foster E, et al. The impact of a school-based nutrition education intervention on dietary intake and cognitive and attitudinal variables relating to fruits and vegetables. Pub Health Nutr 2005;8:650–6.

490. He M, Beynon C, Bouck MS, et al. Impact evaluation of the northern fruit and vegetable pilot programme--a clustered randomised controlled trial. Pub Health Nutr 2009;12:2199–208.
491. Dunton GF, Lagloire R, Robertson T. Using the RE-AIM framework to evaluate the statewide dissemination of a school-based physical activity and nutrition curriculum: "exercise your options." Am J Health Promot 2009;23:229–32.
492. Hoelscher DM, Evans A, Parcel GS, Kelder SH. Designing effective nutrition interventions for adolescents. J Am Diet Assoc 2002;102 (Suppl 3):S52–63.
493. Perez-Rodrigo C, Klepp KI, Yngve A, Sjostrom M, Stockley L, Aranceta J. The school setting: an opportunity for the implementation of dietary guidelines. Public Health Nutr 2001;4:717–24.
494. Perez-Rodrigo C, Aranceta J. School-based nutrition education: lessons learned and new perspectives. Public Health Nutr 2001;4:131–9.
495. Lavin AT. Comprehensive school health education: barriers and opportunities. J Sch Health 1993;63:24–7.
496. Rickard KA, Gallahue DL, Gruen GE, Tridle M, Bewley N, Steele K. The play approach to learning in the context of families and schools: an alternative paradigm for nutrition and fitness education in the 21st century. J Am Diet Assoc 1995;95:1121–6.
497. Contento IR, Kell DG, Keiley MK, Corcoran RD. A formative evaluation of the American Cancer Society changing the course nutrition education curriculum. J Sch Health 1992;62:411–6.
498. American Academy of Pediatrics Council on Sports Medicine and Fitness and Council on School Health. Active healthy living: prevention of childhood obesity through increased physical activity. Pediatrics 2006;117:1834–42.
499. Killen JD, Robinson TN. School-based research on health behavior change: the Stanford Adolescent Heart Health Program as a model for cardiovascular disease risk reduction [Chapter 4]. In: Rothkopf EZ, ed. Review of research in education. Washington, DC: American Education Research Association; 1988:171–200.
500. Howison D, Niedermyer F, Shortridge R. Field testing a fifth-grade nutrition education program designed to change food-selection behavior. J Nutr Educ 1988;20:82–6.
501. King AC, Saylor K, Foster S, et al. Promoting dietary change in adolescents: a school-based approach for modifying and maintaining healthful behavior. Am J Prev Med 1988;4:68–74.
502. Perry CL. Lessons from planet health. Arch Pediatr Adolesc Med 2005;159:292–3.
503. Long JD, Stevens KR. Using technology to promote self-efficacy for healthy eating in adolescents. J Nurs Scholarsh 2004;36:134–9.
504. Perez-Rodrigo C, Wind M, Hildonen C, et al. The pro children intervention: applying the intervention mapping protocol to develop a school-based fruit and vegetable promotion programme. Ann Nutr Metab 2005;49:267–77.
505. President's Council on Physical Fitness and Sports. The President's challenge. Washington, DC: President's Council on Physical Fitness and Sports; 2006.
506. Food and Nutrition Information Center. Database of food and nutrition software and multimedia programs [Database]. Beltsville, MD: US Department of Agriculture, National Agricultural Library, Food and Nutrition Information Center; 2005. Available at http://fnic.nal.usda.gov/nal_display/index.php?info_center=4&tax_level=1&tax_subject=253. Accessed July 15, 2011.

507. US Department of Agriculture. myPyramid.gov. [Internet site]. Alexandria, VA: US Department of Agriculture, Center for Nutrition Policy and Promotion; 2007. Available at http://www.choosemyplate.gov. Accessed July 15, 2011.
508. CDC. Healthy youth! Coordinated school health program. Atlanta, GA: US Department of Health and Human Services, CDC; 2008. Available at http://www.cdc.gov/healthyyouth/cshp. Accessed July 15, 2011.
509. American Academy of Pediatrics Council on School Health. Role of the school nurse in providing school health services. Pediatrics 2008;121:1052–6.
510. Brener ND, Wheeler L, Wolfe LC, Vernon-Smiley M, Caldart-Olson L. Health services: results from the School Health Policies and Programs Study 2006. J Sch Health 2007;77:435–63.
511. National Association of School Nurses. Position statement: education, licensure, and certification of school nurses. Silver Spring, MD: National Association of School Nurses; 2002. Available at http://www.nasn.org/PolicyAdvocacy/PositionPapersandReports/NASNPositionStatementsArticleView/tabid/462/ArticleId/26/Education-Licensure-and-Certification-of-School-Nurses-Adopted-2002. Accessed July 15, 2011.
512. National Association of School Nurses. Resolution: access to a school nurse. Silver Spring, MD: National Association of School Nurses; 2003. Available at http://www.nasn.org/Portals/0/statements/resolutionaccess.pdf . Accessed July 15, 2011.
513. National Association of School Nurses. Position statement: overweight children and adolescents. Silver Spring, MD: National Association of School Nurses, Inc; 2002. Available at http://www.nasn.org/PolicyAdvocacy/PositionPapersandReports/NASNPositionStatementsFullView/tabid/462/smid/824/ArticleID/39/Default.aspx. Accessed July 15, 2011.
514. Vessey JA. Coordinated school health. Pediatr Nurs 2000;26:303–7.
515. National Association of School Nurses. Position Statement: role of the school nurse. Silver Spring, MD: National Association of School Nurses, Inc; 2002. Available at http://www.nasn.org/PolicyAdvocacy/PositionPapersandReports/NASNPositionStatementsFullView/tabid/462/ArticleId/87/Role-of-the-School-Nurse-Revised-2011. Accessed July 15, 2011.
516. Broussard BA, Sugarman JR, Bachman-Carter K, et al. Toward comprehensive obesity prevention programs in Native American communities. Obes Res 1995;3(Suppl 2):S289–97.
517. Small ML, Majer LS, Alensworth D, Farquhar BK, Kann L, Pateman B C. School health services. J Sch Health 1995;65:319–26.
518. Nihiser AJ, Lee SM, Wechsler H, et al. Body mass index measurement in schools. J Sch Health 2007;77:651–71.
519. American Academy of Pediatrics Committee on School Health. School health: policy & practice. 6th ed. Elk Grove, IL: American Academy of Pediatrics; 2004.
520. Davis MM, Gance-Cleveland B, Hassink S, Johnson R, Paradis G, Resnicow K. Recommendations for prevention of childhood obesity. Pediatrics 2007;120:S229–53.
521. National Association of School Nurses. S.C.O.P.E. School Nurse Childhood Obesity Prevention Education. Silver Spring, MD: National Association of School Nurses; 2009. Available at http://www.nasn.org/ContinuingEducation/LiveContinuingEducationPrograms/SCOPE. Accessed July 15, 2011.

522. American Academy of Pediatrics. Pediatric obesity clinical decision support chart. Elk Grove Village, IL: American Academy of Pediatrics; 2008.
523. Strong WB, Malina RM, Blimkie CJ, et al. Evidence based physical activity for school-age youth. J Pediatr 2005;146:732–7.
524. Taras HL, American Academy of Pediatrics Committee on School Health. School-based mental health services. Pediatrics 2004;113:1839–45.
525. Griffiths LJ, Wolke D, Page AS, Horwood JP, the ALSPAC Study Team. Obesity and bullying: different effects for boys and girls. Arch Dis Child 2006;91:121–5.
526. Robinson S. Victimization of obese adolescents. J Sch Nurs 2006;22:201–6.
527. Schwimmer JB, Burwinkle TM, Varni JW. Health-related quality of life of severely obese children and adolescents. JAMA 2003;289:1813–9.
528. Sjoberg RL, Nilsson KW, Leppert J. Obesity, shame, and depression in school-aged children: A population-based study. Pediatrics 2005;116:389–92.
529. Swallen KC, Reither EN, Haas SA, Meier AM. Overweight, obesity, and health-related quality of life among adolescents: The National Longitudinal Study of Adolescent Health. Pediatrics 2005;115:340–7.
530. Killen JD, Taylor CB, Hayward C, et al. Pursuit of thinness and onset of eating disorder symptoms in a community sample of adolescent girls: a three-year prospective analysis. Int J Eat Disord 1994;16:227–338.
531. Linde JA, Wall MM, Haines J, Neumark-Sztainer D. Predictors of initiation and persistence of unhealthy weight control behaviours in adolescents. Int J Behav Nutr Phys Act 2009;29:72.
532. Eaton DK, Lowry R, Brener ND, Galuska DA, Crosby AE. Associations of body mass index and perceived weight with suicide ideation and suicide attempts among U.S. high school students. Arch Pediatr Adolesc Med 2005;159:513–9.
533. Carmack BK. School NPs as advocates. Adv Nurse Pract 1997;5:74.
534. Nabors L, Troilette A, Nash T, Masiulis B. School nurse perceptions of barriers and supports for children with diabetes. J Sch Health 2005;75:119–24.
535. Rose BL, Mansour M, Kohake K. Building a partnership to evaluate school-linked health services: the Cincinnati School Health Demonstration Project. J Sch Health 2005;75:363–9.
536. Barrett Clayton J, Goodwin D, Kendrick O. Nursing, food service, and the child with diabetes. J Sch Nurs 2002;18:150–6.
537. Davidson M. Teaching teens to cope: coping skills training for adolescents with insulin-dependent diabetes mellitus. J Soc Pediatr Nurs 1997;2:65–72.
538. Erickson CD, Splett PL, Mullett SS, Heiman MB. The healthy learner model for student chronic condition management—part 1. J Sch Nurs 2006;22:310–8.
539. Spear BA, Barlow SE, Ervin C, et al. Recommendations for treatment of child and adolescent overweight and obesity. Pediatrics 2007;120(Suppl 4):S254–88.
540. Nader PR, Kaczorowski J, Benioff S, Tonniges T, Schwartz D, Palfrey J. Education for community pediatrics. Clin Pediatr 2004;43:505–21.
541. Puskar KR, Weaver P, DeBlassio K. Nursing research in a school setting. J Sch Nurs 1994;10:8, 10–4.
542. Bradley BJ. The school nurse as health educator. J Sch Health 1997;67:3–8.

543. Barlow SE, Dietz WH. Obesity evaluation and treatment: expert committee recommendations. J Pediatr 1998;102:E29. Epub Sept. 1, 1998. Available at http://pediatrics.aappublications.org/content/102/3/e29.full.html. Accessed July 15, 2011.
544. Himes JH, Dietz WH. Guidelines for overweight in adolescent preventive services: recommendations from an expert committee. The Expert Committee on Clinical Guidelines for Overweight in Adolescent Preventive Services. Am J Clin Nutr 1994;59:307–16.
545. Whitlock E, Williams S, Gold R, Smith P, Shipman S. Screening and interventions for childhood overweight: a summary of evidence for the U.S. Preventive Services Task Force. Pediatrics 2005;116:E125–44. Epub July 1, 2005. Available at http://pediatrics.aappublications.org/content/116/1/e125.short. Accessed July 15, 2011.
546. Howard KR. Childhood overweight: parental perceptions and readiness for change. J Sch Nurs 2007;23:73–9.
547. Downie J. The everyday realities of the multi-dimensional role of the high school community nurse. Aust J Adv Nurs 2002;19:15–24.
548. Lightfoot J. Working to keep school children healthy: the complementary roles of school staff and school nurses. J Public Health Med 2000;22:74–80.
549. National Association of School Nurses. The role of the school nurse in school based health centers: position statement. Silver Spring, MD: National Association of School Nurses, Inc.; 2001. Available at http://www.nasn.org/PolicyAdvocacy/PositionPapersandReports/NASNPositionStatementsArticleView/tabid/462/ArticleId/46/School-Based-Health-Centers-The-Role-of-the-School-Nurse-and-Revised-2011. Accessed July 19, 2011.
550. Barnes M. School based youth health nurses' role in assisting young people access health services in provincial, rural and remote areas of Queensland, Australia. Rural Remote Health 2004;4:279.
551. Barnett S, Duncan P, O'Connor KG. Pediatricians' response to the demand for school health programming. Pediatrics 1999;103:1–7.
552. Stang J, Story M, Kalina B. School-based weight management services: perceptions and practices of school nurses and administrators. Am J Health Promot 1997;11:183–5.
553. Moyers P, Bugle L, Jackson E. Perceptions of school nurses regarding obesity in school-age children. J School Nurs 2005;21:86–93.
554. Wehling Weepie A, McCarthy A. A healthy lifestyle program: promoting child health in schools. J Sch Nurs 2002;18:322–8.
555. Broussard L. School nursing: not just band-aids any more! J Spec Pediatr Nurs 2004;9:77–83.
556. Epstein JL, Sanders MG, Sheldon SB, et al. School, family, and community partnerships: your handbook for action. 3rd ed. Thousand Oaks, CA: Corwin Press; 2009.
557. Epstein J. School, family, and community partnerships: preparing educators and improving schools. Boulder, CO: Westview Press; 2001.
558. Henderson AL, Mara P. A new wave of evidence: the impact of school, family, and community connections on student achievement. Austin, TX: Southwest Educational Development Laboratory; 2002.
559. Gerne KM, Epstein JL. The power of partnerships: school, family, and community collaborations to improve children's health. RMC Health Educator 2004;4:1–7.

560. American Academy of Pediatrics. Family pediatrics: report of the task force on the family. Pediatrics 2003;111:1541–71.
561. Golan M, Weizman A. Familial approach to the treatment of childhood obesity: conceptual model. J Nutr Educ 2001;33:102–7.
562. Golan M, Crow S. Parents are key players in the prevention and treatment of weight-related problems. Nutr Rev 2004;62:39–50.
563. Baranowski T, Baranowski JC, Cullen KW, et al. The Fun, Food, and Fitness Project (FFFP): the Baylor GEMS pilot study. Ethn Dis 2003;13(Suppl 1):S30–9.
564. Davis SM, Clay T, Smyth M, et al. Pathways curriculum and family interventions to promote healthful eating and physical activity in American Indian schoolchildren. Prev Med 2003;37(6 Pt 2):S24–34.
565. Fitzgibbon M, Stolley MR, Schiffer L, Van Horn L, KauferChristoffel K, Dyer A. Two-year follow-up results for Hip-Hop to Health Jr.: a randomized controlled trial for overweight prevention in preschool minority children. J Pediatr 2005;146:618–25.
566. Hopper CA, Gruber MB, Munoz KD, Herb RA. Effect of including parents in a school-based exercise and nutrition program for children. Res Q Exerc Sport 1992;63:315–21.
567. Hopper C, Munoz KD, Gruber MB, Nguyen KP. The effects of a family fitness program on the physical activity and nutrition behaviors of third-grade children. Res Q Exerc Sport 2005;76:130–9.
568. Nader PR, Sallis JF, Patterson T, et al. A family approach to cardiovascular risk reduction: results from the San Diego Family Health Project. Health Educ Q 1989;16:229–44.
569. Nader PR, Sellers DE, Johnson CC, et al. The effect of adult participation in a school-based family intervention to improve Children's diet and physical activity: the Child and Adolescent Trial for Cardiovascular Health. Prev Med 1996;25:455–64.
570. Perry CL, Luepker RV, Murray DV, et al. Parent involvement with children's health promotion: The Minnesota home team. Am J Public Health 1988;78:1156–60.
571. Ransdell LB, Taylor A, Oakland D, Schmidt J, Moyer-Mileur L, Shultz B. Daughters and mothers exercising together: effects of home- and community-based programs. Med Sci Sports Exerc 2003;35:286–96.
572. Steckler A, Ethelbah B, Martin CJ, et al. Pathways process evaluation results: a school-based prevention trial to promote healthful diet and physical activity in American Indian third, fourth, and fifth grade students. Prev Med 2003;37(6 Pt 2):S80–90.
573. Stolley MR, Fitzgibbon ML. Effects of an obesity prevention program on the eating behavior of African American mothers and daughters. Health Educ Behav 1997;24:152–64.
574. Story M, Sherwood NE, Himes JH, et al. An after-school obesity prevention program for African-American girls: The Minnesota GEMS pilot study. Ethn Dis 2003;13(Suppl 1):S54–64.
575. Trevino RP, Hernandez AE, Yin Z, Garcia OA, Hernandez I. Effect of the Bienestar Health Program on physical fitness in low-income Mexican American children. Hisp J Behav Sci 2005;27:120–32.
576. Beech BM, Klesges RC, Kumanyika SK, et al. Child- and parent-targeted interventions: the Memphis GEMS pilot study. Ethn Dis 2003;13(Suppl 1):S40–53.

577. Weeks K, Levy SR, Gordon AK, Handler A, Perhats C, Flay BR. Does parental involvement make a difference? The impact of parent interactive activities on students in a school-based AIDS prevention program. AIDS Educ Prev 1997;9(Suppl 1):90–106.
578. Golan M, Crow S. Targeting parents exclusively in the treatment of childhood obesity: long-term results. Obes Res 2004;12.
579. Golan M, Fainaru M, Weizman A. Role of behaviour modification in the treatment of childhood obesity with the parents as the exclusive agents of change. Int J Obes Relat Metab Disord 1998;22:1217–24.
580. McGarvey E, Keller A, Forrester M, Williams E, Seward D, Suttle DE. Feasibility and benefits of a parent-focused preschool child obesity intervention. Am J Public Health 2004;94:1490–5.
581. McLean N, Griffin S, Toney K, Hardeman W. Family involvement in weight control, weight maintenance and weight-loss interventions: a systematic review of randomised trials. Int J Obes Relat Metab Disord 2003;27:987–1005.
582. Epstein LH, Voloski A, Wing RR, McCurley J. Ten-year outcomes of behavioral family-based treatment for childhood obesity. Health Psych 1994;13:373–83.
583. Coleman KJ, Tiller CL, Sanchez J, et al. Prevention of the epidemic increase in child risk of overweight in low-income schools: the El Paso coordinated approach to child health. Arch Pediatr Adolesc Med 2005;159:217–24.
584. Elder JP, Campbell NR, Candelaria JI, et al. Project salsa: development and institutionalization of a nutritional health promotion project in a Latino community. Am J Health Promot 1998;12:391–401.
585. Good TL, Wiley AR, Thomas RE, et al. Bridging the gap between schools and community: organizing for family involvement in a low-income neighborhood. JEPC 1997;8:277–96.
586. Landis SE, Janes CL. The Claxton Elementary School Health Program: merging perceptions and behaviors to identify problems. J Sch Health 1995;65:250–4.
587. Kakli Z, Kreider H, Little P, Buck T, Coffey M. Focus on families! How to build and support family-centered practices in after school. Boston, MA: United Way of Massachusetts Bay; Harvard Family Research Project; Build the Out-of-School Time Network; 2006. Available at http://www.hfrp.org/family-involvement/publications-resources/focus-on-families!-how-to-build-and-support-family-centered-practices-in-after-school. Accessed July 22, 2011.
588. Pate RR, Saunders RP, Ward DS, Felton G, Trost SG, Dowda M. Evaluation of a community-based intervention to promote physical activity in youth: lessons from Active Winners. Am J Health Promot 2003;17:171–82.
589. Economos CD, Hyatt RR, Goldberg JP, et al. A community intervention reduces BMI z-score in children: Shape Up Somerville first year results. Obesity Res 2007;15:1325–36.
590. Pentz MA. The school-community interface in comprehensive school health education. In: Allensworth D, Lawson E, Nicholson L, Wyche J, eds. Schools and health. Washington, DC: National Academy Press; 1997. 305–36.
591. Margolis PA, Stevens R, Bordley C, et al. From concept to application: the impact of a community-wide intervention to improve the delivery of preventive services to children. Pediatrics 2001;108:42–52.

592. Policy Leadership for Active Youth. Addressing overweight: interventions tailored to the rural south. Atlanta, GA: Georgia State University; 2005.
593. Michael S, Dittus P, Epstein J. Family and community involvement in schools: results from the school health policies and programs study 2006. J Sch Health 2007;77:567–79.
594. Gittelsohn J, Davis SM, Steckler A, et al. Pathways: lessons learned and future directions for school-based interventions among American Indians. Prev Med 2003;37(6 Pt 2):S107–12.
595. Lytle LA, Kubik MY, Perry C, Story M, Birnbaum AS, Murray DM. Influencing healthful food choices in school and home environments: results from the TEENS study. Prev Med 2006;43:8–13.
596. Cohen L, Baer N, Satterwhite P. Developing effective coalitions: an eight step guide. In: Wurzbach J, ed. Community health education and promotion: a guide to program design and evaluation. 2nd ed. Gaithersburg, MD: Aspen Publishers Inc; 2002:144–61.
597. Felton G, Saunders RP, Ward DS, Dishman RK, Dowda M, Pate RR. Promoting physical activity in girls: a case study of one school's success. J Sch Health 2005;75:57–62.
598. Lopez R, Campbell R, Jennings J. The Boston schoolyard initiative: a public-private partnership for rebuilding urban play space. J Health Polit Policy Law 2008;33:617–38.
599. Story M, Nanney MS, Schwartz MB. Schools and obesity prevention: creating school environments and policies to promote healthy eating and physical activity. Milbank Q 2009;87:71–100.
600. White House Task Force on Childhood Obesity. Childhood Obesity Task Force unveils action plan. Solving the problem of childhood obesity within a generation: report to the president. Washington, DC: Executive Office of the President of the United States; 2010. Available at http://www.whitehouse.gov/the-press-office/childhood-obesity-task-force-unveils-action-plan-solving-problem-childhood-obesity-. Accessed July 22, 2011.
601. National Policy and Legal Analysis Network to Prevent Childhood Obesity. Joint use agreement 3: opening school facilities for use during non-school hours and authorizing third parties to operate programs. Oakland, CA: National Policy and Legal Analysis Network to Prevent Childhood Obesity; 2009. Available at http://www.whitehouse.gov/the-press-office/childhood-obesity-task-force-unveils-action-plan-solving-problem-childhood-obesity-. Accessed July 22, 2011.
602. Fothergill K, Ballard E. The school-linked health center: a promising model of community-based care for adolescents. J Adolesc Health 1998;23:29–38.
603. Juhn G, Tang J, Piessens P, Grant U, Johnson N, Murray H. Community learning: the reach for health nursing program-middle school collaboration. J Nurs Educ 1999;38:215–21.
604. Strelow JS, Larsen JS, Sallis JF, Conway TL, Powers HS, McKenzie TL. Factors influencing the performance of volunteers who provide physical activity in middle schools. J Sch Health 2002;72:147–51.
605. Agron P, Berends V, Cole N, Gooley J, Hawksworth K, Martinez N. Engaging parents and stakeholders in school wellness: formative research report. Los Angeles, CA: The California Endowment; 2008. Available at http://www.californiapro-

jectlean.org/docuserfiles//Parent%20Formative%20Research%20Report.pdf . Accessed July 22, 2011.
606. Pate RR, O'Neill JR. After-school interventions to increase physical activity among youth. Br J Sports Med 2009;43:14–8.
607. Robinson TN, Killen JD, Kraemer HC, et al. Dance and reducing television viewing to prevent weight gain in African-American girls: the Stanford GEMS pilot study. Ethn Dis 2003;13(Suppl 1):S65–77.
608. Marschall M. Parent involvement and educational outcomes for Latino students. Rev Policy Res 2006;23:1053–76.
609. Davis SM, Going SB, Helitzer DL, et al. Pathways: a culturally appropriate obesity-prevention program for American Indian schoolchildren. Am J Clin Nutr 1999;69(Suppl 4):S796–802.
610. Snyder TD, Tan AG. Digest of education statistics, 2004. NCES 2006005. Washington, DC: National Center for Education Statistics; 2005. Available at http://nces.ed.gov/pubsearch/pubsinfo.asp?pubid=2006005. Accessed July 22, 2011.
611. Aldana SG. Financial impact of health promotion programs: a review of the literature. Am J Health Promot 2001;15:296–320.
612. Davis L, Loyo K, Glowka A, et al. A comprehensive worksite wellness program in Austin, Texas: partnership between Steps to a Healthier Austin and Capital Metropolitan Transportation Authority. Prev Chronic Dis 2009;6:A60.
613. Wisconsin Department of Health and Family Services, Division of Public Health, Nutrition and Physical Activity Program, Wisconsin Partnership for Activity and Nutrition. Wisconsin worksite resource kit to prevent obesity and related chronic diseases. Madison, WI: Wisconsin Department of Health and Family Services; 2007.
614. Partnership for Prevention. Healthy workforce 2010: an essential health promotion sourcebook for employers large and small. Washington, DC: Partnership for Prevention; 2001. Available at http://www.acsworkplacesolutions.com/documents/Healthy_Workforce_2010.pdf . Accessed July 22, 2011.
615. Aldana SG, Pronk NP. Health promotion programs, modifiable health risks, and employee absenteeism. J Occup Environ Med 2001;43:36–46.
616. Allegrante JP, Michela JL. Impact of a school-based workplace health promotion program on morale of inner-city teachers. J Sch Health 1990;60:25–8.
617. Blair SN, Collingwood TR, Reynolds K, Smith M, Hagan RD, Sterling CL. Health promotion for educators: impact on health behaviors, satisfaction, and general well-being. Am J Public Health 1984;74:147–9.
618. Cullen KW, Baranowski T, Herbert D, deMoor C, Hearn MD, Resnicow K. Influence of school organizational characteristics on the outcomes of a school health promotion program. J Sch Health 1999;69:376–80.
619. Galemore CA. Initiation of a school employee wellness program: applying the comprehensive health education model. J Sch Nurs 2000;16:39–46.
620. Galemore CA. Worksite wellness in the school setting. J Sch Nurs 2000;16:42–5.
621. Galaif ER, Sussman S, Bundek N. The relations of school staff smokers' attitudes about modeling smoking behavior in students and their receptivity to no-smoking policy. J Drug Educ 1996;26:313–22.
622. Kumar R, O'Malley PM, Johnston LD, Schulenberg JE, Gachman JG. Effects of school-level norms on student substance use. Prev Sci 2002;3:105–24.

623. Trinidad DR, Gilpin EA, Pierce JP. Compliance and support for smoke-free school policies. Health Educ Res 2005;20:466–75.
624. Eaton DK, Marx E, Bowie SE. Faculty and staff health promotion: results from the School Health Policies and Programs Study 2006. J Sch Health 2007;77:557–66.
625. Directors of Health Promotion and Education. School employee wellness: a guide for protecting the assets of our nation's schools. Washington, DC: Directors of Health Promotion and Education; 2007. Available at http://www.whf.org/documents/coordinated-school-health-docs/School%20Employee%20Wellness%20-%20Establishing%20Wellness.pdf . Accessed July 22, 2011.
626. Engbers LH, van Poppel MN, Chin AP, van Mechelen W. Worksite health promotion programs with environmental changes: a systematic review. Am J Prev Med 2005;29:61–70.
627. Marshall AL, Owen N, Bauman A. Mediated approaches for influencing physical activity: update of the evidence on mass media, print, telephone and website delivery of interventions. J Sci Med Sport 2004;7:74–80.
628. Brissette I, Fisher B, Spicer DA, King L. Worksite characteristics and environmental and policy supports for cardiovascular disease prevention in New York State. Prev Chronic Dis 2008;5:A37.
629. Hawkins C, O'Garro MA, Wimsett K. Engaging employers to develop healthy workplaces: the WorkWell initiative of Steps to a Healthier Washington in Thurston County. Prev Chronic Dis 2009;6:A61.
630. Oldenburg B, Sallis JF, Harris D, Owen N. Checklist of health promotion environments at worksites (CHEW): development and measurement characteristics. Am J Health Promot 2002;16:288–99.
631. Zunker C, Cox TL, Wingo BC, Knight B, Jefferson WK, Ard JD. Using formative research to develop a worksite health promotion program for African American women. Women Health 2008;48:189–207.
632. Bearden JB. Maine school district goes all out for employee wellness. School Business Affairs 2005;71:26–7.
633. CDC. Public health strategies for preventing and controlling overweight and obesity in school and worksite settings. A report on recommendations of the Task Force on Community Preventive Services. MMWR 2005;54:1–12.
634. Taylor WC. Transforming work breaks to promote health. Am J Prev Med 2005;29:461–5.
635. Yancey A, McCarthy W, Taylor W, et al. The Los Angeles Lift Off: a sociocultural environmental change intervention to integrate physical activity into the workplace. Prev Med 2004;38:848–56.
636. Chan CB, Ryan DA, Tudor-Locke C. Health benefits of a pedometer-based physical activity intervention in sedentary workers. Prev Med 2004;39:1215–22.
637. Matson-Koffman DM, Brownstein NJ, Neiner JA, Greaney ML. A site-specific literature review of policy and environmental interventions that promote physical activity and nutrition for cardiovascular health: what works? Am J Health Promot 2005;19:167–93.
638. Patterson R, Kristal AR, Biener L, et al. Durability and diffusion of the nutrition intervention in the Working Well Trial. Prev Med 1998;27:668–73.

639. White JL, Ransdell LB. Worksite intervention model for facilitating changes in physical activity, fitness, and psychological parameteres. Percept Mot Skills 2003;97:461–6.
640. Auld G, Romaniello C, Heimendinger J, Hambidge C, Hambidge M. Outcomes from a school-based nutrition education program using resource teachers and cross-disciplinary models. J Nutr Educ 1998;30:268–80.
641. Davis K, Burgeson CR, Brener ND, McManus T, Wechsler H. The relationship between qualified personnel and self-reported implementation of recommended physical education practices and programs in U.S. schools. Res Q Exerc Sport 2005;76:202–11.
642. Fulkerson JA, French SA, Story MA, Syder P, Paddock M. Foodservice staff perceptions of their influence on student food choices. J Am Diet Assoc 2002;102:97–9.
643. Dwyer JJ, Allison KR, Barrera M, Hansen B, Goldenberg E, Boutilier MA. Teachers' perspective on barriers to implementing physical activity curriculum guidelines for school children in Toronto. Can J Public Health 2003;94:448–52.
644. Kelder SH, Mitchell PD, McKenzie TL, et al. Long-term implementation of the CATCH physical education program. Health Educ Behav 2003;30:463–75.
645. Kulinna PH, Silverman S. Teachers' attitudes toward teaching physical activity and fitness. Res Q Exerc Sport 2000;71:80–4.
646. Davis M, Baranowski T, Resnicow K, et al. Gimme 5 fruit and vegetables for fun and health: process evaluation. Health Educ Behav 2000;27:167–76.
647. National Association for Sport and Physical Education. National standards for beginning physical education teachers. 2nd ed. Reston, VA: National Association for Sport and Physical Education; 2009.
648. National Association for Sport and Physical Education. Opportunity to learn standards for elementary school physical education. Reston, VA: National Association for Sport and Physical Education; 2000.
649. National Association for Sport and Physical Education. Opportunity to learn standards for high school physical education. Reston, VA: National Association for Sport and Physical Education; 2004.
650. National Association for Sport and Physical Education. Opportunity to learn standards for middle school physical education. Reston, VA: National Association for Sport and Physical Education; 2004.
651. Kealey KA, Peterson AV Jr, Gaul MA, Dinh KT. Teacher training as a behavior change process: principles and results from a longitudinal study. Health Educ Behav 2000;27:64–81.
652. Pateman B, Grunbaum JA, Kann L. Voices from the field—a qualitative analysis of classroom, school, district, and state health education policies and programs. J Sch Health 1999;69:258–63.
653. Stang J, Story M, Kalina B. Nutrition education in Minnesota public schools: perceptions and practices of teachers. J Nutr Educ 1998;30:396–404.
654. American Association for Health Education. AAHE/NCATE health education standards and key elements. Reston, VA: American Association for Health Education; 2001.
655. Coalition of National Health Education Organizations. The health education profession in the 21st century: setting the stage. J Sch Health 1996;66:291–8.

656. Cater JM, Carr DH. Competencies, knowledge, and skills of effective school nutrition managers. R-66-03. University, MS: National Food Service Management Institute; 2004.
657. Rainville AJ, Carr DH. Competencies, knowledge, and skill statements for district school nutrition directors/supervisors. R-50-01. University, MS, National Food Service Management Institute; 2001.
658. Gross S, Cinelli B. Coordinated school health program and dietetics professionals: partners in promoting healthful eating. J Am Diet Assoc 2004;104:793–8.
659. Wei RC, Darling-Hammond L, Andree A, Richardson N, Orphanos S. Professional learning in the learning profession: a status report on teacher development in the United States and abroad. Dallas, TX: National Staff Development Council; 2009. Available at http://www.nsdc.org/news/NSDCstudy2009.pdf . Accessed July 22, 2011.
660. National Association for Sport and Physical Education. Physical activity and fitness recommendations for physical activity professionals. Reston, VA: National Association for Sport and Physical Education; 2002.
661. Wiecha JL, El Ayadi AM, Fuemmeler BF, et al. Diffusion of an integrated health education program in an urban school system: planet health. J Pediatr Psychol 2004;29:467–74.
662. Weiler R, Pigg RM Jr. An evaluation of client satisfaction with training programs and technical assistance provided by Florida's Coordinated School Health Program Office. J Sch Health 2000;70:361–7.
663. McKenzie TL, Sallis JF, Kolody B, Faucette FN. Long-term effects of a physical education curriculum and staff development program: SPARK. Res Q Exerc Sport 1997;68:280–91.
664. Fairclough S, Stratton G. Improving health-enhancing physical activity in girls' physical education. Health Educ Res 2005;20:448–57.
665. State of Michigan Department of Education. Fully qualified teachers of health education. Lansing, MI: State of Michigan Department of Education; 2005.
666. Peregrin T. Take 10! Classroom-based program fights obesity by getting kids out of their seats. J Am Diet Assoc 2001;101:1409.
667. Edmundson E, Parcel GS, Feldman HA, et al. The effects of the Child and Adolescent Trial for Cardiovascular Health upon psychosocial determinants of diet and physical activity behavior. Prev Med 1996;25:442–54.
668. Johnson CC, Galati T, Pedersen S, Smyth M, Parcel GS. Maintenance of the classroom health education curricula: results from the CATCH-ON study. Health Educ Beh 2003;30:476–88.
669. Geiger BF, Petri CJ, Myers O, et al. Using technology to teach health: a collaborative pilot project in Alabama. J Sch Health 2002;72:401–7.
670. Jones Everett S, Brenner N, McManus T. The relationship between staff development and health instruction in schools in the United States. J health Educ 2004;35:2.
671. Bauer KW, Patel A, Prokop LA, Austin Bryn S. Swimming upstream: faculty and staff members from urban middle schools in low-income communities describe their experience implementing nutrition and physical activity initiatives. Prev Chronic Dis 2006;3:A37–45.

672. Sullivan K, Harper M, West CK. Professional development needs reported by school food service directors and recommendations for meeting directors' needs. Oxford, MS: National Food Service Management Institute; 2000.
673. Osganian SK, Ebzery MK, Montgomery DH, et al. Changes in the nutrient content of school lunches: results from the CATCH Eat Smart Food service Intervention. Prev Med 1996;25:400–12.
674. Halpern R. After-school programs for low-income children: promise and challenges. Future child 1999;9:81–95.
675. Neighbors M, Barta K. School nurse summer institute: a model for professional development. J Sch Nurs 2004;20:134–8.
676. Saaranen T, Tossavainen K, Turunen H. School staff members' and occupational health nurses' evaluation of the promotion of occupational well-being—with good planning to better practice. J Interprof Care 2005;19:465–79.
677. Brener ND, Weist M, Adelman H, Taylor L, Vernon-Smiley M. Mental health and social services: results from the School Health Policies and Programs Study 2006. J Sch Health 2007;77:464–85.
678. US Department of Agriculture, Food and Nutrition Service. The power of choice: helping youth make healthy eating and fitness decisions. Washington, DC: US Department of Agriculture; 2003.
679. Libman S. Adult participation in youth sports. A developmental perspective. Child Adolesc Psychiatr Clin N Am 1998;7:725–44.
680. Wiersma LD, Sherman CP. Volunteer youth sport coaches' perspectives of coaching education/certification and parental codes of conduct. Res Q Exerc Sport 2005;76:324–38.

There are several supplemental files that are not available in this version of the article. To view this additional information, please use the citation on the first page of this chapter.

AUTHOR NOTES

CHAPTER 3

Competing Interests

The authors declare that they have no competing interests.

Author Contributions

WP and AT were co-principal investigators on this study. They led the design of the study and obtained funding. WP was the chief investigator and oversaw all aspects; whilst AT led the development of the school component. John Smyth was also a co-principal investigator on the study and led the ethnographic fieldwork, which has been reported elsewhere. MC was the project manager and was responsible for data collection, implementation, and analysis. AT and AM designed the intervention materials and provided professional development to schools. JH oversaw statistical design, analysis and reporting; whilst RE and AM provided expertise in sport and recreation and physical education respectively. All authors contributed to the design of the study, critically commented on the manuscript, and read and approved the final manuscript.

Acknowledgments

Funding for this research was provided by the Australian Research Council (ARC; LP0990206). Financial and/or in-kind support was also provided by industry partners, including the Victorian Health Promotion Foundation (VicHealth), Department of Planning and Community Development–Sport and Recreation Victoria, Tennis Victoria, Football Federation Victoria, YMCA Victoria, Ballarat Aquatic Centre, and the Helen Macpherson Smith Trust. The authors wish to thank the program advisory committee, secondary schools and their staff and students, sports coaches and clubs, and the YMCA and their managers and instructors for their participation and contribution to the program and research.

CHAPTER 4

Author Contributions

Conceived and designed the experiments: KR GS. Performed the experiments: GS KR DC. Analyzed the data: KR GS CW. Contributed reagents/materials/analysis tools: GS KR CW. Wrote the paper: GS KR JB CW JP DC.

CHAPTER 5

Funding

This study was funded by the Swiss Federal Office of Sports (grant number SWI05-013), the Swiss National Science Foundation (grant number PMPDB-114401). The funders had no role in study design, data collection and analysis, decision to publish, or preparation of the manuscript.

Acknowledgments

The authors thank all children, teachers and parents for taking part in the study. Appreciation is expressed to Ralf Roth, Marco Schmid, Martin Knöpfli, Regula Guldimann, Eliane Peterhans, and Tamara Blösch for their assistance with data collection.

Author Contributions

Conceived and designed the experiments: LZ HH WvM HPBLR NPH JP SK. Performed the experiments: UM LZ DE SK. Analyzed the data: UM CS SK. Wrote the paper: UM SK.

CHAPTER 6

Funding

The Healthy Passages Study is funded by the Centers for Disease Control and Prevention, Prevention Research Centers (cooperative agreements U48DP000046, U48DP000057, and U48DP000056). Tracy Richmond is funded by the National Institutes of Health (NIH) Career Development award (NICHD K01 HD058042). The funders had no role in study design, data collection and analysis, decision to publish, or preparation of the manuscript.

Author Contributions

Conceived and designed the experiments: TKR MNE MAS IK FF CEW. Analyzed the data: TKR MNE MAS IK CEW. Wrote the paper: TKR CEW MNE MAS. Helped conceive of, design, and recruit for the cohort from which this study is designed: MOC MJG FAF SWP RL LF. Reviewed and edited the manuscript: MOC MJG FAF SWP RL LF.

CHAPTER 7

Competing Interests

The following authors declared no conflicts of interests: PSM, GW, DR, JH. This study was funded by a Robert Wood Johnson Foundation – Active Living Research grant.

Author Contributions

PSM performed the statistical analysis and drafted the manuscript. GW participated in the design of the study and drafted the manuscript. DR participated in the statistical analysis and helped drafted the manuscript. JH conceived of the study, and was responsible for coordination and design. She also helped draft the manuscript. All authors approved the final manuscript.

Acknowledgments

The authors would like to acknowledge the graduate assistants Erin Johnson, Sara Wolfe, and Alison Jergenson for their hard work during data collection and entry.

Source of Funding

The following authors PSM, GW, DR, JH also disclose any commercial associations, current and over the past 5 years, that might pose a conflict of interest. These include but are not limited to consultancies, including those for investment companies; stock or other equity ownership; stock options; patent licensing arrangements; and payments for conducting or publicizing the study.

CHAPTER 8

Acknowledgments

CATCH is supported by the National Heart, Lung, and Blood Institute; Texas Department of State Health Services; Bexar County Community Health Collaborative; Paso del Norte Health Foundation; Houston Endowment Inc; Michael and Susan Dell Foundation; and CDC Prevention Research Centers program cooperative agreement U48/CCU 609653.

Planet Health is supported by the National Institutes of Child Health and Human Development grant HD-30780 and CDC Prevention Research Centers program cooperative agreement U48/CCU 115807.

Not-On-Tobacco is supported by CDC Prevention Research Centers program cooperative agreements U48/CCU 310831 and 1-U48-DP-000052; American Legacy Foundation; American Lung Association; West Virginia Bureau for Public Health, Division of Tobacco Prevention; and West Virginia Department of Education.

Footnotes

The opinions expressed by authors contributing to this journal do not necessarily reflect the opinions of the U.S. Department of Health and Human Services, the Public Health Service, Centers for Disease Control and Prevention, or the authors' affiliated institutions. Use of trade names is for identification only and does not imply endorsement by any of the groups named above.

CHAPTER 9

Acknowledgments

The SPEEDY study is funded by the National Prevention Research Initiative consisting of the following funding partners: British Heart Foundation; Cancer Research UK; Chief Scientist Office, Scottish Government Health Directorates; Department of Health; Diabetes UK; Economic and Social Research Council; Health and Social Care Research and Development Office for Northern Ireland; Medical Research Council; Welsh Assembly Government and World Cancer Research Fund. Additional funding for the collection, data acquisition, and analysis of the 4-day diet diaries was provided by Norwich Medical School. The work of E.M.F.v.S. and S.J.G. was supported by the Centre for Diet and Activity Research, a UKCRC Public Health Research: Centre of Excellence.

CHAPTER 10

Competing Interests

Production of this paper has been made possible through a financial contribution from the Public Health Agency of Canada. The views expressed herein do not necessarily represent the views of the Public Health Agency of Canada. I Janssen has received honoraria, speaker fees, and consulting fees from several non-profit organizations, including the Public Health Agency of Canada, that have an interest in physical activity and health.

Author Contributions

IJ designed the methods, assisted with the completion of the systematic review, and drafted the manuscript. AB lead most of the components of the systematic review and helped drafts some of the methodology sections of the paper. All authors have read and approved the final manuscript.

Acknowledgments

Production of this paper has been made possible through a financial contribution from the Public Health Agency of Canada. The views expressed herein do not necessarily represent the views of the Public Health Agency of Canada. The leadership and administrative assistance was provided by the Canadian Society for Exercise Physiology.

CHAPTER 12

Competing Interests

The authors declare that they have no competing interests.

Author Contributions

CF conducted the analyses and wrote the manuscript. PJV conceived and supervised the study. SK, CL, MP, KS, and MS advised on the analyses and contributed to the development of the manuscript. All authors read and approved the final manuscript.

Acknowledgments

We thank all of the grade five students, parents and schools for their participation in the REAL Kids Alberta evaluation and APPLE Schools program, and the evaluation assistants, health promotion coordinators and school health facilitators for their contributions in data collection. The REAL Kids Alberta evaluation was funded through a contract with Alberta Health and Wellness. The APPLE Schools program was funded through a donation to the School of Public Health at the University of Alberta. The research was funded through a Canada Research Chair in Population Health and Alberta Innovates Health Solutions Health Scholarship to Dr. Paul J. Veugelers. All interpretations and opinions in the present study are those of the authors.

INDEX

B

C

D

J

K

L

M

N

R

T

U

V

W